An Introduction to the Psychology of Hearing

Third Edition

Brian C. J. Moore

Reader in Auditory Perception,
Department of Experimental Psychology,
University of Cambridge, UK

ACADEMIC PRESS

Harcourt Brace Jovanovich, Publishers

London · San Diego · New York · Berkeley · Boston
Sydney · Tokyo · Toronto

This book is printed on acid-free paper.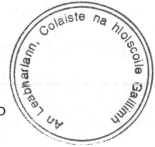

ACADEMIC PRESS LIMITED.
24/28 Oval Road
London NW1 7DX

United States Edition published by
ACADEMIC PRESS INC.
San Diego, CA 92101

British Library Cataloguing in Publication Data
is available

ISBN 0-12-505623-0 Hardback
ISBN 0-12-505624-9 Paperback

Typeset by Paston Press, Loddon, Norfolk
and printed in Great Britain by St Edmundsbury Press Limited,
Bury St Edmunds, Suffolk

Preface to the First Edition

In 1971 I gave my first course of lectures on auditory perception, as part of the psychology course at the University of Reading. Anyone who had attempted to give or attend lectures on auditory perception will be aware of two major problems which I encountered. Firstly, there is no textbook which is both up to date and at a level suitable for undergraduate use. Secondly, scientific papers on hearing in psychological and physiological journals are almost incomprehensible to the beginner in this area. I became increasingly frustrated at having to say to my students "I'm sorry, but there is no book I can recommend," and finally I decided that the only solution to the problem was to write such a book myself.

This book, then, is primarily intended as an undergraduate textbook to accompany courses in auditory perception or hearing. To this end it contains a chapter introducing the basic physics of sound and describing the most important anatomical and physiological features of the auditory system. Some very basic knowledge is assumed (for example, the terms 'neurone' and 'nerve firings' are not explained), but the approach is very much to start from first principles.

As it turned out, the book contains very much more material than I would normally get through in a single course of lectures, so that it could also serve as a text to accompany advanced undergraduate or graduate courses in auditory perception. The general approach throughout the book is to relate the psychological and perceptual aspects of sound to the underlying physiological mechanisms. Thus the book should also be of use and interest to sensory physiologists, physicians and audiologists.

Although the emphasis throughout the book is on laboratory experiments performed under carefully controlled conditions, I have been careful to point out, wherever possible, the real-life or applied relevance of the problems under discussion. Indeed the final chapter of the book is mainly concerned with practical applications. In addition, there is a chapter on speech perception in which links with psychoacoustic phenomena are emphasized. Thus the book should also have something of interest for phoneticians, speech researchers, speech pathologists, linguists, and engineers concerned with problems of the recording, transmission and reproduction of sound or with problems of automatic speech recognition and speaker identification.

My major aim in writing this book was that it should be reasonably up to date, but at the same time not too technical for the novice. Inevitably this has resulted in the omission of some details and the simplification of some concepts. I hope that I have managed to do this without too much distortion, and that the essential flavour of current trends in auditory research has been preserved. Many areas which are traditionally discussed in textbooks on hearing have been omitted entirely; for example, volume and density as attributes of pure tones are not mentioned, nor is the mel scale of pitch. This reflects my own prejudices to some extent, but the basis for omission has generally been the lack of use of these concepts in the last ten years or so.

Perhaps the hardest thing about writing this book was to stop writing it! Almost every day I came across new papers with exciting results which ought to have been mentioned. However, one has to draw the line somewhere, and the book was never intended to be a complete review. I apologize to those whose work has been omitted or mentioned too briefly. The balance of space has inevitably been influenced by my own interests, and I hope that I will be forgiven for devoting so much space to the role of 'timing' information in nerve impulses.

Auditory perception has been a sadly neglected area in British psychology although this is much less true in the United States and Holland. I hope that this book will help to correct the balance, and that those who teach in this area will find the book of some use.

Finally, I would like to thank all those colleagues and friends who read parts of the manuscript and provided helpful comments. The manuscript was written while I was a lecturer in Psychology at the University of Reading. Thanks are due particularly to: Mark Haggard, Max Coltheart, Bernard Moulden, Alan Allport, David Raab, Roy Davis, Wynford Bellin, Mark Terry, Peter Bailey, Arthur Summerfield, Dave Martin, John Gundry, Carol Moore and Pat Sheldon. The responsibility for mistakes is of course mine. Mrs P. Williams typed the manuscript accurately and quickly through many drafts to its final form; I am very grateful to her. Susan and Paul Scott, and my wife Carol, provided valuable help in sorting out the references.

Reading, 1977   B.C.J.M.

Preface to the Second Edition

I have had three main aims in writing the second edition of this book: firstly to clarify certain sections which students and colleagues have told me were difficult to follow in the first edition; secondly to describe some of the most important experimental results which have appeared since the first edition was completed; finally to introduce new material in areas which were thought by colleagues to be important, but which were not covered in the first edition. In this final category, the most important change is a new chapter on 'Auditory pattern and object perception'. I hope that this chapter will go some way towards answering the complaints of those who thought that the first edition did not contain enough on 'perception' or 'psychology'. I have been careful, in this chapter, to emphasize links with other areas of psychology, and particularly that of selective attention.

I wish to clarify which students the book is appropriate for. In the UK the book is suitable for advanced undergraduate, and Master's level courses in psychology, speech and hearing sciences, and audiology. In the USA the book might be found a little difficult for undergraduate psychologists, but it would be well suited to graduate courses in perception. The book is suitable for those in the USA taking undergraduate and graduate level courses in subjects with a greater emphasis on hearing, such as audiology, and speech and hearing science.

Finally, I wish to thank all those who helped in the preparation of the second edition. The following people provided valuable comments, criticisms and suggestions: Bernard O'Loughlin, Robert Milroy, Brian Glasberg, Michael Shailer, Roy Patterson, Robert Peters, Paul Whittle and Tony Marcel. Kay Knights quickly and patiently typed many drafts of the revised manuscript, and Roy Hammans helped in the preparation of new figures.

Cambridge, 1982   B.C.J.M.

Preface to the Third Edition

The most obvious change in the third edition is the addition of a new chapter on the temporal resolution of the ear. However, all of the other chapters have been extensively revised and updated. The most substantial changes are the following: Chapter 1 includes new data on active processes in the cochlea; Chapter 3 describes the phenomena of comodulation masking release and profile analysis; Chapter 6 includes new data on binaural sluggishness and binaural adaptation; Chapter 8 describes several new phenomena in speech perception, including duplex perception, sinewave speech and audiovisual integration. Where new material has been added, I have tried to remove an equivalent amount of old material. Mostly I have removed: experiments or theories shown to have been wrong or to have a doubtful interpretation by more recent work; material of marginal interest judged by (the lack of) references to it over the last decade; material found too 'difficult' by a majority of readers.

I would like to thank my colleagues and students who have read drafts of revised chapters and made many helpful comments. These include Tom Baer, Peter Bailey, Mahnaz Baldry, Dave Emmerich, Larry Feth, Brian Glasberg, Sarah Hawkins, Chris Plack, Gregory Schooneveldt, Anne Sherman, Michael Shailer, Andrew Simpson and Michael Stone. I am very grateful to them all. I would also like to thank Ian Cannell, Brian Glasberg, Chris Plack and Gregory Schooneveldt for help in producing new figures and Mahnaz Baldry for much help with word processing.

Cambridge, 1989   B.C.J.M.

To Mahnaz and my parents

Contents

1

The nature of sound and the structure and function of the auditory system

1 INTRODUCTION

One of the general aims of this book is to specify, as far as possible, the relationships between the characteristics of the sounds which enter the ear and the sensations which they produce. Wherever possible these relationships will be specified in terms of the underlying mechanisms. In other words, we will be trying to understand what the auditory system does and how it works. It is not always possible to fulfil both of these objectives. While some aspects of auditory perception can be explained by reference to the anatomy or physiology of the auditory system, our knowledge in this respect is not usually as precise or as far reaching as we would like. Often the results of behavioural studies (generally psychophysical experiments) provide us with evidence as to the kinds of things that are occurring in the auditory system, but we may not be able to specify the detailed physiological mechanisms which are involved. Sometimes we can use the results of psychophysical experiments to determine if a particular type of neural coding (see later), which in principle could convey information about a sound, is actually involved in the perception or discrimination of that sound. Before we can begin to specify underlying mechanisms, however, we must know something of the physical nature of sounds, and of the basic anatomy and physiology of the auditory system. That is the purpose of this chapter.

2 THE PHYSICAL CHARACTERISTICS OF SOUNDS

A The nature of sound

Sound originates from the motion or vibration of an object. This motion is impressed upon the surrounding medium (usually air) as a pattern of changes in pressure. What actually happens is that the atmospheric particles, or molecules, are squeezed closer together than normal (called condensation), and then pulled farther apart than normal (called rarefaction). The sound wave moves outwards from the vibrating body, but the molecules do not advance with the wave: they vibrate about an average resting place. The sound wave generally weakens as it moves away from the source, and also may be subject to reflections and refractions caused by walls or objects in its path. Thus the sound 'image' reaching the ear will differ somewhat from that initially generated.

One of the simplest types of sound is the sine wave, also known as a sinusoid, which has the waveform (pressure variation plotted against time) shown in Fig. 1.1. This wave is simple both from the physical and mathematical point of view and from the point of view of the auditory system. It happens that sinusoids produce particularly simple responses in the auditory system, and that they have a very clean or 'pure' sound, like that of a tuning fork. Thus they are also called simple tones or pure tones. To describe a sinusoid we need to specify three things: the frequency, or the number of times per second the waveform repeats itself (specified in Hertz, where 1 Hertz (Hz) = 1 cycle/s); the amplitude, or the amount of pressure variation about the mean; and the phase, or the portion of the cycle through which the

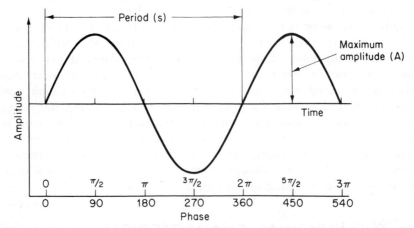

FIG. 1.1   The waveform of a sine wave or sinusoidal vibration. Only 1.5 cycles are shown, although the waveform should be pictured as repeating indefinitely. The instantaneous amplitude is given by the expression $A.\sin(2\pi ft)$, where t = time, f = frequency and A = maximum amplitude. Phase is indicated along the bottom, using as a reference point the first zero-crossing of the wave. Phase may be measured in degrees or in radians. One complete cycle corresponds to 360° or 2π radians.

wave has advanced in relation to some fixed point in time. For continuous sinusoids, phase is only important when we are interested in the relationship between two or more different waves. The time taken for one complete cycle of the waveform is called the period, which is the reciprocal of the frequency.

A sine wave is not the only kind of sound which repeats regularly. Many of the sounds which we encounter in everyday life, such as those produced by musical instruments, and certain speech sounds, also show such regularity, and hence are called periodic sounds. Although these sounds are generally more complex than sinusoids, they share a common subjective characteristic with sinusoids in that they have pitches. Pitch may be defined as that attribute of auditory sensation in terms of which sounds may be ordered on a musical scale. In other words, variations in pitch create a sense of melody. A sound that evokes a pitch is often called a 'tone', especially when the pitch has a clear musical quality. In general, tones are periodic, but, as we shall see later, this is not always the case.

The pitch of a sound is related to its repetition rate and, hence, in the case of a sinusoid, to its frequency. It should be emphasized that pitch is a subjective attribute of a stimulus, and as such cannot be measured directly. However, for a sinusoid, the pitch is closely related to the frequency; the higher the frequency, the higher the pitch. For a more complex sound, the pitch is often investigated by asking the subject to adjust a sinusoid so that it has the same pitch as the complex sound. The frequency of the sinusoid is then taken as a measure of the pitch of the complex sound.

B Fourier analysis and spectral representations

Although all sounds can be specified in terms of variations in sound pressure occurring over time, it is often more convenient, and more meaningful, to specify them in a different way when the sounds are complex. This method is based on a theorem by Fourier, who proved that any complex waveform (with certain restrictions) can be analysed, or broken down, into a series of sinusoids with specific frequencies, amplitudes and phases. Such an analysis is called Fourier analysis, and each sinusoid is called a (Fourier) component of the complex sound. We may thus define a complex tone as a tone composed of a number of simple tones, or sinusoids.

The simplest type of complex tone to which Fourier analysis can be applied is one which is periodic. Such a tone is composed of a number of sinusoids, each of which has a frequency that is an integral multiple of the frequency of a common (not necessarily present) fundamental component. The fundamental component thus has the lowest frequency of any of the components in the complex tone, and it may be said to form the 'foundation' for the other components. The fundamental component has a frequency equal to the repetition rate of the complex waveform as a whole. The frequency components of the complex tone are known as harmonics and are numbered, the fundamental being given harmonic number 1. Thus, for example, a note of A_3 played on the piano would have a fundamental component or first harmonic of frequency 220 Hz, a second harmonic of frequency 440 Hz, a third harmonic of frequency 660 Hz, etc. The nth harmonic has a frequency which is n times that of the fundamental. An illustration of how a complex tone can be built up from a series of sinusoids is given in Fig. 1.2. Sometimes musicians refer to harmonics above the fundamental as 'overtones'. The first overtone is the second harmonic, the second overtone is the third harmonic, and so on.

One of the reasons for representing sounds in this way is that humans do seem to be able to hear the harmonics of a periodic sound wave individually to a limited extent. For example, Mersenne (1636) stated that "the string, struck and sounded freely makes at least five sounds at the same time, the first of which is the natural sound of the string and serves as the foundation for the rest ...". The fact that we can hear pitches corresponding to the individual sinusoidal components of a complex tone is known as Ohm's Acoustical Law, after the German physicist Georg Ohm. Normally, when we are presented with a complex tone, we do not listen in this way; rather we hear a single pitch corresponding to the repetition rate of the whole sound. Nevertheless we do appear to be able to hear out the lower harmonics of a complex sound to some extent (see Chapters 3 and 5 for further discussion of this). When we are presented with two simultaneous pure tones, whose frequencies are not too similar, then these will often be heard as two separate tones each with its own pitch rather than as a single complex sound. Thus, our perception corresponds to the analysis of the sound in terms of its Fourier components. Notice that our perception of colour is quite different; if lights of two different frequencies (or wavelengths) are mixed, we see a single colour corresponding to the mixture, rather than seeing two component hues.

The structure of a sound, in terms of its frequency components, is often represented by its magnitude spectrum, a plot of sound amplitude, energy or power as a function of frequency. In these cases we would talk of the amplitude spectrum, energy spectrum or power spectrum (see section C for a description of the relationship between amplitude, energy and power). Examples of magnitude spectra are given in Fig. 1.3. For periodic sounds of long duration, the energy falls at specific discrete frequencies and the spectrum is known as a line spectrum. The first three examples are of this type. The sinusoid, by definition, consists of a single frequency component. The square wave, as shown in Fig. 1.2, consists of the odd harmonics of the fundamental component (1 kHz in our example), and the amplitudes of the harmonics decrease with increasing harmonic number. The train of brief pulses, or clicks, contains all the harmonics of the fundamental at equal amplitude. However, since each pulse contains only a small amount of energy, and since there are many harmonics, each harmonic has a low amplitude.

For sounds which are not periodic, such as white noise (a hissing sound), the spectrum tends to be more complex, and is obtained by use of a mathematical device known as the Fourier transform. Nonperiodic sounds

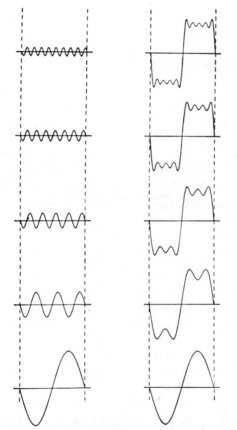

FIG. 1.2 An illustration of how a complex waveform (a square wave) can be built up from a series of sinusoidal components. The square wave is composed of odd harmonics only, and the 1st, 3rd, 5th, 7th and 9th harmonics are shown on the left. The series on the right shows progressive changes from a simple sine wave as each component is added. If enough additional harmonics, with appropriate amplitudes and phases, were added, the composite wave would approach a perfectly square shape. From Newman (1948), by permission of John Wiley, New York.

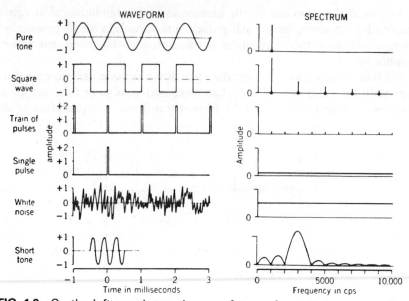

FIG. 1.3 On the left are shown the waveforms of some common auditory stimuli, and on the right are the corresponding spectra. The periodic stimuli (pure tone, square wave and train of pulses) have line spectra, while the nonperiodic stimuli (single pulse, white noise and short tone burst) have continuous spectra.

can still have line spectra, for example a mixture of two nonharmonically related sinusoids. The term partial is used to describe any discrete sinusoidal component of a complex sound, whether it is a harmonic or not. More commonly, nonperiodic sounds have continuous spectra; the energy is spread over certain frequency bands, rather than being concentrated at particular frequencies. Our last three examples are of this type. The single pulse, or click, and the white noise both have flat amplitude spectra; the amplitude does not vary as a function of frequency (this is only true for very brief clicks). Although the pulse and the noise have spectra of the same shape, the amplitude of the spectrum of the pulse is lower, since it contains much less energy than the noise. The pulse and the noise differ in their phase spectra, which represent the phases of the components as a function of frequency (not shown in the figure). For the noise the phases of the components are randomly distributed. For the pulse the components all have a phase of 90° at time zero. This is known as cosine phase, and it means that each component is at its peak amplitude at time zero. The result is that at this time the components all add, whereas at other times they cancel.

The final example shows a short burst of a sinusoid, often called a tone pulse or tone burst. The magnitude spectrum of a sinusoid is only a line if the sinusoid lasts an extremely long time. For tone pulses of short duration, the magnitude spectrum contains energy over a range of frequencies around the nominal frequency of the sinusoid. This spread of energy increases as the duration of the tone pulse is shortened. Corresponding changes occur in our perception of such tone pulses; as a tone pulse is shortened in duration it sounds less tone-like and more click-like.

The mathematical techniques used in calculating spectra by Fourier analysis or the Fourier Transform require integration over infinite time. In practical situations, this is impossible, since we cannot sample a waveform over infinite time. Also, it is obvious that the ear does not integrate over infinite time. In many situations it is useful to take a sample of a sound and assume that the waveform has zero value outside the time limits of the sample. This process is often described as applying a 'window' to the sound; only the portion of the waveform falling within the window is 'seen'. The Fourier transform of the windowed sample can then be calculated, giving what is called the short-term spectrum of the sound. Typical window lengths are between 5 ms and 200 ms. For a complex sound such as speech, it is useful to analyse the speech using a succession of windows, which may overlap in time, so that changes in the short-term spectrum with time can be calculated. Examples of this approach will be given in Chapter 8.

We noted above that the spectrum of continuous white noise is, in theory, flat. However, in practice, the Fourier transform has to be calculated for a particular sample of the noise. Any such sample of 'white' noise may not have a flat amplitude spectrum. It is only when the spectrum is averaged over a long period of time that it becomes flat.

Whenever a stimulus is changed abruptly (e.g. by a change in intensity or a change in frequency), a spread in spectral energy occurs. For example, the short-term spectrum of a continuous sinusoid has a single narrow peak corresponding to the frequency of the sinusoid. However, if the frequency or intensity of the sinusoid are changed abruptly, the short term spectrum for a window centred on the change is much broader. This spreading of spectral energy over frequency is often called 'energy splatter'. Energy splatter can be reduced by slowing down the changes (e.g. by switching tones on and off gradually), but it cannot be completely eliminated.

C The measurement of sound level

The instruments used to measure the magnitudes of sounds, such as microphones, normally respond to changes in air pressure. However, sound magnitudes are often specified in terms of intensity, which is the sound energy transmitted per second through a unit area in a sound field. For a medium such as air there is a simple relationship between the pressure variation of a plane (flat-fronted) sound wave in a free field (i.e. in the absence of reflected sound) and the acoustic intensity; intensity is proportional to the square of the pressure variation.

It turns out that the auditory system can deal with a huge range of sound intensities (see Chapter 2). This makes it inconvenient to deal with sound intensities directly. Instead a logarithmic scale expressing the ratio of two intensities is used. One intensity, I_0, is chosen as a reference and the other intensity, I_1, is expressed relative to this. One Bel corresponds to a ratio of intensities of $10:1$. Thus the number of Bels corresponding to a given intensity ratio is obtained by taking the logarithm to the base 10 of the intensity ratio. For example, an intensity ratio of $100:1$ corresponds to 2 Bels. Unfortunately, the Bel is a rather large unit for everyday use, and to obtain units of convenient size the Bel is divided into 10 decibels (dB). Thus the number of decibels corresponding to a given ratio of acoustic intensity is:

$$\text{number of decibels} = 10 \, \log_{10} \, (I_1/I_0).$$

When the magnitude of a sound is specified in decibels, it is customary to use the word 'level' to refer to its magnitude. Notice that a given number of decibels represents an intensity or power ratio, not an absolute intensity. In order to specify the absolute intensity of a sound it is necessary to state that the intensity (or power) of the sound, I_1, is n dB above or below some reference intensity, I_0. The reference intensity most commonly used is 10^{-12} watts per square metre (W/m^2), which is equivalent to a pressure of 2×10^{-5} N/m^2 or 20 μPa (micropascal). A sound level specified using this reference level is referred to as a sound pressure level (SPL). Thus a sound at 60 dB SPL is 60 dB higher in level than the reference level of 0 dB, and has an intensity of $10^{-6} \, \text{W/m}^2$. Notice that multiplying (or dividing) the ratio of intensities by 10 increases (or decreases) the number of decibels by 10. It is also convenient to remember that a two-fold change in intensity corresponds to a change in level of 3 dB.

The reference sound level, 0 dB SPL, is a low sound level which was chosen to be close to the average human absolute threshold for a 1000 Hz sinusoid. The absolute threshold is the minimum detectable level of a sound in the absence of any other external sounds (the manner of presentation of the sound and method of determining detectability must be specified). In fact the average human absolute threshold at 1000 Hz is about 6.5 dB SPL. Sometimes it is convenient to choose as a reference level the threshold of a subject for the sound being used. A sound level specified in this way is referred to as a sensation level (SL). Thus, for a given subject, a sound at 60 dB SL will be 60 dB above the absolute threshold of that subject for that sound. The physical intensity corresponding to a given sensation level will, of course, differ from subject to subject and from sound to sound.

Finally, it is useful to adapt the decibel notation so that it expresses ratios of pressure as well as ratios of intensity. This may be done by recalling that intensity is proportional to the square of pressure. If one sound has an intensity of I_1 and a pressure P_1, and a second sound has an intensity I_2 and pressure P_2, then the difference in level between them is:

$$\text{number of decibels} = 10 \log_{10}(I_1/I_2) = 10 \log_{10}(P_1/P_2)^2 = 20 \log_{10}(P_1/P_2).$$

Thus a ten-fold increase in pressure corresponds to a 100-fold increase in intensity and is represented by +20 dB. Table 1.1 gives some examples of intensity and pressure ratios expressed in decibels, and also indicates sound levels, in dB SPL, corresponding to various common sounds.

For sounds with discrete spectra, or line spectra, the sound level can be specified either as the overall (total) level or in terms of the levels of the individual components. The total level can be calculated from the total power of the sound, which in turn is proportional to the mean square pressure (measured as the deviation from normal atmospheric pressure). If we wish to calculate levels in terms of pressure, then we have to express the pressure of the sound as its root-mean-square (RMS) value.

For sounds with continuous spectra we can also specify the overall level, but if we wish to indicate how the energy is distributed over frequency, we need some other measure. This measure is obtained by specifying the total

Table 1.1. The relationship between decibels, intensity ratios and pressure ratios. Sound levels in dB SPL are expressed relative to a reference intensity I_0 of 10^{-12} W/m^2. This is equivalent to a pressure of 20 μPa.

Sound level, dB SPL	Intensity ratio I/I_0	Pressure ratio P/P_0	Typical example
140	10^{14}	10^7	Gunshot at close range
120	10^{12}	10^6	Loud rock group
100	10^{10}	10^5	Shouting at close range
80	10^8	10^4	Busy street
70	10^7	3.16×10^3	Normal conversation
50	10^5	316	Quiet conversation
30	10^3	31.6	Soft whisper
20	10^2	10	Country area at night
6.5	4.5	2.1	Mean absolute threshold at 1 kHz
3	2	1.4	
0	1	1	Reference level
−10	0.1	0.316	

energy or power between certain frequency limits, i.e. over a certain band of frequencies. Conventionally, a bandwidth of 1 Hz is chosen. The energy in this one-cycle-wide band, at a given frequency, is known as the energy density. For a continuous noise, we may also specify the energy per unit time (i.e. the power or intensity) in this one-cycle-wide band, and this is known as the noise power density. When the noise power density is expressed in decibels relative to the standard reference intensity of 10^{-12} W/m^2 (equivalent to 20 μPa), it is known as the spectrum level. Thus a noise may be characterized by its spectrum level as a function of frequency. A white noise has a uniform spectrum level.

D   Beats

When two sinusoids with slightly different frequencies are added together, they resemble a single sinusoid, with frequency equal to the mean frequency of the two components, but whose amplitude fluctuates at a regular rate. These fluctuations in amplitude are known as 'beats'. Beats occur because of the changing phase relationship between the two sinusoids, which causes them alternately to reinforce and cancel one another. The resulting amplitude fluctuations occur at a rate equal to the frequency difference between the two tones. For example, if two sinusoids with frequencies 1000 Hz and 1002 Hz are added together, two beats will occur each second. Slow beats like this result in audible loudness fluctuations. We will see in Chapters 2 and 3 that beats sometimes play a role in psychoacoustic experiments.

3   THE CONCEPT OF LINEARITY

One concept which is widely used in auditory research is that of linearity. The auditory system is often conceived as being made up of successive stages, the output of a given stage forming the input to the next. Each of these stages can be considered as a device or system, with an input and an output. For a system to be linear, certain relationships between the input and output must hold true. The following two conditions must be satisfied. (1) The output of the system in response to a number of independent inputs presented simultaneously should be equal to the sum of the outputs that would have been obtained if each input were presented alone. For example, if the response to input A is X, and the response to input B is Y, then the response to A and B together is simply $X + Y$. (2) If the input to the system is changed in magnitude by a factor k, then the output should also change in magnitude by a factor k, but be otherwise unaltered. For example, if the input is doubled, then the output is doubled, but without any change in the form of the output. These two conditions are known as superposition and homogeneity, respectively.

The output of a linear system never contains frequency components that were not present in the input signal. Thus, a sinusoidal input gives rise to a sinusoidal output of the same frequency (the amplitude and phase may, however, be changed). This is not necessarily true for other types of waveforms. For example, if the input to a linear system is a square wave, the output is not necessarily a square wave. This provides another reason for the popularity of sinusoids in auditory research; sinusoids are the only waveforms which are always 'preserved' by a linear system.

If a system is linear, then its analysis and characterization become relatively simple. If we measure its response to a sinusoidal input, as a function of frequency, then that response tells us all that we need to know about the system. To predict the response to any arbitrary complex input, we first need to perform a Fourier analysis of the input. We already have the information to calculate the response to each of the sinusoidal components comprising the input. The response to the whole complex can then be calculated as the sum of the responses to its individual sinusoidal components. This is a powerful method, and it gives another reason for using sinusoids as stimuli. We shall see later that some parts of the auditory system behave as though they were approximately linear, while others behave in a grossly nonlinear way. When a system is nonlinear, the response to complex inputs cannot generally be predicted from the responses to the sinusoidal components comprising the inputs. Thus the characteristics of the system must be investigated using both sinusoidal and complex inputs.

4 FILTERS AND THEIR PROPERTIES

In many psychoacoustic experiments the experimenter may wish to manipulate the spectra of the stimuli in some way. For example, it may be desired to remove certain frequency components from a complex stimulus, while leaving other components unchanged. In practice this is usually achieved by altering the electrical signal before it is converted into sound by a loudspeaker or headphone. The electronic devices which may be used to manipulate the spectrum of a signal are known as filters. They are generally linear devices, so that in response to a sinusoidal input, the output is a sinusoid of the same frequency. However, they are designed so that at their outputs some frequencies are attenuated more than others. A highpass filter removes all frequency components below a certain cutoff frequency, but does not affect components above this frequency. A lowpass filter does the reverse. A bandpass filter has two cutoff frequencies, passing components between those two frequencies, and removing components outside this passband. A bandstop filter also has two cutoff frequencies, but it removes components between these two frequencies, leaving other components intact. Such filters may be used not only for manipulating stimuli, but also for analysing them.

Bandpass filters will be of particular interest to us, not only because of their widespread use for signal analysis, but also because one stage of the peripheral auditory system is often likened to a bank of bandpass filters, each of which has a different centre frequency, so that the whole range of audible frequencies is covered. This concept will be used extensively later in the book, so it is instructive to consider the properties of filters in some detail.

In practice it is not possible to design filters with perfectly sharp cutoffs. Instead there will be a range of frequencies over which some components will be reduced in level, but not entirely removed. Thus in order to specify a filter we have to define both the cutoff frequency (or frequencies) and the slope of the filter response curve. Some typical filter characteristics are illustrated in Fig. 1.4. The cutoff frequency is usually defined as the frequency at which the output of the filter has fallen by 3 dB relative to the output in the passband. This corresponds to a reduction in power or intensity by a factor of two, and a reduction in amplitude (or voltage for an electronic filter) by a factor of $\sqrt{2}$ (see Table 1.1). For a bandpass filter, the range of frequencies between the two cutoffs defines the bandwidth of the filter. This is called the -3 dB bandwidth, the 3 dB down bandwidth or (equivalently) the half-power bandwidth. Sometimes, for simplicity, it is just called the 3 dB bandwidth. When a bandwidth is given without specifying dB limits, it is generally assumed that the 3 dB down points were used.

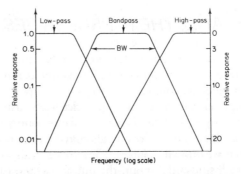

FIG. 1.4 Typical characteristics for three types of filters: lowpass, bandpass and highpass. The input to each filter is a sinusoid of variable frequency but constant magnitude. The output of each filter is plotted relative to the input, as a function of frequency. The left ordinate gives the ratio of the output to the input in linear power units. The right ordinate gives that ratio in dB.

An alternative measure of bandwidth is the equivalent rectangular bandwidth (ERB). The ERB of a given filter is equal to the bandwidth of a perfect rectangular filter which has a transmission in its passband equal to the maximum transmission of the specified filter and transmits the same power of white noise as the specified filter. In other words, if we take a rectangular filter and scale it to have the same maximum height and area as our filter, then the bandwidth of the rectangular filter is the ERB of our filter. The equalization of height and area is done with the filter characteristic plotted in linear power coordinates.

The response characteristics of electronic filters outside their passbands can often be approximated as straight lines when they are plotted on dB versus log-frequency coordinates. Thus, it is useful to express the slopes of filters in units such that equal frequency ratios represent equal amounts. One unit which does this is the octave. An octave corresponds to a frequency ratio of 2:1. Thus if we say that a lowpass filter has a slope of 24 dB/octave, this means that the output outside the passband decreases by 24 dB each time the frequency is doubled. Sometimes it is not possible to measure the response of a filter over a frequency range as large as an octave. Thus we need to be able to work out the proportion of an octave corresponding to any given frequency ratio. Consider two frequencies, f_1 and f_2. Their relative frequency, expressed as a certain number of octaves, n, is given by the relation:

$$f_1/f_2 = 2^n$$

where n may be positive, negative, a fraction or a number of octaves. Taking the logarithm on both sides of this equation, we get:

$$\log_{10}(f_1/f_2) = n \times 0.301$$

from which it is possible to calculate n given f_1/f_2, and vice versa.

Sometimes the bandwidths of bandpass filters are expressed in octaves. In this case the two frequencies involved are the upper and lower cutoffs of the filter, i.e. the 3 dB down points. One type of filter in common use has a bandwidth of 1/3 octave. For such a filter, the upper cutoff has a frequency 1.26 times that of the lower cutoff.

If a signal with a 'flat' spectrum, such as a white noise or a single brief click, is passed through a filter, the magnitude spectrum of the output of the filter will have the same shape (i.e. be the same function of frequency) as the filter characteristic. Thus we can also talk about a highpass noise, a bandpass click, and so on. A stimulus whose spectrum covers the whole audible frequency range is often referred to as broadband. Any alteration of the spectrum of a signal by filtering also produces a corresponding alteration in the waveform of the signal, and usually an alteration in the way it is perceived. For example, if white noise is passed through a narrow bandpass filter, the waveform at the output of the filter resembles a sinusoid which is fluctuating in amplitude from moment to moment. This narrowband noise has a pitch-like quality, the pitch corresponding to its centre frequency.

The response of a filter to a single brief click, or impulse, can be very informative. In fact this response, known as the impulse response, completely defines the filter characteristic. Since a click has a flat magnitude spectrum, the spectrum of the output of the filter, namely the impulse response, will have the same shape as the filter characteristic. Hence the filter characteristic, or shape, can be obtained by calculating the Fourier transform of the impulse response.

Figure 1.5 shows a series of impulse responses from filters having pass-bands centred at 1 kHz, but with various bandwidths. For the narrowest filter (top) the response looks like a sinusoid which builds up and decays smoothly, and which has a frequency close to 1 kHz. This is described as a 'ringing' response, and it is similar to what is heard when a wine glass is tapped with a spoon. The filter 'rings' at its own preferred frequency. As the filter bandwidth increases, the frequency of the ringing becomes less regular, and the duration of the response decreases. For the widest filter bandwidth, the impulse response has a waveform resembling that of the input impulse. For an infinitely wide filter, the output would exactly match the input (provided that the filter delayed all frequency components by an equal time; this is equivalent to saying that the filter has a linear phase response). This figure illustrates a general limitation of analysing sounds with filters. The narrower the bandwidth of a filter, and the steeper its slopes, the longer is its response time. Thus an increase in the resolution of individual frequency components can only be obtained at the expense of a loss of resolution in time.

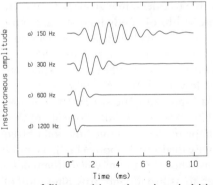

FIG. 1.5   The response of filters with various bandwidths to a brief impulse. All filters had a centre frequency of 1 kHz, and the bandwidth is indicated to the left of each trace. The responses are not drawn to scale. The peak amplitude of the response actually increases as the filter bandwidth increases.

If a filter with a narrow bandwidth is excited with a series of impulses, then the response to one impulse may not have died away before the next impulse occurs. Thus, the impulse responses will merge. If, for example, an impulse occurs every 2 ms (repetition rate 500 pulses/s), then for the narrowest filter in Fig. 1.5, the merged impulse responses will form a continuous sinusoid with a frequency of 1 kHz. In effect, the filter has 'picked out' the second harmonic of the pulse train, and is responding only to that harmonic. Filters with different centre frequencies will respond to different harmonics in the pulse train. However, if the bandwidth of the filter is not sufficiently narrow, it will respond to more than one harmonic. The waveform at the output will not be sinusoidal, but will fluctuate at a rate equal to the repetition rate of the pulse train. When the filter bandwidth is very wide, then a series of isolated impulse responses will be observed. These phenomena are illustrated in Figs 1.10 and 5.5, and we will discuss them more fully later in this chapter and in Chapter 5.

5 BASIC STRUCTURE AND FUNCTION OF THE AUDITORY SYSTEM

A The outer and middle ear

The peripheral part of the auditory system of most mammals is rather similar. In this section we will start by considering the human auditory system, but later will draw examples from studies of other mammals. Figure 1.6 shows the structure of the peripheral part of the human auditory system. The outer ear is composed of the pinna (the part we actually see) and the auditory canal or meatus. The pinna has generally been considered a rather unimportant part of the auditory system, but it does in fact significantly modify the incoming sound, particularly at high frequencies, and this is important in our ability to localize sounds (see Chapter 6). Sound travels down the meatus and causes the eardrum, or tympanic membrane, to vibrate. These vibrations are transmitted through the middle ear by three small bones, the ossicles, to a membrane-covered opening in the bony wall of the spiral-shaped structure of the inner ear – the cochlea. This opening is called the oval window. The three bones are called the malleus, incus and stapes, the stapes being the lightest and smallest of these and the one which actually makes contact with the oval window. The popular names for these bones are the hammer, anvil and stirrup, and they are noteworthy for being the smallest bones in the body.

The major function of the middle ear is to ensure the efficient transfer of sound from the air to the fluids in the cochlea. If the sound were to impinge directly onto the oval window, most of it would simply be reflected back, rather than entering the cochlea. This happens because the resistance of the

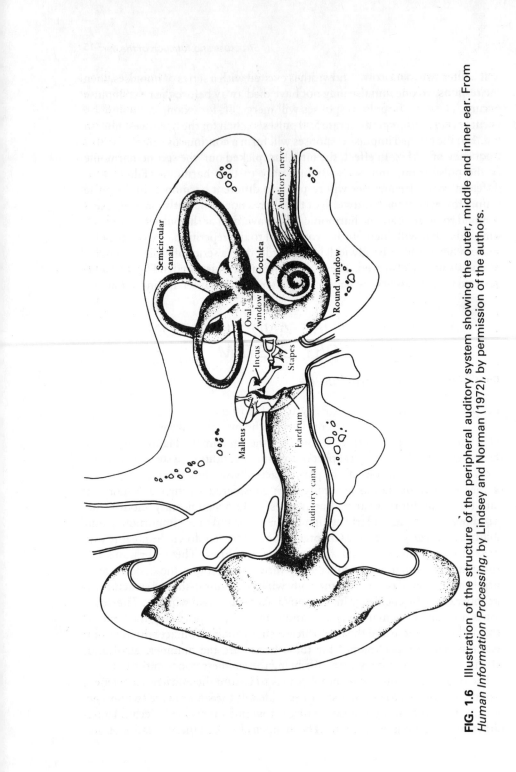

FIG. 1.6 Illustration of the structure of the peripheral auditory system showing the outer, middle and inner ear. From *Human Information Processing*, by Lindsey and Norman (1972), by permission of the authors.

Semicircular canals

Cochlea

Auditory nerve

Oval window

Round window

Incus

Stapes

Malleus

Eardrum

Auditory canal

oval window to movement is very different to that of air. Technically, this is described as a difference in acoustical impedance. The middle ear acts as an impedance-matching device or transformer that improves sound transmission and reduces the amount of reflected sound. This is accomplished mainly by the difference in effective areas of the eardrum and the oval window, and to a small extent by the lever action of the ossicles. Transmission of sound through the middle ear is most efficient at middle frequencies (500–4000 Hz).

The ossicles have minute muscles attached to them which contract when we are exposed to intense sounds. This contraction, known as the middle ear reflex, is probably mediated by neural centres in the brain stem, but its anatomical basis is not fully known. The reflex reduces the transmission of sound through the middle ear, but only at low frequencies, and it may help to prevent damage to the delicate structures of the cochlea. However, the activation of the reflex is too slow to provide any protection against impulsive sounds, such as gun shots or hammer blows. Two other functions have been suggested for the reflex. The first is the reduction of the audibility of self-generated sounds, particularly speech. It has been shown that the reflex is activated just before vocalization. The second is a reduction of the masking of middle and high frequencies by lower ones, a function which is particularly important at high sound levels (see Fig. 3.10, and the associated discussion of the 'upward spread of masking' in Chapter 3, section 4).

B The inner ear and the basilar membrane

The cochlea is the most important part of the ear from our point of view, and an understanding of what goes on in the cochlea can provide a key to many aspects of auditory perception. The cochlea is filled with almost incompressible fluids, and it also has bony rigid walls. It is divided along its length by two membranes, Reissner's membrane and the basilar membrane (see Fig. 1.12). It is the motion of the basilar membrane in response to sound which is of primary interest to us. The start of the cochlea, where the oval window is situated, is known as the base; while the other end, the inner tip, is known as the apex. It is also common to talk about the basal end and the apical end. At the apex there is a small opening (the helicotrema) between the basilar membrane and the walls of the cochlea, which connects the two outer chambers of the cochlea, the scala vestibuli and the scala tympani. Inward movement of the oval window results in a corresponding outward movement in a membrane covering a second opening in the cochlea – the round window.

When the oval window is set in motion by an incoming sound, a pressure difference occurs across the basilar membrane. The pressure wave travels almost instantaneously through the incompressible fluids of the cochlea. Consequently, the pressure difference is applied essentially simultaneously along the whole length of the basilar membrane. The pattern of motion on the basilar membrane, however, takes some time to develop. The pattern which occurs does not depend on which end of the cochlea is stimulated. Sounds which reach the cochlea via the bones of the head rather than through the air (e.g. our own voices) do not produce atypical responses.

The response of the basilar membrane to sinusoidal stimulation takes the form of a travelling wave which moves along the basilar membrane from the base towards the apex. The amplitude of the wave increases at first and then decreases rather abruptly. The basic form of the wave is illustrated in Fig. 1.7, which shows the instantaneous displacement of the basilar membrane (derived from a cochlear model) for two successive instants in time, in response to a 200 Hz sinusoid. This figure also shows the line joining the amplitude peaks, which is called the envelope. The distance between peaks or zero-crossings in the wave decreases as the wave travels along, and the envelope shows a peak at a particular position on the basilar membrane.

The response of the basilar membrane to sounds of different frequencies is strongly affected by its mechanical properties, which vary considerably from base to apex. At the base it is relatively narrow and stiff, while at the apex it is wider and much less stiff. As a result, the position of the peak in the pattern of vibration differs according to the frequency of stimulation. High frequency sounds produce a maximum displacement of the basilar membrane near the oval window, so that there is little movement on the remainder of the membrane. Low frequency sounds produce a pattern of vibration which

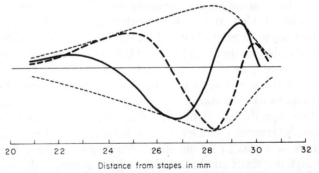

Distance from stapes in mm

FIG. 1.7 The instantaneous displacement of the cochlear partition at two successive instants in time, derived from a cochlear model. The pattern moves from left to right, building up gradually with distance, and decaying rapidly beyond the point of maximal displacement. The dotted line represents the envelope traced out by the amplitude peaks in the waveform. From von Békésy (1947), by permission of *J. Acoust. Soc. Am.*

extends all the way along the basilar membrane, but which reaches a maximum before the end of the membrane. Figure 1.8 shows the envelopes of the patterns of vibration for several different low frequency sinusoids (from von Békésy, 1960). Although it is now known that responses on the basilar

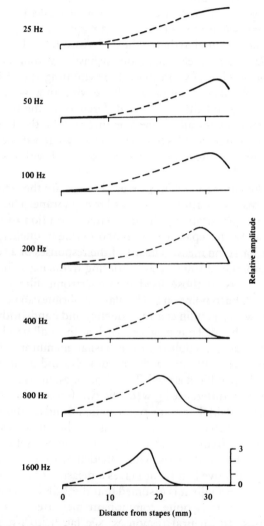

FIG. 1.8 Envelopes of patterns of vibration on the basilar membrane for a number of low frequency sounds. Solid lines indicate the results of actual measurements, while the dashed lines are von Békésy's extrapolations. From *Experiments in Hearing*, by von Békésy (1960), used with the permission of McGraw-Hill.

membrane are more sharply tuned than shown in this figure, the figure does illustrate the important point that sounds of different frequencies produce maximum displacement at different places along the basilar membrane. In effect the cochlea is behaving like a Fourier analyser, although with a less than perfect frequency analysing power.

It is worth noting that, in response to steady sinusoidal stimulation each point on the basilar membrane vibrates in an approximately sinusoidal manner with a frequency equal to that of the input waveform. For example, if we apply a 1000 Hz pure tone, each point on the basilar membrane for which there is a detectable amount of vibration will be vibrating at that frequency. Some parts of the basilar membrane will be vibrating with a greater amplitude than others, and there will be differences in the phases of the vibration at different points along the membrane, but the frequency of vibration of each point will be the same. This is true whatever the frequency of the input waveform, provided it is a single sinusoid within the audible range of frequencies.

A number of different methods may be used to specify the 'sharpness' of tuning of the patterns of vibration on the basilar membrane. These methods allow us to describe quantitatively the frequency resolution of the basilar membrane, i.e. its ability to separate sounds of differing frequencies. Most of the recent data are based on measurements of the responses of a single point on the basilar membrane to sinusoids of differing frequency. The measures obtained are analogous to those used with electronic filters, which we discussed in section 4. Each point on the basilar membrane can be considered as a bandpass filter with a certain centre frequency and bandwidth, and with slopes outside the passband. Thus measures such as the 3 dB bandwidth, and slopes in dB/octave, can be applied to the basilar membrane. Often it is difficult to measure the 3 dB bandwidth accurately, and a measure taken further down from the passband is used. The commonest measure is the 10 dB bandwidth, which is the difference between the two frequencies at which the response has fallen by 10 dB. For many types of filters, and for the response of the basilar membrane, the bandwidth is not constant, but increases roughly in proportion with centre frequency. Thus it is sometimes useful to use the relative bandwidth, which is the bandwidth divided by the centre frequency. The reciprocal of the relative bandwidth gives a measure of the sharpness of tuning, known as Q. Normally it is assumed that the 3 dB bandwidth is used to define Q. However, it is quite common in measurements of basilar membrane responses, and neural responses (see later), to use the 10 dB bandwidth. In this case the measure of sharpness of tuning is described as $Q_{10\,dB}$.

Most of the pioneering work on patterns of vibration along the basilar membrane was done by von Békésy (1928, 1942). His technique involved the use of a light microscope and stroboscopic illumination to measure the vibration amplitude at many points along the basilar membrane in human cadaver ears. For practical reasons his measurements were limited to the apical end of the basilar membrane, so that he measured mainly low frequency responses. The 'tuning curves' found by von Békésy were rather broad. The relative bandwidth was about 0.6 in the frequency range observed. This has presented a considerable problem for auditory theorists, since the observed frequency selectivity appeared to be insufficient to explain either our psychoacoustically observed frequency resolving power (e.g. the ability to 'hear out'.partials in a complex tone), or the selectivity observed in individual neurones in the auditory nerve (see later on in this Chapter). However, there are a number of difficulties associated with the technique used by von Békésy, and these render his results untrustworthy. Firstly, the vibration amplitudes had to be at least of the order of one wavelength of visible light, which required very high sound levels – about 140 dB SPL. The vibration of the basilar membrane is now believed to be nonlinear, so that it is not valid to extrapolate from these high levels to more normal sound levels. Secondly, the frequency analysing mechanism is now known to be physiologically vulnerable, so that cadaver ears give markedly atypical responses.

Recent measurements of basilar membrane vibration, using different techniques in living animals, have shown that the basilar membrane is much more sharply tuned than found by von Békésy. In one technique, using an effect called the Mössbauer effect, a radioactive source of gamma rays, of very small mass and physical dimensions, is placed upon the basilar membrane. Changes in the velocity of this source, produced by motion of the basilar membrane, can be detected as a change in the wavelength of the emitted radiation. This is an example of a Doppler shift, like the drop in pitch of a train whistle as it passes you. The sensitivity of this method increases with increasing frequency; at 1000 Hz a peak deflection of about 20 nanometres (nm) (1 nm is a ten millionth of a centimetre) can be measured, while at 10 kHz the limit is about 2 nm. This corresponds to a SPL of 70–80 dB. Thus this method has been used mainly at high frequencies, where sound levels much lower than those used by von Békésy can be utilized. A second technique involves placing a small mirror on the surface of the basilar membrane and shining a laser beam onto the mirror. The interference between the incident and reflected light can be used to determine the motion of the mirror; hence the name 'laser interferometry'.

Results using these techniques in live animals have shown that the sharpness of tuning of the basilar membrane depends critically on the physiological condition of the animal; the better the condition, the sharper is the tuning (Khanna and Leonard, 1982; Sellick *et al.*, 1982; Leonard and Khanna, 1984; Robles *et al.*, 1986). Nowadays, the physiological status of the cochlea is often monitored by placing an electrode in or near the auditory nerve, and measuring the combined responses of the neurones to tone bursts or clicks; this response is known as the compound action potential (AP or CAP). The lowest sound level at which an AP can be detected is called the AP threshold. Usually, the basilar membrane is sharply tuned when the AP threshold is low, indicating good physiological condition.

An example is given in Fig. 1.9, which shows the input sound level (in dB SPL) required to produce a constant velocity of motion at a particular point on the basilar membrane, as a function of stimulus frequency (data from Sellick *et al.*, 1982). This is sometimes called a 'constant velocity tuning curve'. At the start of the experiment, when AP thresholds were low, a very sharp tuning curve was obtained (solid circles). As the condition of the animal deteriorated, the tuning became broader, and the sound level required to produce the criterion response increased markedly around the tip.

It now seems clear that in a normal, healthy ear each point on the basilar membrane is sharply tuned, responding with high sensitivity to a limited

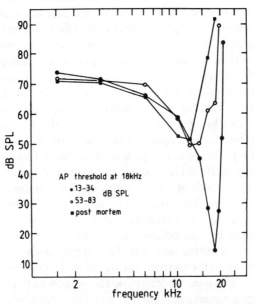

FIG. 1.9 Tuning curves measured at a single point on the basilar membrane. Each curve shows the input sound level required to produce a constant velocity on the basilar membrane, plotted as a function of stimulus frequency. The curve marked by solid circles was obtained at the start of the experiment when the animal was in good physiological condition. From Sellick *et al.* (1982), by permission of the authors and *J. Acoust. Soc. Am.*

range of frequencies, and requiring higher and higher sound intensities to produce a response as the frequency is moved beyond that range. $Q_{10\,dB}$ values are typically in the range 3–10. It also seems likely that the sharp tuning and high sensitivity reflect an *active* process; that is, they do not result simply from the mechanical properties of the basilar membrane and surrounding fluid, but depend on biological structures actively influencing the mechanics (for reviews, see Yates, 1986; Pickles, 1986, 1988). The most likely structures to play this role are the outer hair cells, which will be described later.

Recent work has also shown that the basilar membrane vibration is nonlinear; the magnitude of the response does not grow directly in proportion with the magnitude of the input (Rhode, 1971; Rhode and Robles, 1974; Sellick *et al.*, 1982). The nonlinearity causes the peak in the pattern of vibration to flatten out at high sound levels, which partly accounts for the broad tuning observed by von Békésy. The nonlinearity decreases as the physiological condition of the cochlea worsens, and after death the responses are linear. This suggests that the active process responsible for sharp tuning and high sensitivity on the basilar membrane is also responsible for the nonlinearity. The nonlinearity has aroused considerable theoretical interest and may provide a key to the understanding of certain combination tones which occur in the auditory system (see section 5D).

So far we have described the responses of the basilar membrane to steady sinusoidal stimulation. While there are some disagreements about the details of patterns of vibration, it is now beyond doubt that pure tones produce patterns with single maxima, whose positions depend upon frequency. In other words, there is a frequency-to-place conversion. The situation with other types of sounds is somewhat more complex. Consider first the case of two sinusoids, of different frequencies, presented simultaneously. The kind of pattern that will occur depends on the frequency separation of the two tones. If this is very large, then the two tones will produce two, effectively separate, patterns of vibration. Each will produce a maximum at the place on the basilar membrane which would have been excited most had that tone been presented alone. Thus the response of the basilar membrane to a low frequency tone will be essentially unaffected by a high frequency tone, and vice versa. In this kind of situation the basilar membrane behaves like a Fourier analyser, breaking down the complex sound into its sinusoidal components. When the two tones are relatively closer together in frequency, however, the patterns of vibration on the basilar membrane will interact, so that some points on the basilar membrane will be responding to both of the tones. At those points the displacement of the basilar membrane as a function of time will not be sinusoidal, but will be a complex waveform resulting from the interference of the two tones. When the two tones are sufficiently close in frequency, there will no longer be a separate maximum in the pattern of vibration for each of the component tones; instead there will be a single, broader, maximum. Thus, in a sense, the basilar membrane has failed to resolve the individual frequency components. We shall see, in Chapter 3, that the frequency resolving power of the auditory system, as observed psychoacoustically, is also limited.

The position of the basilar membrane which is excited most by a given frequency varies approximately with the logarithm of frequency, for frequencies above 500 Hz. Further, the relative bandwidths of the patterns of vibration on the basilar membrane in response to sinusoidal stimulation are approximately constant in this frequency range. This means that the frequency separation necessary for the resolution of two tones is proportional to centre frequency. Consider how this applies to the kind of complex sound which might be produced by a musical instrument, namely a harmonic complex tone. The frequency separation between adjacent harmonics is constant (and equal to the fundamental frequency). Thus the patterns of vibration for the higher harmonics will overlap much more than those for the lower harmonics. This is illustrated schematically in Fig. 1.10, which shows

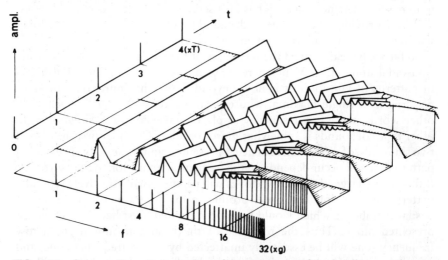

FIG. 1.10 Schematic representation of the response of the basilar membrane to a series of periodic impulses. Time is plotted along the *t* axis on a linear scale. The frequency (*f*) and amplitude (ampl.) scales are logarithmic. The waveform of the stimulus is indicated on the top left and its spectrum is at the bottom left. For the central part of the figure the frequency axis may be considered as equivalent to a position axis, indicating distance along the basilar membrane. This part of the figure shows the envelopes of the travelling wave patterns as a function of time and position. From Duifhuis (1972), by permission of the author.

responses to a periodic pulse train; this stimulus is composed of harmonics which all have the same amplitude (Fig. 1.3). The figure shows idealized envelopes of the patterns of vibration as a function of time (linear scale) and frequency (logarithmic scale). The lower harmonics are separated out to some extent, while at the same time the envelopes corresponding to those harmonics fluctuate relatively little as a function of time. The response as a function of time to a low harmonic is similar to the response which would have been observed if the harmonic had been presented alone. For the higher harmonics, the patterns of vibration overlap to a considerable extent. The individual harmonics are no longer resolved. At points on the basilar membrane where this happens, the envelopes of the patterns of vibration fluctuate strongly as a function of time. For the higher harmonics, the time pattern of the envelope on the basilar membrane is like that of the stimulus as a whole. We shall see in Chapters 3 and 5 that these factors play a crucial role in our perception of complex tones.

The response of the basilar membrane to a sudden change in sound pressure (a step function) or to a short impulse (a single click) is somewhat different. The spectra of these stimuli contain a wide range of frequencies, so that we can expect to see responses all along the basilar membrane. What happens is that a 'travelling bulge', looking like a short decaying wave train, is set up on the basilar membrane, and travels all the way along it. A number of workers have investigated the response of a single point on the basilar membrane in response to a brief click; this is called the impulse response function of that point. Figure 1.11 shows an impulse response function computed from the data of Wilson and Johnstone (1972). It looks like a damped, or decaying, sinusoidal oscillation, and resembles the impulse response of a bandpass filter (see Fig. 1.5). The frequency of this oscillation depends on which part of the basilar membrane is being studied. The basal end of the basilar membrane, which responds best to high frequencies, will show a high-frequency oscillation, while the apical end, which responds best to low frequencies, will show a low-frequency oscillation. Thus, the waveform as a function of time will vary continuously with position along the basilar membrane, according to the frequency which excites that position most. We shall see in Chapter 6 that this pattern of responses affects our ability to localize sounds of a transient character.

C The transduction process and the hair cells

So far we have been concerned with the mechanical responses of the basilar membrane to sound stimulation. We have seen that the basilar membrane acts as a kind of spectrum analyser, or Fourier analyser, but with a limited

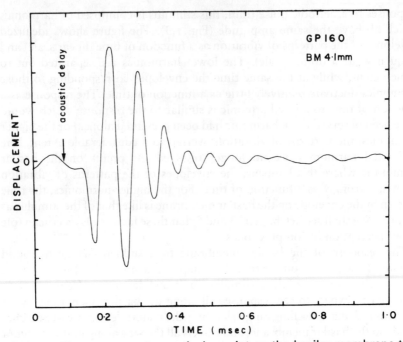

FIG. 1.11 The response at a particular point on the basilar membrane to a short impulse. From Wilson and Johnstone (1972), by permission of the authors.

resolving power. Let us consider how the information about frequency, amplitude and time, which is carried in the vibration patterns of the basilar membrane, is converted or coded into neural signals in the auditory nervous system.

Between the basilar membrane and the tectorial membrane are hair cells, which form part of a structure called the organ of Corti (see Fig. 1.12). The hair cells are divided into two groups by an arch known as the tunnel of Corti. Those on the side of the arch closest to the outside of the cochlea are known as outer hair cells, and are arranged in three rows in the cat and up to five rows in humans. The hair cells on the other side of the arch form a single row, and are known as inner hair cells. There are about 25 000 outer hair cells, each with about 140 hairs protruding from it, while there are about 3500 inner hair cells, each with about 40 hairs. The tectorial membrane, which has a gelatinous structure, lies above the hairs. It appears that the hairs of the outer hair cells actually make contact with the tectorial membrane, but this may not be true for the inner hair cells. The tectorial membrane appears to be effectively hinged at one side (the left in Fig. 1.12), so that when the basilar

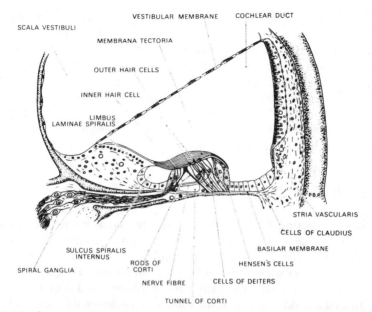

FIG. 1.12 Cross-section of the cochlea, showing the organ of Corti. The actual receptors are the hair cells lying on either side of the tunnel of Corti. From Hamilton, *Textbook of Human Anatomy*, Macmillan (1976).

membrane moves up and down, a shearing motion is created between the basilar membrane and the tectorial membrane. As a result the hairs at the tops of the hair cells are displaced. It is thought that this leads to excitation of the inner hair cells, which leads in turn to the generation of action potentials in the neurones of the auditory nerve. Thus the inner hair cells act to transduce mechanical movements into neural activity.

There are many details of the transduction process which remain poorly understood. However, it now seems clear that the inner and outer hair cells have very different functions. The great majority of afferent neurones, which carry information from the cochlea to higher levels of the auditory system, connect to inner hair cells; each inner hair cell is contacted by about 20 neurones (Spoendlin, 1970). Thus, most, if not all, information about sounds is conveyed via the inner hair cells. The main role of the outer hair cells may be actively to influence the mechanics of the cochlea, so as to produce high sensitivity and sharp tuning. There is even evidence that the outer hair cells have a motor function, changing their length and shape in response to electrical stimulation (for a review see Pickles, 1988). Supporting the idea that the outer hair cells play an active role in influencing cochlear mechanics, drugs or other agents which selectively affect the operation of the outer hair cells result in a loss of sharp tuning and a reduction of sensitivity of the basilar membrane. Furthermore, it is likely that this action of the outer hair cells is partly under the control of higher centres of the auditory system. There are about 1800 efferent nerve fibres which carry information from the auditory system to the cochlea, most of them originating in the superior olivary complex of the brain stem (see section 7). Many of these efferent fibres make contact with the outer hair cells, and thus can affect their activity. It appears that even the earliest stages in the analysis of auditory signals are partly under the control of higher centres.

D   Cochlear echoes

Evidence supporting the idea that there are active biological processes influencing cochlear mechanics has come from a remarkable phenomenon first reported by Kemp (1978). If a low-level click is applied to the ear, then it is possible to detect sound being reflected from the ear, using a microphone sealed into the ear canal. The early part of this reflected sound appears to come from the middle ear, but some sound can be detected for delays from 5 to 60 ms following the instant of click presentation. These delays are far too long to be attributed to the middle ear, and thus they almost certainly result from activity in the cochlea itself. Hence the reflected sounds are known as 'evoked oto-acoustic emissions' although they have also been called 'Kemp echoes' and 'cochlear echoes'.

Since Kemp's original discovery, there has been a considerable amount of work studying this phenomenon. We do not have space to report in detail on this work, and we will restrict ourselves to certain aspects of it. Although the input click in Kemp's experiment contained energy over a wide range of frequencies, only certain frequencies were present in the reflected sound. Kemp suggested that the reflections are generated at points on the basilar membrane, or in the transduction mechanism, where there is a gradient or discontinuity in the mechanical or electrical properties. The response is nonlinear, in that the reflected sound does not have an intensity in direct proportion to the input intensity. In fact, the relative level of the reflection is greatest at low sound levels; the echo grows about 3 dB for each 10 dB increase in input level. This nonlinear behaviour can be used to distinguish the response arising from the cochlea from the middle ear response; the latter behaves in a linear manner. Sometimes the amount of energy reflected from the cochlea at a given frequency may exceed that which was present in the input click. This has led Kemp and others to suggest that the echo reflects an active process of biological amplification.

Cochlear echoes can be very stable in a given individual, both in waveform and frequency content, but each ear gives its own characteristic response. Responses tend to be strongest between 500 and 2500 Hz, probably because transmission from the cochlea back through the middle ear is most efficient in this range. Cochlear echoes can be measured for brief tone bursts as well as clicks, and it is even possible to detect a reflected component in response to continuous stimulation with pure tones. The echo response to a particular component in a stimulus can be suppressed if the ear is stimulated more strongly at a neighbouring frequency (compare section 6F). By presenting neighbouring tones at a variety of frequencies, and adjusting their levels, it is possible to map out equal suppression contours. These contours have the same general shape as tuning curves on the basilar membrane (Fig. 1.9). This lends strong support to the notion that the echoes are generated within the cochlea.

Cochlear echoes are only observed in ears which are in good physiological condition. Thus human ears with even moderate pathology of cochlear origin show no detectable echoes. The echo is also abolished in ears which have been exposed to intense sounds or to drugs which adversely affect the operation of the cochlea. In the former case, the echo may return after a period of recovery. This suggests that the echo is linked to a physiologically vulnerable process, just like the process which is responsible for the sharp tuning and high sensitivity of the basilar membrane. The measurement of cochlear echoes may provide a sensitive way of monitoring the physiological state of the cochlea.

When the ear is stimulated with two tones, having frequencies f_1 and f_2 (where $f_2 > f_1$), then an echo may be detected with frequency $2f_1 - f_2$ (Kim *et al.*, 1980). It turns out that subjects often also report hearing a tone with a pitch corresponding to the frequency $2f_1 - f_2$. Such a tone is called a combination tone. This particular combination tone has been frequently observed in auditory research (see Chapters 3 and 5) and it indicates the presence of a significant nonlinearity in the auditory system. Its presence as a cochlear echo implies that it is present as a mechanical disturbance in the cochlea, probably as a travelling wave on the basilar membrane. The level of the combination tone, relative to the level of the primary tones in the ear canal, can be reversibly reduced by exposing the ear to a fatiguing tone of 80–90 dB SPL at a frequency near or slightly below the primary frequencies (see Chapter 2, section 7, for a discussion of fatigue). Again this indicates that the nonlinear aspect of cochlear function is physiologically vulnerable.

Sometimes the transient stimulation induces a sustained oscillation at a particular frequency, and the subject may report hearing this oscillation as a tonal sensation. The phenomenon of hearing sound in the absence of external stimulation is known as tinnitus. It appears that tinnitus may arise from abnormal activity at several different points in the auditory system, but in a few cases it corresponds to mechanical activity in the cochlea. Many ears emit sounds in the absence of any input and these can be detected in the ear canal (Zurek, 1981). Such sounds are called 'spontaneous oto-acoustic emissions', and their existence indicates that there is a source of energy within the cochlea which is capable of generating sounds.

In summary, while the exact mechanism by which the cochlear echo is generated is not understood, there is agreement that it is connected with active processes occurring inside the cochlea. These processes have a strong nonlinear component, they are biologically active, they are physiologically vulnerable and they appear to be responsible for the sensitivity and sharp tuning of the basilar membrane.

6   NEURAL RESPONSES IN THE AUDITORY NERVE

Most of the recent studies of activity in the auditory nerve have used electrodes with very fine tips, known as microelectrodes. These record the nerve impulses, or spikes, in single auditory nerve fibres (often called single units). Three general results have emerged, which seem to hold for most mammals. Firstly, the fibres show background or spontaneous firing in the absence of sound stimulation. Spontaneous firing rates range from close to 0 per second up to about 150 per second. Secondly, the fibres respond better to some frequencies than to others; they show frequency selectivity. Finally, the fibres show phase locking; neural firings tend to occur at a particular phase of the stimulating waveform, so that there is a temporal regularity in the firing pattern of a neurone in response to a periodic stimulus. We will consider each of these phenomena in more detail.

A   Spontaneous firing rates and thresholds

Liberman (1978) presented evidence that auditory nerve fibres could be classified into three groups on the basis of their spontaneous rates. About 61% of fibres have high spontaneous rates (18 to 250 spikes per second); 23% have medium rates (0.5 to 18 spikes per second); and 16% have low spontaneous rates (less than 0.5 spike per second). The spontaneous rates are correlated with the position and size of the synapses on the inner hair cells. High spontaneous rates are associated with large synapses, primarily located on the side of the inner hair cells facing the outer hair cells. Low spontaneous rates are associated with smaller synapses on the opposite side of the hair cells. The spontaneous rates are also correlated with the thresholds of the neurones. The threshold is the lowest sound level at which a change in response of the neurone can be measured. High spontaneous rates tend to be associated with low thresholds and vice versa. The most sensitive neurones may have thresholds close to 0 dB SPL, whereas the least sensitive neurones may have thresholds of 80 dB SPL or more.

B Tuning curves and iso-rate contours

The frequency selectivity of a single nerve fibre is often illustrated by a tuning curve, which shows the fibre's threshold as a function of frequency. This curve is also known as the frequency-threshold curve (FTC). The stimuli are usually tone bursts, rather than continuous tones, so that changes in activity are more easily detected. The frequency at which the threshold of the fibre is lowest is called the characteristic frequency (CF). Some typical tuning curves are presented in Fig. 1.13. It may be seen that, on the logarithmic frequency

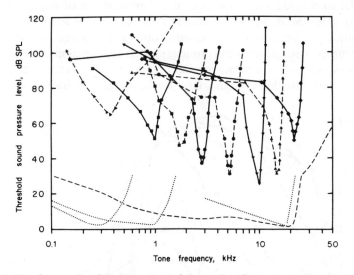

FIG. 1.13 A sample of tuning curves (also called frequency-threshold curves) obtained from single neurones in the auditory nerve of anaesthetized cats. Each curve shows results for one neurone. The sound level required for threshold is plotted as a function of the stimulus frequency (logarithmic scale). The dotted and dashed curves at the bottom are tuning curves for particular points on the basilar membrane (shifted downwards by an arbitrary amount), but these curves are now believed to be broader than would be found in an animal in pristine physiological condition. From Evans (1975), by permission of the author.

scale used, the tuning curves are generally steeper on the high-frequency side than on the low-frequency one. It is generally assumed that the frequency selectivity in single auditory nerve fibres occurs because those fibres are responding to activity at restricted regions of the basilar membrane. In other words, a single nerve fibre is assumed to derive its output from a particular part of the basilar membrane. Experiments tracing single neurones whose tuning curves had been determined directly confirm this supposition (Liberman, 1982). Furthermore, CFs are distributed in an orderly manner in the auditory nerve. Fibres with high CFs are found in the periphery of the nerve bundle, and there is an orderly decrease in CF towards the centre of the nerve bundle (Kiang *et al.*, 1965). This kind of organization is known as tonotopic organization and it indicates that the place representation of frequency along the basilar membrane is preserved as a place representation in the auditory nerve. It appears that the sharpness of tuning of the basilar membrane is essentially the same as the sharpness of tuning of single neurones in the auditory nerve (Khanna and Leonard, 1982; Sellick *et al.*, 1982; Robles *et al.*, 1986).

In order to provide a description of the characteristics of single fibres at levels above threshold, iso-rate contours can be plotted. To determine an iso-rate contour the intensity of sinusoidal stimulation required to produce a predetermined firing rate in the neurone is plotted as a function of frequency. The resulting curves are generally similar in shape to tuning curves, although they sometimes broaden at high sound levels. An alternative method is to

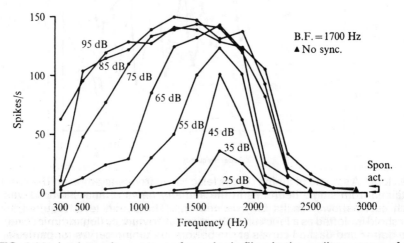

FIG. 1.14   Iso-intensity contours for a single fibre in the auditory nerve of an anaesthetized squirrel monkey. Note that the frequency producing maximal firing varies as a function of level. From Rose *et al.* (1971), by permission of the authors.

record firing rates at equal sound levels as a function of tone frequency. The resulting curves (iso-intensity contours) generally vary in shape according to the sound level chosen and differ considerably from tuning curves (see Fig. 1.14). The interpretation of iso-intensity contours is difficult, because their shape depends upon how the rate of firing of the nerve fibre varies with intensity; this is not usually a linear function (see later). However, it is of interest that for some fibres the frequency that gives maximal firing varies as a function of level. This poses some problems for one of the theories of pitch perception which will be discussed in Chapter 5.

C Rate versus level functions

Figure 1.15 shows how the rate of discharge of an auditory nerve fibre changes as a function of stimulus level. The stimulus was a continuous tone at

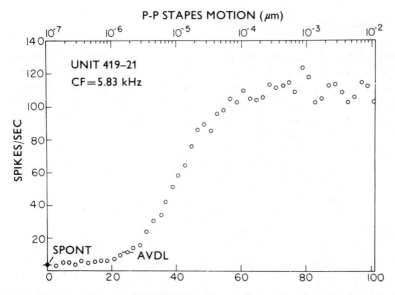

FIG. 1.15 An example of how the discharge rate of a single auditory nerve fibre varies as a function of stimulus level, for a continuous stimulating tone at the CF of the neurone. The threshold of the neurone is the lowest sound level at which there is a detectable change in firing rate and is indicated by the letters AVDL (audio visual detection level). Above a certain sound level increases in level do not produce increases in firing rate; the neurone is saturated. The range of levels between threshold and saturation is known as the 'dynamic range' and is typically 30-40 dB. The sound level is specified in dB with an arbitrary reference level. The level at the point marked AVDL corresponds to about 2 dB SPL. From Kiang (1968), by permission of the author.

the CF of the unit. The general shape of the curve is typical of most auditory nerve fibres, although there is considerable variability in both the spontaneous firing rate and the maximum firing rate. Notice that above a certain sound level the neurone no longer responds to increases in sound level with an increase in firing rate; the neurone is said to be saturated. The range of sound levels between threshold and the level at which saturation occurs is called the dynamic range. This range is correlated with the threshold and spontaneous rate of the neurone; high spontaneous rates and low thresholds are associated with small dynamic ranges. For most neurones the dynamic range is between 20 and 50 dB, but a few neurones do not show complete saturation; instead the firing rate continues to increase gradually with increasing sound level even at high sound levels. This has been called 'sloping saturation' (Sachs and Abbas, 1974) and it occurs particularly for neurones with low spontaneous rates.

D   Neural excitation patterns

Although the technique of recording from single auditory neurones has provided very valuable evidence about the coding of sounds in the auditory system, it is lacking in one very fundamental respect: it does not tell us anything about the pattern of neural responses over different auditory neurones, or about possible interactions or mutual dependencies in the firing patterns of different auditory neurones. A considerable advance has come recently from studies of the responses of a great many single neurones within one experimental animal to a limited set of stimuli (Pfeiffer and Kim, 1975; Kim and Molnar, 1979; Sachs and Young, 1980). These studies have shown, as we would expect, that in response to a single, low level, pure tone there is a high level of activity in neurones with CFs close to the tone frequency, with activity dropping off for CFs on either side of this. However, at higher sound levels the picture is more complicated. As a result of neural saturation there may be a more or less uniform high level of neural activity over a wide range of CFs, with activity only falling off at CFs far removed from the stimulus frequency. We will discuss some of the implications of this in Chapters 2 and 3.

The distribution of neural activity as a function of CF is sometimes called the 'excitation pattern'. However, the definition of an appropriate measure of 'activity' is difficult, since both spontaneous and maximum firing rates vary considerably, even in neurones with similar CFs. Thus, at best we could only represent what was happening in an 'average' neurone at a given CF. This last problem can be partially overcome by representing excitation patterns in a

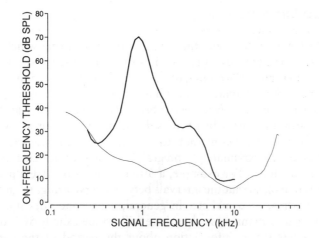

FIG. 1.16 An excitation pattern for a 1 kHz sinusoid with a level of 70 dB SPL, determined from the responses of single neurones in the auditory nerve of the cat. The sinusoid at 1 kHz was alternated with a 'signal' whose frequency was varied. For each 'signal' frequency, the level of the signal was determined at which the response to the signal was just greater than the response to the fixed 1 kHz tone. This level is referred to as the 'on-frequency threshold' and it is plotted as a function of frequency (thick curve), giving the desired excitation pattern. The thin curve indicates the threshold at CF of the most sensitive neurones as a function of CF. The origin of the small 'bump' around 3 kHz is not clear; it may reflect some characteristic of the transmission of sound through the outer and middle ear. From B. Delgutte (personal communication).

different way; instead of determining the amount of neural activity at each CF, we determine what the level of a pure tone with frequency equal to that CF would have to be in order to produce an equal amount of neural activity. Thus the excitation pattern becomes a representation of the effective amount of excitation produced by a stimulus as a function of CF, and is plotted as effective level (in dB) against CF. Normally the CF is plotted on a logarithmic scale, roughly in accord with the way that frequency appears to be represented on the basilar membrane. Excitation patterns have been determined in this way by Bertrand Delgutte (personal communication). An example is shown in Fig. 1.16. We shall see in Chapter 3 that psychoacoustic techniques have been developed which, given certain assumptions, allow the determination of excitation patterns like this for man, and that such excitation patterns can be considered as an internal representation of the spectrum of the stimulus.

E   Phase locking

So far we have described only the changes in rate of firing which occur in response to a given stimulus. However, information about the stimulus is also carried in the temporal patterning of the neural firings. In response to a pure tone the nerve firings tend to be phase locked or synchronized to the stimulating waveform. A given nerve fibre does not necessarily fire on every cycle of the stimulus but, when firings do occur, they occur at roughly the same phase of the waveform each time. Thus the time intervals between firings will be (approximately) integral multiples of the period of the stimulating waveform. For example, a 500 Hz tone will have a period of 2 milliseconds (2 ms), so that the intervals between nerve firings might be 2 ms, or 4 ms, or 6 ms, or 8 ms, etc. In general, a neurone does not fire in a completely regular manner, so that there will not be exactly 500, or 250 or 125 spikes/s. However, information about the period of the stimulating waveform is carried unambiguously in the temporal pattern of firing of a single neurone, and if we consider the responses over an ensemble of fibres, then there will be some nerve spikes on every cycle of the stimulus. Phase locking is just what we would expect to occur as a result of the transduction process. Deflection of the hairs on the outer hair cells towards the outside of the cochlea, produced by movement of the basilar membrane towards the tectorial membrane, leads to neural excitation. No excitation occurs when the basilar membrane moves in the opposite direction. (This description is somewhat over-simplified; see, for example, Ruggero *et al.*, 1986.) Thus, nerve firings tend to occur on a deflection of the basilar membrane towards the tectorial membrane produced by the rarefaction phase of the signal.

One way to demonstrate phase locking in a single auditory nerve fibre is to plot a histogram of the time intervals between successive nerve firings. Several such interspike interval histograms are shown in Fig. 1.17, for a neurone with a CF of 1.6 kHz. For each of the different stimulating frequencies (from 0.408 to 2.3 kHz in this case) the intervals between nerve spikes lie predominantly at integral multiples of the period of the stimulating tone. These intervals are indicated by dots below each abscissa. Thus, although the neurone does not fire on every cycle of the stimulus, the distribution of time intervals between nerve firings depends closely on the frequency of the stimulating waveform.

Phase locking does not occur over the whole range of audible frequencies. The upper frequency limit seems to lie at about 4–5 kHz (Rose *et al.*, 1968). This upper limit is not determined by the maximum firing rates of neurones. Rather it is determined by the precision with which the initiation of a nerve impulse is linked to a particular phase of the stimulus. It turns out that there is variability in the exact instant of initiation of a nerve impulse. At high frequencies this variability becomes comparable with the period of the

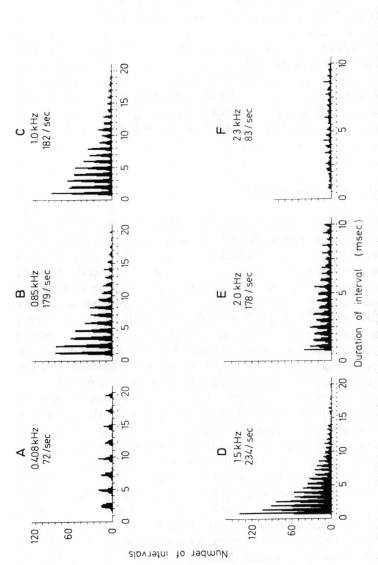

FIG. 1.17 Interspike interval histograms for a single auditory neurone (in the squirrel monkey) with a CF of 1.6 kHz. The frequency of the stimulating tone and the mean response rate in spikes per second are indicated above each histogram. All tones were at 80 dB SPL and of duration 1 s. Notice that the time scales in E and F differ from those in A to D. From Rose *et al.* (1968), by permission of the authors.

waveform, so that above a certain frequency the spikes will be 'smeared out' over the whole period of the waveform, instead of occurring primarily at a particular phase. It is this smearing which is responsible for the loss of phase locking above 4–5 kHz.

There is still considerable controversy over the extent to which information carried in the timing of neural impulses is actually used in perceptual processes. Most workers accept that our ability to localize sounds depends in part on a comparison of the temporal information from the two ears, but the relevance of temporal information in masking and in pitch perception is still hotly debated. These problems will be discussed more fully in Chapters 3 and 5.

F   Two-tone suppression

So far we have discussed the responses of auditory neurones to single pure tones. One of the reasons for using pure tones as stimuli is that given earlier: if the peripheral auditory system could be characterized as approximately linear, then the response to a complex stimulus could be calculated as the linear sum of the responses to the sinusoidal (Fourier) components of the stimulus (see section 3). Although neural responses themselves are clearly nonlinear (showing, for example, thresholds and saturation), they sometimes behave as though the system driving them were linear. In other situations the behaviour is clearly nonlinear, so that it is necessary to investigate directly the neural responses to complex stimuli, if we are to understand how the properties of these complex stimuli are coded in the auditory system.

Auditory nerve responses to two tones have been investigated by a number of workers. One striking finding which has emerged is that the tone-driven activity of a single fibre in response to one tone can be suppressed by the presence of a second tone. This was originally called two-tone inhibition (Sachs and Kiang, 1968), although the term 'two-tone suppression' is now generally preferred, since the effect does not appear to involve neural inhibition. Typically the phenomenon is investigated by presenting a tone at, or close to, the CF of a neurone. A second tone is then presented, its frequency and intensity are varied, and the effects of this on the response of the neurone are noted. When the frequency and intensity of the second tone fall within the excitatory area bounded by the tuning curve, it usually produces an increase in firing rate. However, when it falls just outside that area, the response to the first tone is reduced or suppressed. The effect is usually greatest in two suppression regions at frequencies slightly above or below the area of the unit's excitatory response to a single tone (see Fig. 1.18). The suppression effects begin and cease very rapidly, within a few milliseconds of the onset

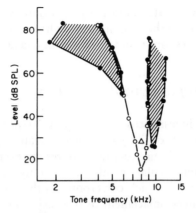

FIG. 1.18 The open circles show the tuning curve (threshold versus frequency) of a single neurone with a CF at 8 kHz. The neurone was stimulated with a tone at CF, and just above threshold (indicated by the open triangle). A second tone was then added and its frequency and intensity varied. Any tone within the shaded areas bounded by the solid circles would reduce the response to the tone at CF by 20% or more. These are the suppression areas. Data from Arthur *et al.* (1971).

and termination of the second tone (Arthur *et al.*, 1971). Thus it is unlikely that the suppression is established through any elaborate neural interconnections. It is likely that it is related to the nonlinearities of the basilar membrane (Legouix *et al.*, 1973; Rhode and Robles, 1974).

The effects of two-tone stimulation on temporal patterns of neural firing have also been studied. For tones which are nonharmonically related, Hind *et al.* (1967) found that discharges may be phase locked to one tone, or the other, or to both tones simultaneously. Which of these occurs is determined by the intensities of the two tones and their frequencies in relation to the 'response area' of the fibre. When phase locking occurs to only one tone of a pair, each of which is effective when acting alone, the temporal structure of the response may be indistinguishable from that which occurs when that tone is presented alone. Further, the discharge rate may be similar to the value produced by that tone alone. Thus the dominant tone appears to 'capture' the response of the neurone. We will discuss in Chapter 3 the possibility that this 'capture effect' underlies the masking of one sound by another. Notice that the 'capture effect' is probably another manifestation of two-tone suppression. The tone which is suppressed ceases to contribute to the pattern of phase locking, and the neurone responds as if only the suppressing tone were present. Suppression measured by phase locking can be shown even if the suppressor is within the excitatory response area of the neurone. However suppression of response rate is normally seen only when the suppressor is outside or at the edges of the response area. Otherwise the suppressor itself evokes an excitatory response, and produces an increase in firing rate.

G   Phase locking to complex sounds

Brugge *et al.* (1969) investigated auditory nerve responses to pairs of tones with simple frequency ratios (i.e. harmonically related tones). They drew the following conclusions: (1) auditory nerve fibres are excited by deflections of the cochlear partition (basilar membrane) in only one direction; (2) the discharges occur at times which correspond to the positive pressure of the stimulating waveform (displacement of the basilar membrane towards the tectorial membrane); (3) the effective stimulating waveform can be approximated by addition of the component sinusoids, although the required amplitude and phase relations usually cannot be taken directly from the actual stimulus parameters. The results of Brugge *et al.* (1969) indicate that interactions between two tones may take place even when their frequencies are quite widely separated (frequency ratios between the two tones of up to 7:1 were used).

Javel (1980) investigated the responses of single auditory neurones to stimuli consisting of three successive high harmonics of a complex tone. He showed that a portion of the neural activity in the neurones responding to the component frequencies was phase locked to the overall repetition rate of the stimulus (equal to the absent fundamental frequency). We will discuss in Chapter 5 the possibility that such temporal coding is responsible for the pitch of complex tones.

The responses of auditory neurones to clicks are closely related to the corresponding patterns of vibration which occur on the basilar membrane (see section 5). Such responses are often plotted in the form of post-stimulus time (PST) histograms. To determine a PST histogram, the click is presented many times, and the numbers of neural impulses occurring at various times after the instant of click presentation are counted. These are then plotted in the form of a histogram, with the instant of click presentation being taken as time zero (see Fig. 1.19). It may be seen that spikes tend to occur at certain preferred intervals after the presentation of the click, as indicated by the peaks in the histogram. The multiple peaks presumably occur because the response of the basilar membrane to a click is a damped or decaying oscillation (see Fig. 1.11). Nerve firings tend to occur at a particular phase of this damped oscillation. The time intervals between the peaks correspond to the reciprocal of the CF of the neurone. If the polarity of the click is reversed (e.g. from rarefaction to condensation) the pattern is shifted in time, so that

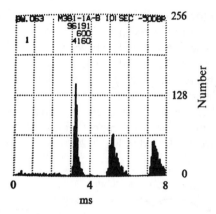

FIG. 1.19 A post-stimulus time (PST) histogram showing the number of nerve spikes occurring in response to a click, presented repeatedly, as a function of the time delay from the instant of presentation of the click. The time interval between peaks in the histogram corresponds to the reciprocal of the CF of the neurone (540 Hz). From Kiang *et al.* (1965), by permission of the author and MIT Press.

peaks now appear where dips were located. The latency of the first peak is shortest for rarefaction clicks, again indicating that the excitation of hair-cells occurs when the basilar membrane is deflected towards the tectorial membrane. These factors are particularly relevant to our ability to locate sounds of a transient character (see Chapter 6).

7 NEURAL RESPONSES AT HIGHER LEVELS IN THE AUDITORY SYSTEM

In the visual system it is known that neurones respond preferentially to certain features of the stimulus, such as lines of a particular orientation, movement or colour. There seems to be a hierarchy of specialized neural detectors (sometimes called feature detectors), ranging from centre-surround units to hypercomplex cells (Hubel and Wiesel, 1968). The information in the optic nerve is recoded and processed at different points in the visual system, so that the responses of cortical units are very different from those in the optic nerve.

Much the same thing seems to happen in the auditory system, except that it is much less clear what the crucial features of the stimulus are which will produce responses from a given neurone or set of neurones. In addition, the anatomy of the auditory system is exceedingly complex, so that many of the neural pathways within and between the various nuclei in the auditory system have yet to be investigated in detail. It is beyond the scope of this book to give more than the briefest description of recent research on the neurophysiology of higher centres in the auditory system. We will content ourselves with describing some properties of cortical neurones, and will introduce other data later in the book, when they have some relevance to the mechanism or process under discussion. Some of the more important neural centres or nuclei in the auditory pathway are illustrated in Fig. 1.20.

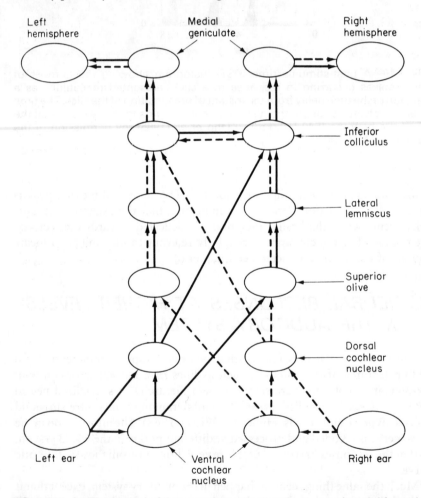

FIG. 1.20 An illustration of the most important pathways and nuclei from the ear to the auditory cortex. The nuclei illustrated are located in the brain stem.

It is likely that the cortex is concerned with analysing more complex aspects of stimuli than simple frequency or intensity. Many cortical neurones will not respond to steady pure tones at all, and the tuning properties of those which do respond to pure tones tend to differ from those found in primary auditory neurones. Abeles and Goldstein (1972) found three different types of tuning properties: narrow, broad and multirange (responding to a number of preferred frequencies). They considered that this suggested a hierarchical organization, with several narrow range units converging on to one multi-range unit. There is some dispute whether the tonotopic organization which is found at lower levels in the auditory system persists at the cortex. Merzenich *et al.* (1973a), using CF determinations in the anaesthetized cat, reported a highly ordered tonotopic organization; the CF changed in an orderly way according to the place of penetration of the electrode. On the other hand, Evans (1968), using unanaesthetized, unrestrained cats, found only a very general trend in the location of unit CFs. He considered that what little trend there was represented a residuum of anatomical arrangement from subcortical levels, rather than a property which had a functional significance for frequency analysis. A number of studies have indicated that anaesthetics do considerably alter the responses of cortical neurones, so that data obtained using anaesthetics must be interpreted with considerable caution.

Evans (1968), using mostly unanaesthetized cats, reported that 20% of cortical neurones respond only to complex stimuli such as clicks, bursts of noise or 'kissing' sounds. Of those neurones which would respond to tonal stimuli 10% would only do so if the tone frequency was changing. Whitfield and Evans (1965) reported that frequency-modulated tones (see Fig. 3.7) were very effective stimuli for the majority of neurones responding to tones. Many neurones exhibited responses which were preferential to certain directions of frequency change. These neurones have been called 'frequency sweep detectors'. Some neurones respond preferentially to particular rates of modulation or to particular rates of frequency sweep. For other neurones repetition rate and duration of tonal stimuli were critical parameters. Of all units studied 17% responded only to the onset of a tonal stimulus, while 10% responded only to the termination and 2% responded to both onset and termination. Over 50% of neurones were preferentially or specifically sensitive to particular locations of the sound source. This general finding has been confirmed and extended by Brugge and Merzenich (1973) for res-trained, unanaesthetized monkeys. They found that many units were sensitive to interaural (between the ears) time or intensity differences. At low frequencies spike count was a periodic function of interaural time delay. In several penetrations neighbouring cells were most sensitive to the same interaural delay. Some cells were sensitive to small interaural shifts in sound pressure levels over a range of about 20 dB. We shall see in Chapter 6 that the features of the stimuli to which these cells are responsive are crucial in our ability to localize sounds.

8   GENERAL SUMMARY AND CONCLUSIONS

Sound consists of variations in pressure as a function of time. It is often convenient to analyse a complex pressure wave into its sinusoidal frequency components. Periodic sounds can be shown by Fourier analysis to have line spectra containing harmonics of the fundamental component. This component has a frequency equal to the repetition rate of the whole complex. Nonperiodic sounds can be analysed using the Fourier transform. They have continuous spectra, in which the energy is distributed over a frequency range, rather than being concentrated at discrete frequencies.

Sound levels are usually measured using the decibel (dB) scale. This is a logarithmic measure which expresses the ratio of two intensities. When the reference intensity is chosen to be 10^{-12} W/m^2 (equivalent to a sound pressure of 20 μPa), the level has units of dB sound pressure level (dB SPL). When the reference intensity is the absolute threshold for a given sound and a given subject, the units are dB sensation level (dB SL).

The auditory system is often conceived as being composed of a series of successive stages. A stage is linear if it satisfies the conditions of superposition and homogeneity. The response of a linear system to a complex input can be calculated as the sum of the responses to the individual sinusoidal components of that input. Some stages of the auditory system appear to be roughly linear (e.g., the middle ear) but others are distinctly nonlinear.

A filter is a device which passes certain frequency components, but attenuates others. Filters can be used both for the manipulation of stimuli, and for their analysis. Filters can be characterized by their cutoff frequencies, usually measured at the 3 dB down points, and by their slopes in dB/octave. The bandwidth of a bandpass filter is equal to the frequency range between the two 3 dB down points.

The peripheral auditory system is composed of the outer, middle and inner ear. The middle ear acts as an impedance-matching transformer, to improve the efficiency of the transfer of energy between the air and the fluid-filled cochlea. A membrane called the basilar membrane runs along the length of the cochlea, dividing it into two chambers. Sounds produce travelling waves along the basilar membrane, and for each frequency there is a maximum in the pattern of vibration at a different place. Low frequencies produce maximum vibration close to the apex and high frequencies produce maximum vibration close to the base. The basilar membrane thus acts as a crude

Fourier analyser, or filter bank, splitting complex sounds into their component frequencies. The sharp tuning of the basilar membrane is physiologically vulnerable.

Movement of the basilar membrane causes a displacement of the hairs at the tips of the hair cells which lie within the organ of Corti on the basilar membrane, and this leads to action potentials within the nerve fibres of the auditory nerve. Most afferent nerve fibres contact the inner hair cells. The outer hair cells probably actively influence the vibration patterns on the basilar membrane, contributing to the sharp tuning and high sensitivity. They also seem to be involved in producing certain nonlinearities in the response, and in the production of cochlear emissions. The action of the outer hair cells may be influenced by efferent neurones carrying signals from the brain stem.

The nerve fibres of the auditory nerve show spontaneous activity in the absence of sound, and each nerve fibre has a threshold and a saturation level, above which increases in intensity produce no change in response. High spontaneous rates tend to be associated with low thresholds and low dynamic ranges. The threshold of a given fibre is lowest for one frequency, called the characteristic frequency (CF), and increases for frequencies on either side of this. The plot of threshold versus frequency is called the frequency-threshold curve or tuning curve. Single nerve fibres give tuning curves which are similar to those measured for single points on the basilar membrane.

The temporal pattern of the firing within a given neurone can also carry information about the stimulus. Nerve firings tend to occur at a particular phase of the stimulating waveform, a process known as phase locking. Phase locking breaks down above 4–5 kHz.

Sometimes the response of a single neurone to a sinusoidal tone may be reduced by a second tone, even when the second tone alone produces no response in the neurone. This is known as two-tone suppression, and it is an example of a nonlinear process in the peripheral auditory system.

The responses of neurones at higher levels of the auditory system have not been studied as thoroughly as responses in the auditory nerve. Some neurones in the auditory cortex appear to respond only to complex stimuli, or stimuli with time varying characteristics.

FURTHER READING

The following books contain useful chapters on the physics of sound as related to hearing:

Green, D. M. (1976). *An Introduction to Hearing*. Erlbaum, New Jersey.
Van Bergeijk, W. A., Pierce, J. R. and David E. E. (1961). *Waves and the Ear*. Heinemann, London.

The physiology of the auditory system is comprehensively reviewed in: Pickles, J. O. (1988). *An Introduction to the Physiology of Hearing*, Second Edition. Academic Press, London and New York.

Recent reviews are also provided by:

Haggard, M. P. and Evans, E. F. (eds) (1987). *Hearing. Brit. Med. Bull.* 43, 774–1042. The papers by Hackney, Russell, Wilson, Palmer and D. R. Moore are especially relevant.

A compact disc (CD) of auditory demonstrations has been produced by A. J. M. Houtsma, T. D. Rossing and W. M. Wagenaars (1987). The disc can be obtained through the Acoustical Society of America, 500 Sunnyside Blvd., Woodbury, NY 11797-2999, USA. The cost is 20 dollars, payable in advance. Demonstrations 4, 5, 6 and 32 are especially relevant to this chapter.

2
The perception of loudness

1 INTRODUCTION

The human ear is remarkable both in terms of its absolute sensitivity and in terms of the range of sound intensities to which it can respond. The most intense sound we can hear without damaging our ears has a level about 120 dB above that of the faintest sound we can detect. This corresponds to a ratio of intensities of 1 000 000 000 000 : 1. One aim of this chapter is to discuss the possible ways in which such a range could be coded.

Loudness is defined as that attribute of auditory sensation in terms of which sounds can be ordered on a scale extending from quiet to loud. A second aim of this chapter is to discuss how the loudness of sounds depends upon frequency and intensity, and to relate this to the way in which the sounds are coded. A problem which arises in studying the loudness of sounds, particularly when these are complex or of a transient nature, is that loudness is a subjective quantity, and as such cannot be measured directly. This problem has been tackled in a number of different ways: sometimes subjects are asked to match the loudness of a sound to that of some standard comparison stimulus (often a 1000 Hz tone); in other experiments subjects are asked to rate loudness on a numerical scale, a technique known as magnitude estimation. As we shall see, there are problems associated with each of these methods.

A third area of discussion will be that of loudness adaptation, fatigue and damage risk. In general, adaptation and fatigue in the auditory system are much less marked than in the visual system, and the effects also have different time courses. In certain types of hearing loss, adaptation effects become more marked. We will discuss how this, and the phenomenon of recruitment (see below), can be used in the differential diagnosis of hearing disorders.

2 ABSOLUTE THRESHOLDS

The absolute threshold of a sound is the minimum detectable level of that sound in the absence of any other external sounds. There have been several determinations of absolute thresholds as a function of frequency. It is important to define very carefully the way in which the physical intensity of the threshold stimulus is measured, and two methods have been in common use. One method requires the measurement of the sound pressure at some point close to the entrance of the ear canal or inside the ear canal, using a small 'probe' microphone. Ideally, the measurement is made very close to the eardrum. In all cases it is necessary to specify the exact position of the probe, since small changes in position can markedly affect the results at high frequencies. The threshold so determined is called the minimum audible pressure (MAP). The sounds are usually, but not always, delivered by headphone.

The other method uses tones delivered by loudspeaker, usually in a large anechoic chamber (a room whose walls are highly sound absorbing). The measurement of sound level is made after the listener is removed from the sound field, at the point which had been occupied by the centre of the listener's head. The threshold determined in this way is called the minimum audible field (MAF). The two methods give somewhat different results since the head, the pinna and the meatus do have an influence on the sound field. The MAP also depends on exactly where the microphone is placed.

A typical set of results for MAP is shown in Fig. 2.1. These were obtained

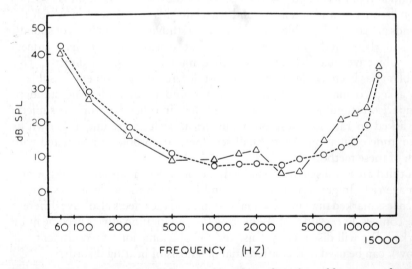

FIG. 2.1   The minimum audible sound level as a function of frequency for two positions close to the entrance of the ear canal (meatus). The solid curve gives sound levels measured 0.3 cm inside the entrance to the meatus, and the dashed curve gives levels measured 0.7 cm outside the entrance to the meatus. Redrawn from Dadson and King (1952), by permission of the authors and the Director of the National Physical Laboratory, UK.

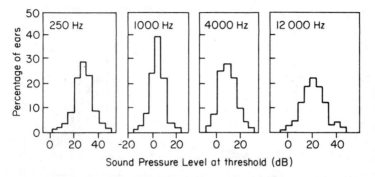

FIG. 2.2 The distribution of sound levels at threshold for 198 ears at four frequencies. Redrawn from Dadson and King (1952), by permission of the authors and the Director of the National Physical Laboratory, UK.

by Dadson and King (1952), using a sample of 198 ears, with sound pressures measured at two positions close to the entrance of the meatus. The distribution of thresholds for the same group of subjects at four different frequencies is shown in Fig. 2.2. Although the subjects were 'otologically normal', with ages between 18 and 25 years, it is clear that there is a large variability among different subjects. Part of this may be attributable to criterion differences; subjects may have varied in their willingness to report a signal on the basis of minimal sensory evidence (see section 10 of this Chapter). However, the range of thresholds is too large to be explained in this way. Tumarkin (1972) has suggested that the majority of the ears tested in this sample may have been biologically subnormal, and he cites evidence from Bredberg (1968) showing that the number of hair cells in the inner ear is diminishing almost from the day we are born. It is certainly puzzling that a considerable number of subjects had thresholds 20 dB or more below the mean.

The general shape of the curve relating threshold to frequency (often called the audibility curve) is now well established. We are most sensitive to frequencies in the range 1000–5000 Hz, while thresholds increase rapidly at very high and very low frequencies. At least part of our sensitivity to middle frequencies derives from the action of the pinna and ear canal. Figure 2.3, from Djupesland and Zwislocki (1972), shows the sound pressure transformation between the eardrum and a point 1 cm outside the tragus (the small projection at the entrance to the ear canal). The outer ear enhances the sound pressure at the eardrum for frequencies in the range 1–9 kHz, with a maximum enhancement at 3 kHz of about 15 dB. Another factor which contributes to the shape of the audibility curve is the transmission character-

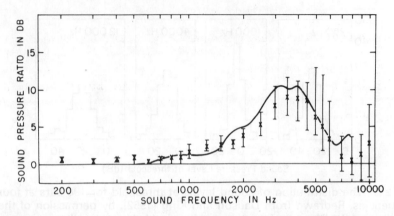

FIG. 2.3   The transformation in sound pressure between the eardrum and the entrance to the ear canal. Crosses indicate the means, vertical bars the interquartile ranges. The solid line reproduces earlier data of Wiener and Ross (1946). From Djupesland and Zwislocki (1972), by permission of the authors.

istic of the middle ear. Transmission is most efficient for midrange frequencies and drops off markedly for very low and very high frequencies. This can account for the rapid rise in threshold at the low- and high-frequency ends of the audibility curve.

The amplitudes of vibration corresponding to the SPLs at threshold are remarkably small. For example, the data of Dadson and King (1952) show that the root-mean-square pressure variation at threshold for a 3000 Hz tone is about 40 μPa. This corresponds to a displacement amplitude, at the entrance to the ear canal, of 6.25×10^{-12} m, or 0.00625 nm. The action of the ear canal will increase the threshold displacement at the eardrum to about 0.03 or 0.04 nm, but this is still a very small value.

At low frequencies, MAPs, measured under headphones, are greater than MAFs, by between 5 and 10 dB. A number of workers have shown that this is due to physiological noise of vascular origin, which is produced within the meatus when earphones are worn (Anderson and Whittle, 1971; Soderquist and Lindsey, 1972). The detectability of low-frequency tones can be shown to vary according to their temporal position within the cardiac cycle (heart beat). The level of this low-frequency 'physiological noise' varies with the leakage of air around the headphone (this will depend in part on headband pressure), with the volume of the subject's meatus, and with the strength of their heart beat. These sources of variance are lessened when circumaural headphones (which fit around the pinnae) rather than supra-aural headphones (which lie over and flatten the pinnae) are used. Thus circumaural headphones are preferable for use at low frequencies. However, at high frequencies these headphones are less reliable, and more difficult to calibrate than supra-aural headphones. 'Open-ear' headphones can considerably reduce low-frequency physiological noise.

The highest frequency audible varies considerably with the age of the subject. Young children can often hear tones as high as 20 kHz, but for most adults threshold rises rapidly above about 15 kHz. The loss of sensitivity with increasing age (presbyacusis) is much greater at high frequencies than at low, and the variability between different observers is also greater at high frequencies. At the other end of the scale there seems to be no particular low frequency limit to our hearing. Whittle *et al.* (1972) measured thresholds for frequencies from 50 Hz down to 3.15 Hz, and showed that their results formed a continuum with the results at higher frequencies. However, for the 3.15 Hz tone, the threshold level was about 120 dB SPL! It has been suggested (Johnson and von Gierke, 1974) that sounds below about 16 Hz are not heard in the normal sense, but are detected by virtue of the distortion products (harmonics) which they produce after passing through the middle ear. In addition, very intense low-frequency tones can sometimes be felt as vibration before they are heard. The low-frequency limit for the 'true' hearing of pure tones probably lies about 16 Hz. This is close to the lowest frequency which evokes a pitch sensation.

In many practical situations our ability to detect faint sounds is limited not by our absolute sensitivity to those sounds but by the level of ambient noise. In other words, detection will depend upon the masked threshold rather than the absolute threshold. In such cases the threshold as a function of frequency will depend upon the character of the ambient noise (e.g. frequency content, level, and whether intermittent or continuous). The effects of these variables are discussed more fully in Chapter 3.

Before finishing our discussion of absolute thresholds, we should mention that, in audiology, thresholds are usually specified relative to the average threshold at each frequency for young, healthy listeners with 'normal' hearing. Thresholds specified in this way have units dB HL (hearing level) in Europe or dB HTL (hearing threshold level) in the USA. Thus, for example, a threshold of 40 dB HL at 1 kHz would mean that the patient had a threshold which was 40 dB higher than 'normal' at that frequency. Threshold in this case would correspond to about 46 dB SPL. In psychoacoustic work thresholds are normally plotted with threshold increasing upwards, as in Fig. 2.1. However, in audiology, threshold elevations are shown as hearing losses, plotted downwards. The average 'normal' threshold is represented as a horizontal line at the top of the plot, and the degree of hearing loss is indicated by how much the threshold falls below this line. This type of plot is called an 'audiogram'.

3   *EQUAL-LOUDNESS CONTOURS*

There are many occasions when engineers and acousticians require a subjective scale corresponding to the loudness of a sound. Since complex sounds are often analysed in terms of their individual frequency components, a useful first step is to derive such a scale for pure tones. One way of doing this is to use the technique of magnitude estimation in order to determine the relationship between physical intensity and judged loudness. However, the validity of this technique has been questioned, and before discussing it (section 4) we will consider an alternative measure of loudness which is not at first sight as straightforward, but which nevertheless has proved useful in practice and which is not so controversial. The alternative is the loudness level, which tells us not how loud a tone is, but rather how intense a 1000 Hz tone must be in order to sound equally loud. To determine the loudness level of a given sound, the subject is asked to adjust the level of a 1000 Hz tone until it has the same loudness as the test sound. The 1000 Hz tone and the test sound are presented alternately rather than simultaneously. The level of the 1000 Hz tone which gives equal loudness is the loudness level of the test sound, measured in 'phons'. Thus, the loudness level of any sound is the level (in dB SPL) of the 1000 Hz tone to which it sounds equal in loudness and the unit of loudness level is the phon.

In a variation of this procedure, the 1000 Hz tone may be fixed in level, and the test sound adjusted to give a loudness match. If this is repeated for various different frequencies of a sinusoidal test sound, an equal-loudness contour is generated (Fletcher and Munson, 1933). Some typical results are shown in Fig. 2.4 (from Robinson and Dadson, 1956). This figure shows equal-loudness contours for loudness levels from 20 phons to 120 phons, and it also includes the absolute threshold (MAF) curve. The equal-loudness contours are of similar shape to the threshold curve, but tend to become flatter at high loudness levels. This means that the rate of growth of loudness differs for tones of different frequency. For example, the absolute threshold for a 100 Hz tone is about 20 dB above that for a 1000 Hz tone (thresholds at 23 and 3 dB SPL). But for the 100 phon contour, the intensities are nearly the same at 100 and 1000 Hz (102 and 100 dB SPL). For the same range of loudness level, from threshold to 100 phons, the level of the 1000 Hz tone must be increased by 97 dB, while that of the 100 Hz tone must be increased by only 79 dB. Thus the rate of growth of loudness with increasing intensity is greater for low frequencies (and to some extent for very high frequencies) than for middle frequencies.

These findings have certain implications for the reproduction of sound; the

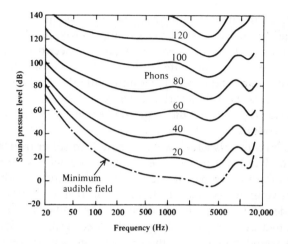

FIG. 2.4 Equal-loudness contours for various loudness levels. The absolute threshold curve is also indicated. Redrawn from Robinson and Dadson (1956), by permission of the authors and the Director of the National Physical Laboratory, UK.

relative loudness of the different frequency components in a sound will change as a function of the overall level, so that unless the sounds are reproduced at the same level as the original, the 'tonal balance' will be altered. This is one of the reasons why human voices often sound 'boomy' when reproduced at high levels via loudspeakers; the ear becomes relatively more sensitive to low frequencies at high intensities. Conversely, at low levels we are less sensitive to the very low and very high frequencies, so that many amplifiers incorporate a 'loudness' control which boosts the bass (and to some extent the treble) at low listening levels. Such controls are of only limited use, since they take no account of loudspeaker efficiency and size of room.

The shapes of equal-loudness contours have been used in the design of sound level meters which attempt to give an approximate measure of the loudness of complex sounds. Such meters contain weighting networks, so that the meter does not simply sum the intensity at all different frequencies, but rather weights the intensity at each frequency according to the shape of the equal-loudness contours. At low sound levels, low-frequency components contribute little to the total loudness of a complex sound, so an 'A' weighting is used which reduces the contribution of low frequencies to the final meter reading. The 'A' weighting is based on the 40 phon equal-loudness contour.

At high levels, all frequencies contribute more or less equally to the loudness sensation (the equal-loudness contours being approximately flat), so that a more nearly linear weighting characteristic, the 'C' network, is used. The 'B' weighting is used for intermediate levels; it is based on the 70 phon equal-loudness contour. Sound levels measured with these meters are usually specified in terms of the weighting used. Thus, a given level might be specified as 35 dBA, meaning that the meter gave a reading of 35 dB when the 'A' weighting was used.

The sound level meters which we have described suffer from a number of problems. Firstly, they can only be reliably used with steady sounds of relatively long duration; the responses to transient sounds do not correspond to the subjective impressions of the loudness of such sounds. Secondly, they do not provide a satisfactory way of summing the loudness of components in widely separated frequency bands. As we shall see in Chapter 3, the loudness of a complex sound with a given amount of energy depends on whether that energy is contained within a narrow range of frequencies or is spread over a wide range of frequencies.

Finally, it should not be assumed that sound level meters give a 'true' estimate of the loudness of a given sound. The readings obtained are closely related to the decibel scale, which is a scale of physical magnitude rather than a scale of subjective sensation. Thus it would be quite wrong to say that a sound giving a reading of 80 dB was twice as loud as a sound giving a reading of 40 dB; the 80 dB sound would actually appear to be about 16 times as loud as the 40 dB sound (see later). However, the meters do enable us roughly to compare the loudness of different complex sounds. We discuss below some of the models which attempt to provide more satisfactory estimates of the loudness of complex sounds.

4   THE SCALING OF LOUDNESS

In this section we will briefly discuss the attempts which have been made to derive scales relating the physical magnitudes of sounds to their subjective loudness. The development of scales of loudness and of other sensory dimensions was pioneered by S. S. Stevens, and the reader is referred to his work for further details (e.g. Stevens, 1957). Two methods have been commonly used to derive scales of loudness. In one, called magnitude estimation, sounds with various different levels are presented, and the subject is asked to assign a number to each one according to its perceived loudness. Sometimes a reference sound (called the 'modulus' or 'standard') is presented, and the subject is asked to judge the loudness of each test sound relative to that of the standard. In a second method, called magnitude production, the subject is presented with a standard sound, and is asked to adjust the level of a test sound until it has a specified loudness relative to that of the standard, for example, twice as loud, four times as loud, half as loud, and so on.

Stevens suggested that loudness, L, was a power function of physical intensity, I:

$$L = kI^{0.3}$$

where k is a constant depending on the subject and the units used. In other words, the loudness of a given sound is proportional to its intensity raised to the power 0.3. A simple approximation to this is that a two-fold change in loudness is produced by a 10 dB step in level. Stevens proposed the 'sone' as the unit of loudness. One sone is defined arbitrarily as the loudness of a 1000 Hz tone at 40 dB SPL. A 1000 Hz tone with a level of 50 dB SPL will usually be judged as about twice as loud as a 40 dB tone, and has a loudness of 2 sones.

Loudness scales have been used by Zwicker and Scharf (1965), Zwicker (1958) and Stevens (1972) in models which allow the calculation of the loudness of complex sounds. We will not present these models in detail, since they are rather complicated. Although there are some differences between the models, in essence they involve splitting the complex stimulus into a number of frequency bands (usually third-octave bands), and the determination of the level in each one. The level in each band is then converted to a 'loudness', using Steven's Power Law, and the loudness in each band is summed to give the total loudness. The effect of the bandwidth of sounds on their loudness is discussed more fully in Chapter 3.

The power-law relationship between intensity and loudness has been confirmed in a large number of experiments using a variety of techniques. However, there have also been criticisms of loudness scaling. The techniques used seem very susceptible to bias effects, so that results are affected by factors such as: (1) the range of stimuli presented; (2) the first stimulus presented; (3) the instructions to the subject; (4) the range of permissible responses; (5) symmetry of the response range (judgements tend to be biased towards the middle of the range available for responses); (6) various other factors related to experience, motivation, training and attention (Poulton, 1979). Very large individual differences are observed, and consistent results are only obtained by averaging many judgements of a large number of subjects. Warren (1970a) attempted to eliminate known bias effects by obtaining just a single judgement from each subject. Only those responses distributed symmetrically about the centre of the available range were considered as bias free. He found that half-loudness corresponds to a 6 dB attenuation, rather than the 10 dB suggested by Stevens. However, considerable variability is also apparent in his data.

There are also theoretical objections to loudness scaling. One of these, pointed out by Treisman (1964), is that there are two stages involved in obtaining a loudness judgement, each of which may be governed by a different function. In the first stage, the stimulus evokes a loudness sensation in the listener. It is the functional relationship between the stimulus magnitude and the sensation which we wish to determine. In the second stage, the listener gives a number which is related in some way to the magnitude of the sensation. It is only if the relation between sensation and number is linear that the responses of the subject will directly indicate the relative magnitude of the sensation. If the listener is used to working with some other scale, such as a logarithmic scale, then the judgements will not give a direct indication of the loudness sensation. Unfortunately there is no easy way to determine what sort of number scale the listener is using.

A second theoretical objection is to the whole concept of asking a listener to judge the magnitude of a sensation. What we do in everyday life is to judge the 'loudness' of sound sources, so that our estimate is affected by the apparent distance of the sound source, the context in which it is heard and the nature of the sound (e.g. whether it is meaningful or not). In other words, we are attempting to make an estimate of the properties of the source itself. Introspection as to the magnitude of the sensation evoked may be an unnatural and difficult process. This point of view has been well expressed by Helmholtz (quoted in Warren, 1981), who said that:

> ... we are exceedingly well trained in finding out by our sensations the objective nature of the objects around us, but we are completely unskilled in observing these sensations per se; and the practice of associating them with things outside of us actually prevents us from being distinctly conscious of the pure sensations.

It is not at all clear that methods of calculating loudness using 'psychological' loudness scales give better agreement with loudness judgements than methods based on a physical analysis of the stimuli. Thus Corliss and Winzer (1964) said:

> The loudness of several complex sounds computed on the basis of Stevens' model did not agree with the results of Zwicker's model. The results were not related in any consistent way and both sets of computations were at variance with the subject's response.

Similarly, Howes (1971) compared the loudness of broadband noise calculated by a method similar to Zwicker's, with the loudness calculated by summing weighted intensities of sub-bands of noise and obtaining the loudness of the sum. This 'power summation' method gave better agreement with actual loudness judgements than did Zwicker's method. Carter (1972) applied five different methods in the calculation of the loudness of repeated acoustic transients. A white noise was used as a comparison stimulus. The method predicting loudness most effectively in the face of variation in rise time and repetition rate of the transients was dBA, a measure obtained using a sound level meter with 'A' weighting (see section 3). This method was clearly superior to methods employing the sone scale.

At present there are a great many competing methods for calculating loudness, and no one method seems to be entirely successful in dealing with the great variety of sounds which are encountered in everyday life. There is certainly room for considerable scepticism when a statement such as 'a Concorde is twice as loud as a Boeing 747' is made.

5 TEMPORAL INTEGRATION

It has been known for many years (Exner, 1876) that both absolute thresholds and the loudness of sounds depend upon duration. The studies of absolute threshold which were described earlier were all carried out with sounds, usually tone bursts, of relatively long duration. For durations exceeding about 500 ms, the sound intensity at threshold is roughly independent of duration. However, for durations less than about 200 ms the sound intensity necessary for detection increases as duration decreases (remember that intensity is a measure of energy per unit time). Many workers have investigated the relation between threshold and duration for tone pulses, over a wide range of frequencies and durations. The early work of Hughes (1946) and Garner and Miller (1947) indicated that, over a reasonable range of durations, the ear appears to integrate the energy of the stimulus over time in the detection of short duration tone bursts. If this were exactly true, the following formula would hold:

$$I \times t = \text{constant}$$

where I is the threshold intensity for a tone pulse of duration t. In other words, the threshold would depend only on the total amount of energy in the stimulus and not on how that energy was distributed over time. In practice the results are fitted better by the expression:

$$(I - I_L) \times t = I_L \times \tau = \text{constant}$$

where I_L is the threshold intensity for a long-duration tone pulse and τ is a constant representing the 'integration time' of the auditory system. Notice that in this formula it is not the product of time and intensity which is constant, but the product of time and the amount by which the intensity exceeds the value I_L. Garner and Miller (1947) interpreted I_L as the minimum intensity which is an effective stimulus for the ear. They assumed that only intensities above this minimum value are integrated linearly by the ear.

Thresholds as a function of duration are often plotted on dB versus log-duration coordinates. When plotted in this way, energy integration is indicated by the data falling on a straight line with a slope of -3 dB per doubling of duration. Although the average data for a group of subjects typically give a slope close to this value, the slopes for individual subjects can differ significantly from -3 dB per doubling. For some hearing-impaired listeners, the slopes can be very shallow. This suggests that it would be unwise to ascribe too much significance to the average slope. It seems very unlikely that the auditory system would actually integrate stimulus energy; it is almost certainly neural activity which is integrated. However, energy integration provides a convenient and conceptually simple way of describing how threshold normally varies with duration.

Plomp and Bouman (1959) found that the time constant of integration, τ, varies according to frequency, being around 375 ms at 250 Hz and 150 ms at 8000 Hz. Other workers have also found time constants which vary with frequency (e.g. Watson and Gengel, 1968), although the actual values of the time constants have not always been in agreement. On the other hand, Olson and Carhart (1966) found, for frequencies of 250, 1000 and 4000 Hz, that changes in threshold with stimulus duration are similar for all stimuli, while Bilger and Feldman (1968) reported that results depend upon the particular method chosen to measure temporal integration.

The limits of energy integration have been studied using tone pulses of various durations but with equal energy (Green *et al.*, 1957). In theory, perfect integration would lead to constant detectability. Green and co-workers used as their measure of detectability the quantity d' (pronounced d-prime), which is derived from the theory of signal detection (see the appendix to Chapter 3). They found that detectability was generally constant over the range of durations from 15 to 150 ms, but fell off for durations smaller or greater than this (see Fig. 2.5). A similar 'plateau' was found by Sheeley and Bilger (1964), although the plateau occurred at longer durations for low frequencies (250 Hz) and shorter durations for high frequencies (4000 Hz). The fall in detectability at longer durations is in line with previous studies, indicating that there is a limit to the time over which the ear can integrate energy (or a lower limit to the intensity which can be effectively integrated). The fall in detectability at very short durations may be connected with the inevitable spread of energy over frequency which occurs for signals of short duration (see Chapter 1, section 2). It may be that energy can only be integrated when it falls within a fairly narrow range of frequencies and that this range is exceeded for signals of very short duration. This idea is closely connected with the concept of the critical band, which is discussed in Chapter 3.

The effect of duration on loudness has also been measured extensively, but

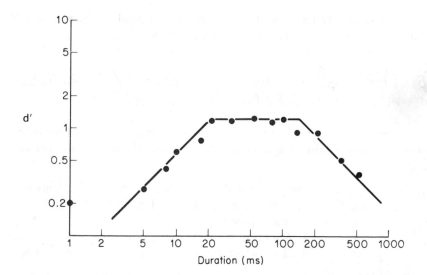

FIG. 2.5   The mean detectability (*d'*) of equal energy tone bursts of frequency 1 kHz as a function of duration. Note the range of durations over which detectability is roughly constant. From Stephens (1973), by permission of the author.

the results show considerable variability except for a general agreement that, at a given intensity, loudness increases with duration. Boone (1973) required subjects to match the loudness of tone bursts to that of a continuous reference tone. He found that, for a frequency of 1000 Hz, the loudness was related to the total energy of the burst. He also found that the silent interval between successive bursts had an effect, and that this effect was frequency dependent. Stephens (1974) investigated the loudness of equal-energy tone bursts of various durations using two different techniques. In the first, subjects were required to give a numerical estimate of the loudness of tone bursts in relation to a standard which was presented initially and stated to have a loudness of 100 arbitrary units. In the second, subjects were required to adjust the intensity of a fixed-duration stimulus so that its loudness matched that of the tone burst being judged. Stephens also investigated the effect of different sets of instructions. He found that, in most cases, there was a plateau for a particular range of durations, indicating that equal energy means equal loudness, but he also found that the experimental technique and the exact wording of instructions affected the results. One reason for this is that listeners find it difficult to separate the loudness and duration aspects of the stimuli when making their judgements. With both techniques the plateau occur at shorter durations for higher frequencies. The influence of duration on loudness is discussed further in Chapter 3.

6 THE DETECTION OF INTENSITY CHANGES AND THE CODING OF LOUDNESS

The smallest detectable change in intensity has been measured for many different types of stimuli by a variety of methods. The three main methods are:

1. *Modulation detection.* The stimulus is amplitude modulated (i.e. made to vary in amplitude) at a slow regular rate (see Fig. 3.7) and the subject is required to detect the modulation.
2. *Increment detection.* A continuous background stimulus is presented, and the subject is required to detect an increment in the level of the background.
3. *Intensity discrimination of gated or pulsed stimuli.* Two separate pulses of sound are presented successively, one being more intense than the other, and the subject is required to indicate which was the more intense. The order of presentation of the two stimuli in a trial (loud–soft or soft–loud) is randomly varied. This type of task is called a two-alternative forced-choice (2AFC) procedure, and the intensity difference limen (DL) is usually defined as that intensity difference which produces 75% correct responses.

Although there are some minor discrepancies in the experimental results for the different types of method, the general trend is similar. Thresholds for detecting intensity changes are usually specified in decibels, i.e. as the change in level at threshold.

For wideband noise, or for bandpass filtered noise, the smallest detectable intensity change is approximately a constant fraction of the intensity of the stimulus. If I is the intensity of a noise band, and ΔI is the smallest detectable change in intensity, then $\Delta I/I$ is roughly constant. This is an example of Weber's Law, which states that the smallest detectable change in a stimulus is proportional to the magnitude of that stimulus. The value of $\Delta I/I$ is called the Weber fraction. If the smallest detectable change is expressed in decibels, i.e. as $10 \log [(I+\Delta I)/I]$, then this, too, is constant. Thus the just-detectable change in level, ΔL, is constant, regardless of the absolute level, and for wideband noise has a value of about 0.5–1 dB (Rodenburg, 1972). This holds from about 20 dB above threshold to 100 dB above threshold (Miller, 1947). The value of ΔL increases for sounds which are close to the absolute threshold.

For pure tones the situation is somewhat different. Riesz's (1928) data for modulated tones, and data from a number of other workers using pulsed tones, show that Weber's Law does not hold (Harris, 1963; Viemeister, 1972; Jesteadt *et al.*, 1977). Instead it is found that if ΔI (in dB) is plotted against I (also in dB), a straight line is obtained with a slope of about 0.9; Weber's law would give a slope of 1.0. Thus discrimination, as measured by the Weber fraction, improves at high levels. This has been termed the 'near miss' to Weber's Law. The data of Riesz for modulation detection show a value of ΔL of 1.5 dB at 20 dB SL, 0.7 dB at 40 dB SL, and 0.3 dB at 80 dB SL (all at 1000 Hz).

Let us consider the implications of these findings in terms of the physiological coding of intensity in the auditory system. The three major phenomena which we have to explain are: (1) the auditory system is capable of detecting changes in level for a range of levels – the dynamic range – of at least 120 dB (Viemeister and Bacon, 1988); (2) Weber's Law holds for the discrimination of bursts of noise; and (3) discrimination of the level of pure tones improves (relative to Weber's Law) at high sound levels.

A   The dynamic range of the auditory system

For many years the wide dynamic range of the auditory system was considered to be difficult to explain in terms of the properties of neurones in the auditory nerve. For example, following a survey of a large number of nerve fibres, Palmer and Evans (1979) concluded that the proportion of nerve fibres with wide dynamic ranges (say 60 dB or more) is only about 10%. Further, at sound levels above about 60 dB SPL, of the small number of fibres which were not saturated, all showed a substantial reduction in the slope of the rate versus intensity function. Thus changes in intensity resulted in only small changes in firing rate. If intensity discrimination were based on changes in the firing rates of neurones with CFs close to the stimulus frequency, we might expect intensity discrimination to worsen at high sound levels, whereas in fact it does not.

These findings suggested that there might be some other mechanism for the coding of intensity changes at high intensities. One possibility lies in the way the excitation pattern of the stimulus would spread with increasing intensity (see Fig. 2.6). At high intensities, the majority of neurones at the centre of the pattern would be saturated, but changes in intensity could still be signalled by changes in the firing rates of neurones at the edges of the pattern.

At first sight it appears that this argument could not hold for the discrimination of wideband stimuli, such as white noise. In theory the excitation pattern for white noise has no edges, so that all fibres ought to be saturated by

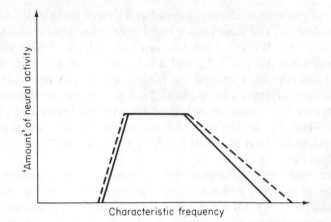

FIG. 2.6 An idealized neural excitation pattern for a tone at a high level (solid line). An increase in level, indicated by the dashed lines, produces no change in activity for the neurones in the centre of the pattern, since these are saturated. However, changes in neural activity do occur at the edges of the pattern. Note the greater growth of activity that occurs on the high frequency side.

a noise of high intensity. However, we are not equally sensitive to all frequencies, as absolute threshold curves and equal-loudness contours indicate. Thus, although the nerve fibres with midrange CFs would be saturated by an intense white noise, this might not be the case for neurones with very low and very high CFs. Furthermore, the stimuli have generally been presented via headphones which only pass a limited range of frequencies (in Miller's, 1947, case the noise spectrum was only flat (+/−5 dB) between 150 and 7000 Hz). Thus the acoustic stimuli would not have been truly wideband, even if the electrical signals were.

We see, then, that changes in firing rate for neurones at the edges of the excitation pattern evoked by the stimulus could provide an explanation for the wide dynamic range of the auditory system. This idea has been tested by measuring intensity discrimination in the presence of background noise chosen to obscure or mask the edges of the excitation pattern of the signal (see Chapter 3 for more information on masking). For example, Viemeister (1972) investigated the intensity discrimination of pulsed 950 Hz sinusoids, in the presence of various types of filtered noise. He found little effect with a lowpass noise, whose cutoff frequency was 800 Hz, but a bandpass noise centred at 1900 Hz or a highpass noise with a cutoff at 1900 Hz both slightly degraded performance at high levels. With the latter stimulus Weber's Law was obtained. Moore and Raab (1974) investigated the intensity discrimination of 1000 Hz tone bursts in the presence of three types of noise: wideband; highpass with cutoff frequency at 2000 Hz; and bandstop with cutoff frequencies at 500 Hz and 2000 Hz. Performance was not impaired by the noise at low levels of the tone and noise, but at high levels performance worsened, the greatest impairment being produced by the bandstop noise and the least by the wideband noise. This experiment confirms that information at CFs remote from the stimulus frequency is important, and it further indicates that information on both the high- and low-frequency sides of the excitation pattern affects intensity discrimination at high levels; the bandstop noise, which disrupts both sides of the pattern, had a greater effect than the highpass noise, which only disrupts information on the high frequency side. It seems then that, at least for tones, information from the edges of the excitation pattern allows improved performance at high levels.

Although these experiments indicate that spread of excitation may play a role in intensity discrimination, they also show that reasonable performance is possible even when the edges of the excitation pattern are masked by noise. In other words, spread of excitation is not *essential* for maintaining the wide dynamic range of the auditory system. For example, in the condition of Moore and Raab using bandstop noise, the edges of the excitation pattern on both the low- and high-frequency sides were disrupted, so that at high levels most neurones at the centre of the pattern should have been saturated. Yet, for this condition Weber's Law was found; performance was equally good at high and low levels. If the neurones in the centre of the excitation pattern were saturated at high levels, then the small effect of masking the edges of the excitation pattern indicates that it may be necessary to invoke some further mechanism for intensity discrimination.

One possibility is that the timing of neural impulses provides a cue to the intensity of a tone in a noise background. When a tone is above threshold but is presented against a noise background, some neurones will be phase locked to the tone, while neurones with CFs far from that of the tone will show a more random pattern of neural firing. When the tone is increased in intensity, more of the neurones will become phase locked, and furthermore the degree of temporal regularity in the firing of neurones which are already phase locked will increase, since the noise will now produce relatively less 'jitter'. Thus, a change in temporal regularity of the patterns of neural firing will signal the intensity change of the tone. Such a mechanism could operate over a wide range of intensities, and would not be affected by saturation effects; temporal patterns of firing can alter even for neurones which are saturated. The mechanism would, however, be limited to frequencies below about 4–5 kHz.

Phase locking might be particularly important for coding the relative levels of components in complex sounds. As described in Chapter 1, section 6, neurones with a given CF tend to phase lock to the stimulus components which are most effective at that CF. When the level of a component is increased relative to the other components, the degree of phase locking to that component will increase. In general, any change in the spectral composition of a complex sound will result in a change in the pattern of phase locking as a function of CF, provided the spectral change is in the frequency region below 4–5 kHz.

The possibility that phase locking plays a role in intensity discrimination has been tested using stimuli containing only frequencies above the range where phase locking occurs. The most critical experiments have presented the stimuli in a background of bandstop noise so that information from the spread of the excitation pattern was also eliminated. Viemeister (1983) measured the intensity discrimination of 200 ms bursts of bandpass noise, with a passband from 6 to 14 kHz. The noise was presented in a background noise with a bandstop in the range 6–14 kHz. He found that intensity discrimination remained relatively good over a wide range of sound levels. This suggests that phase locking is not essential for intensity discrimination. Carlyon and Moore (1984) investigated the intensity discrimination of sinusoidal tone bursts in the presence of a background noise with a bandstop centred on the frequency of the tone. Performance was compared for high-frequency and low-frequency tones. When the tones were of long duration (225 ms), there was little effect of the overall level of the sounds, although there was a slight deterioration in intensity discrimination for high frequency (6500 Hz) tones at moderate sound levels (55–70 dB SPL). When the tones were of short duration (30 ms) the deterioration at high frequencies and moderate sound levels became more pronounced.

Carlyon and Moore (1984) suggested that, at low frequencies, intensity discrimination depends upon both the spread of excitation and phase locking. One or both of these types of information is always available, even in the presence of bandstop noise. At high frequencies, where phase locking does not occur, spread of excitation becomes relatively more important. However, even when the edges of the excitation pattern are masked by bandpass noise, good intensity discrimination is still possible for long duration stimuli. This indicates that information from the small number of unsaturated neurones with CFs close to the stimulus frequency is sufficient for good intensity discrimination. It is only when the stimulus is of short duration that an impairment is observed, and then it is at medium levels rather than at high levels. Carlyon and Moore suggested that the midlevel deterioration could be explained in terms of distinct populations of neurones with different thresholds, as described in Chapter 1. At moderate sound levels the low-threshold neurones might all be saturated, while the high-threshold neurones might be only just starting to respond.

In recent years the 'problem' of the wide dynamic range of the auditory system has been viewed in a rather different way. This new viewpoint has come from studies of the capacity of single neurones to carry information about intensity changes. This capacity depends both upon the shape of the rate versus level function, and upon the statistical properties of the neural responses, and particularly their variability at each level (Teich and Khanna, 1985). Such studies have indicated that information from only a small number of neurones is sufficient to account for intensity discrimination (Delgutte, 1987; Viemeister, 1988). The number required seems to be about 100. Indeed, if the information contained in the firing rates of all the 30 000 neurones in the auditory nerve were used optimally, then intensity discrimination would be much better than it actually is. For example, ΔL for 1000 Hz tone bursts would be less than 0.1 dB at medium to high levels (Delgutte, 1987). Thus the 'problem' of the dynamic range of the auditory system has changed. Rather than having to explain how intensity discrimination is possible over a wide range of sound levels, we have to explain why intensity discrimination is not better than observed. It appears that, for most stimuli, intensity discrimination is not limited by the information carried in the auditory nerve, but by the use made of that information at more central levels of processing (Carlyon and Moore, 1984). It is only when the information in the auditory nerve is highly impoverished that impaired intensity discrimination is observed. This may happen for brief high-frequency tones presented in bandstop noise.

In summary, it seems likely that a number of different mechanisms play a role in intensity discrimination. Intensity changes can be signalled both by changes in the firing rates of neurones at the centre of the excitation pattern, and by the spreading of the excitation pattern, so that more neurones are brought into operation. However, the spread of excitation is not critical for maintaining performance at high sound levels. In addition, cues related to phase locking may play a role in intensity discrimination. This may be particularly important for complex stimuli, for which the relative levels of different components may be signalled by the degree of phase locking to the components. However, phase locking is also not critical, since good intensity discrimination is possible for stimuli whose frequency components are restricted to the range where phase locking does not occur. It appears that the information carried in the firing rates of neurones in the auditory nerve is more than sufficient to account for intensity discrimination. Thus, intensity discrimination appears normally to be limited by the capacity of more central parts of the auditory system to make use of the information in the auditory nerve.

B   Weber's law

At one time it was thought that Weber's law held for bands of noise because the inherent fluctuations in the noise limit performance. For example, in a task involving the intensity discrimination of bursts of noise, a device that chooses the burst containing the greater energy on each trial, would conform to Weber's law (Green, 1960). However, it has been found that Weber's law holds even for 'frozen' noise, i.e. noise which is identical from one trial to the next and which does not have random fluctuations in energy (Raab and Goldberg, 1975). This indicates that Weber's law must arise from the operation of the auditory system, rather than from the statistical properties of the stimuli.

As mentioned earlier, the ability of a single neurone to code changes in intensity depends both upon the shape of the rate versus level function, and upon the variability in the firing rate. For a given neurone, the efficiency of coding of intensity changes is a u-shaped function of sound level. Thus, the information conveyed by a single neurone is optimal over a small range of sound levels, and is poorer above and below that range. The poor coding at low levels occurs because stimuli close to or below the threshold of the neurone result in minimal changes in firing rate. The poor coding at high levels occurs because of neural saturation. Thus, if discrimination were based on the information from single neurones it would not conform to Weber's law.

Weber's law can be predicted by models which combine the firing rate information from a relatively small number of neurones (about 100) whose thresholds and dynamic ranges are appropriately staggered so as to cover the dynamic range of the auditory system (Delgutte, 1987; Viemeister, 1988). In models of this type it is generally assumed that the combination is done on a localized basis. In other words, information from neurones with similar CFs is combined, and there are many independent 'channels' each responding to a limited range of CFs. Weber's law is assumed to hold for each channel. Thus, information about the levels of components in complex sounds can be coded over a wide range of overall sound levels. This assumption, that there are many frequency channels each of which conforms to Weber's law, has been widespread in psychophysics for many years, and we will return to it in Chapters 3 and 4. Chapter 3 also considers the concept of frequency channels in more detail.

C   The near miss to Weber's law

Let us now consider the differences which have been observed in the intensity discrimination of pure tones and of bursts of noise. If we accept that Weber's law reflects the normal mode of operation of a given frequency channel, we have to explain why the intensity discrimination of pure tones deviates from Weber's law.

There are probably at least two factors contributing to the improvement in intensity discrimination of pure tones at high sound levels. The first was described by Zwicker (1956, 1970), who studied modulation detection for pure tones. He suggested that a change in intensity can be detected whenever the excitation pattern evoked by the stimulus changes somewhere by (approximately) 1 dB or more. In other words, he assumed that Weber's law held for all frequency channels, and that the Weber fraction was about 1 dB for each channel. The high-frequency side of the excitation pattern grows in a nonlinear way with increasing intensity; a 10 dB change in stimulus level gives rise to a greater than 10 dB change on the high-frequency side of the pattern. This is deduced from changes in the shapes of masking patterns for tones in noise as a function of intensity (see Chapter 3), and is illustrated in Fig. 2.7. This nonlinear growth in the excitation pattern means that a 1 dB

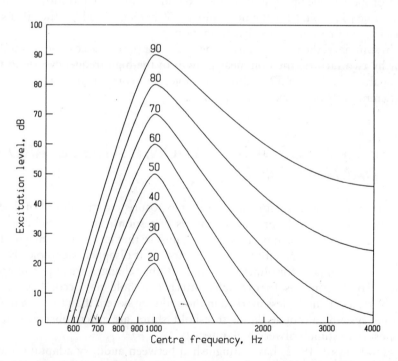

FIG. 2.7 Psychoacoustical excitation patterns for a 1 kHz sinusoid at levels ranging from 20 to 90 dB SPL in 10 dB steps; each excitation pattern is labelled with the corresponding sound level. The patterns were calculated on the basis of psychoacoustic data as described in Chapter 3.

change in excitation on the high-frequency side will be produced by relatively smaller stimulus increments at high levels. As the stimulus level is increased, the excitation pattern spreads more and more. For a given change in stimulus level, the greatest change in excitation level occurs at the highest part of the pattern, since that is the part showing the greatest nonlinearity (see Fig. 2.7). In support of this idea, Zwicker reported that the addition of a highpass noise, which masks the high-frequency side of the excitation pattern but does not actually mask the tone, causes the DL for amplitude modulation at high levels to approach that found at low levels (masking is discussed in detail in Chapter 3).

The second factor contributing to the near miss to Weber's law has been described by Florentine and Buus (1981). They suggested that subjects do not make use of information only from a single channel. Rather, they combine information across all of the excited channels, i.e. across the whole of the excitation pattern. As the level of a tone is increased, more channels become active, and the increase in the number of active channels allows improved performance. They presented a model based on this idea and showed that it was able to account for the near miss to Weber's law and for the effects of masking noise on intensity discrimination.

In summary, the near miss to Weber's law for pure tones can be accounted for by two factors: the nonlinear growth of the high-frequency side of the excitation pattern; and the ability of subjects to combine information from different parts of the excitation pattern.

7   LOUDNESS ADAPTATION, FATIGUE AND DAMAGE RISK

It is a property of all sensory systems that exposure to a stimulus of sufficient duration and intensity produces changes in responsiveness. Some changes occur during the presentation of the stimulus, so that its apparent magnitude decreases (as for exposure to bright lights) or it disappears completely (as sometimes happens for olfactory stimuli). Other changes are apparent after the end of the stimulus; for example, shifts in threshold may occur. In general, such effects are much less marked in the auditory system than they are in the visual system, although large threshold shifts are often observed after exposure to stimuli of very high intensity.

Hood (1950, 1972) has distinguished between auditory adaptation and auditory fatigue, and has emphasized that these are two quite distinct processes. The essential feature of fatigue is that it "results from the application of a stimulus which is usually considerably in excess of that required to sustain the normal physiological response of the receptor, and it is measured after the stimulus has been removed" (Hood, 1972). For example, a subject's absolute threshold at a particular frequency might be measured, after which the subject would be exposed to a fatiguing tone of a particular frequency and intensity for a period of time. The threshold would then be measured again, and the shift in threshold would be taken as a measure of fatigue. Notice that this procedure is concerned with "the effect of an excessive stimulus upon a small and finite group of receptors, namely those which are normally brought into activity at near threshold intensities" (Hood, 1972). Auditory fatigue defined in this way is often referred to as post-stimulatory auditory fatigue, and the shift in threshold is called temporary threshold shift (TTS).

Auditory adaptation has as its essential feature the process of 'equilibration'. The response of a receptor to a steady stimulus declines as a function of time until it reaches a steady value at which the energy expended by the receptor is just balanced by the metabolic energy which is available to sustain it. The psychological counterpart of this is a decline in the apparent magnitude of a stimulus (e.g. its loudness) during the first few minutes of presentation, followed by a period in which the apparent magnitude remains roughly constant.

Although there is a great deal of evidence that fatigue and adaptation are distinct phenomena, at both the physiological and psychological level, they are not always easy to distinguish. As Elliot and Fraser (1970) have pointed out:

> . . . the question continues to plague investigators as to whether, when the ear is stimulated, for example with a 60- or 80-dB tone, the changes observed during stimulation, or immediately after its cessation are primarily indicative of adaptation or of fatigue. Consequently, although the terms are well established, we are using them with the realization that they often do not refer to completely independent physiological processes.

We will not attempt here to give a detailed account of the physiological processes involved in fatigue and adaptation, or of the factors which affect these. For a review of these the reader is referred to Elliot and Fraser (1970). They concluded that ". . . stimulation results in reversible neural changes that indicate neural adaptation, reduction in hair-cell response, and in all probability, a variety of cochlear environmental changes that interfere with both hair-cell and nerve-cell functioning".

A Post-stimulatory auditory fatigue

The most common index of auditory fatigue is TTS, whose measurement was described briefly above. One problem with measuring TTS is that the recovery process may be quite rapid, so that a threshold measurement has to be obtained as quickly as possible; but this in turn can lead to inaccuracies in the measurement. The most common method is to use a motor-driven attenuator, which the subject controls so as to maintain the level of the signal as close as possible to threshold. Sometimes continuous tones are used as signals but, since subjects often have difficulty in tracking these, pulsed tones are generally preferred.

There are five major factors which influence the size of TTS: (1) the intensity of the fatiguing stimulus (I); (2) the duration of the fatiguing stimulus (D); (3) the frequency of the fatiguing stimulus (F_e); (4) the frequency of the test stimulus (F_t); and (5) the time between cessation of the fatiguing stimulus and the post-exposure threshold determination – called the recovery interval (RI). We will briefly summarize the effects of each of these.

TTS generally increases with I, the intensity of the fatiguing stimulus. At low intensities TTS changes relatively slowly as a function of I, the TTS is symmetrically distributed about F_e, and is limited to its immediate neighbourhood. In other words, only test tones with frequencies F_t close to F_e show a TTS. As I increases, the TTS increases, the frequency range over which the effects occur increases, with the greatest increase above F_e, and the frequency of the maximum TTS shifts one half-octave or more above F_e. At high levels, and when F_t is above F_e, TTS grows very rapidly as a function of I. For fatiguing intensities above about 90–100 dB SPL, TTS rises precipitously (see Fig. 2.8), and it has been suggested that this point of inflection indicates a division between fatigue which is physiological and transient in nature and fatigue which is more permanent and pathological in nature (Hood, 1950; Hirsh and Bilger, 1955). The upward frequency shift in F_t at which the maximum TTS occurs is not fully understood, but it may be related to the mechanical properties of the basilar membrane. There is evidence that the vibration envelope on the basilar membrane shifts towards the basal (high-frequency) end of the membrane with increasing amplitude of a sinusoidal stimulus (Rhode, 1971; McFadden, 1986).

Fatigue generally increases with exposure duration, D, and a number of workers have reported that TTS is linearly related to log D (Hood, 1950; Ward *et al.*, 1958). However, for low frequencies, particularly when the fatiguing stimulus is noise or a rapidly interrupted tone (Ward, 1963a), the growth rate is reduced, probably because the middle-ear reflex (see Chapter 1, section 5) reduces sound transmission at low frequencies. The log D function probably does not extend below a D of 5 min.

Fatigue effects are generally more marked at high frequencies, at least up to 4 kHz. Thus, when the fatiguing stimulus is a broadband noise, maximum TTSs occur between 4 and 6 kHz. It is also the case that permanent hearing losses, resulting from exposure to intense sounds or from old age, tend to be

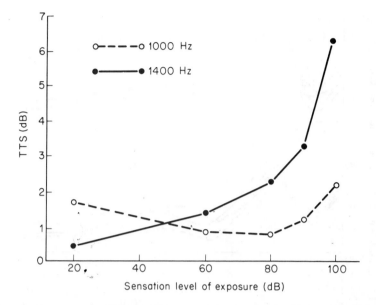

FIG. 2.8 Increases in TTS with increases in the level of the 1 kHz fatiguing tone. Test tones of 1 kHz and 1.4 kHz were used. Note that for high exposure levels the function accelerates, and that the TTS is greater for a frequency above that of the fatiguing tone than for a tone at that frequency. From Hirsh and Bilger (1955), by permission of the authors and *J. Acoust. Soc. Am.*

greatest in this region. Both of these may result from the greater stiffness of the high-frequency portions of the basilar membrane, so that elastic limits are more easily exceeded.

TTS generally decreases with increasing RI, although for many conditions the recovery curve is diphasic; recovery from the large TTS immediately following exposure is often followed by a 'bounce', particularly at high frequencies. Thus, a valley at RI = 1 min is often followed by a bounce at RI = 2 min (see Fig. 2.9). The diphasic nature of the recovery curve has led to the suggestion that two processes are involved; a short-lived recovery process which may correspond to neural activity, and a longer process which involves hair-cell and metabolic changes. For RIs greater than 2 min, recovery is approximately linearly related to log RI. Furthermore, for a given amount of TTS, the recovery proceeds at a similar rate regardless of how that amount of TTS was produced. This seems to hold for RIs from 2 min up to about 112 min (Ward *et al.*, 1958). However, when the TTS at 2 min (denoted TTS$_2$) is greater than 40–50 dB, recovery may be much slower. Even when TTS$_2$ does not exceed 40 dB, recovery times may be as long as 16 h. Recovery over

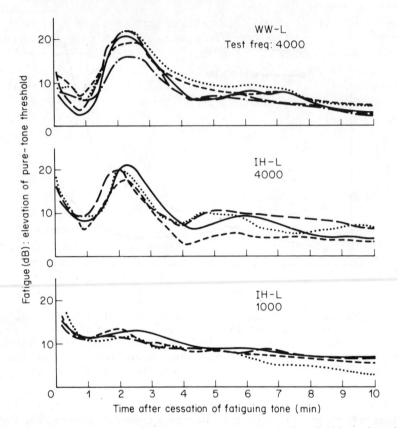

FIG. 2.9   Recovery curves illustrating the elevation in threshold produced by a fatiguing tone of 500 Hz at 120 dB SPL for 3 min. Test tones of 4 kHz (two subjects) and 1 kHz (one subject) were used, and each set of curves represents re-tests under identical conditions. Note the 'bounce' that occurs at 2 min for the 4 kHz test tones. From Hirsh and Ward (1952), by permission of the authors and *J. Acoust. Soc. Am.*

such long time intervals may indicate that tissue alterations, resulting from stimulation that exceeds the tissue's elastic limits, have occurred.

Recently a number of studies have appeared reporting the effects of exposure to environmental noise of various kinds, including rock and roll music. Harris (1972) in a review of these concluded that

> ... the quieter bands may be harmless, but if the amplification/reverberation condition reaches 110 dBA, a sizeable fraction of persons would be adversely affected probably permanently; while a 120 dBA level, at which some music groups have registered, would create havoc with most audiograms.

To a first approximation, the permanent damage caused by exposure to intense sounds is related to the total energy received by the ear over a given period. An exposure to a sound level of 90 dB SPL for 8 h per day is considered in most countries to be just within safety limits, although there are proposals in the EEC to reduce the limit to 85 dB. If the exposure duration is halved, the permissible sound intensity is doubled, corresponding to a 3 dB increase in level. Thus, 93 dB is permissible for 4 h, 96 dB for 1 h, 99 dB for 0.5 h, 102 dB for 15 min, 105 dB for 7.5 min, and so on. Clearly, sound levels over 110 dB can produce permanent damage very quickly.

B Auditory adaptation

Early studies of auditory adaptation made use of loudness balance tests, and in particular a test known as the simultaneous dichotic loudness balance (SDLB). For example, a tone of fixed level, say 80 dB SPL, would be applied to the one ear (the test ear), and a loudness balance made with a comparison tone of the same frequency but variable level applied to the other ear (the control ear). For a normal subject, this balance is obtained with a level of about 80 dB SPL. The tone in the control ear is now removed, but that in the test ear is continued for a further 3 min. Following this adaptation period, a loudness balance is established once again. It is generally found that the tone in the control ear now produces a loudness match at a lower level, say 60 dB SPL. Thus the amount of adaptation corresponds to a change in level of 20 dB. Notice that the measurement of the decrement of response takes place while the adapting stimulus is being applied.

There are several problems associated with this SDLB technique. Firstly, adaptation may occur in the control ear, either by means of central neural effects or by physical crossover of the sound, which occurs at 40–50 dB SL in the frequency range from 100 to 10 000 Hz (von Békésy and Rosenblith, 1951). Secondly, if the comparison tone is presented continuously during a loudness balance, this too may introduce adaptation in the control ear. Thirdly, it is possible that the presentation of the tone in the control ear affects the loudness of the tone in the test ear. Finally, it is not clear whether the balance is made on the basis of loudness per se, or on the basis of the position of the sound image within the head (see Chapter 6).

Several papers have suggested that if the test conditions are designed to eliminate binaural interaction between adapting and comparison tones, then suprathreshold loudness adaptation is essentially absent (e.g. Bray *et al.*, 1973). One technique makes use of a comparison tone whose frequency differs from that of the adapting tone. The adapting tone is presented continuously to one ear, while the comparison tone is presented intermittently to the other. This technique is called a 'simultaneous heterophonic loudness balance technique' (the corresponding name for the case when adapting and comparison tones have the same frequency is 'homophonic'). An alternative is to use a monaural heterophonic technique, where adapting and comparison tones are presented to the same ear, but are sufficiently different in frequency (say, 500 Hz and 10 000 Hz) for adaptation to one to have little effect on the loudness of the other. A third technique requires the subject to adjust the intensity of a continuously presented sound so as to maintain it at constant loudness. If the subject increases the intensity of the sound with increasing duration of presentation, then this indicates that adaptation is occurring. Most of the workers using these techniques have reported that there is no significant loudness adaptation for adapting tones between 50 and 90 dB SPL. This has been taken to indicate that the effects which are observed for the homophonic SDLB test are mediated by central interactions, and should not be interpreted as indicating a genuine decrement in loudness for a continuously presented stimulus. On the other hand, there is at least one report (Weiler and Friedman, 1973) of significant (>20 dB) adaptation obtained using a monaural heterophonic technique, so that not all adaptation phenomena can be attributed to binaural interactions.

In a review of loudness adaptation, Scharf (1981) has presented data obtained with a method of successive magnitude estimation. The listener is required to assign numbers to express the loudness of a sound at successive time intervals (see section 4 for a description of loudness scaling). The results indicate that adaptation occurs only for low-level tones, below about 30 dB SL. Scharf's main conclusions were as follows:

> A sound presented alone adapts only if it is below 30 dB SL. High frequency pure tones adapt more than low-frequency tones or than noises, whether broadband or narrow-band. Steady sounds adapt more than modulated sounds, and if the sound amplitude is modulated sufficiently adaptation may disappear altogether as when two tones beat together. People differ widely with respect to the degree of adaptation they experience. While most people hear the loudness of a high-frequency, low-level tone decline by at least half within one min, some others report no change in loudness and still others report that the tone disappears. No relation has been found, however, between the degree to which a person adapts and such individual characteristics as threshold, age, and sex, although there is some evidence that children under 16 years adapt less than adults. Free field listening may produce less adaptation than earphone listening.

There have been comparatively few studies of the spread of adaptation to frequencies adjacent to that of the adapting tone, and most have used the SDLB technique, which we have seen suffers from difficulties of interpretation. Thwing (1955) used a 1000 Hz tone at 80 dB SL as the adapting stimulus. For 15 s in every 2 min he presented a tone of a different frequency in the opposite ear and, at the same time, adjusted the frequency in the test ear to match that of the comparison stimulus. The level of the comparison stimulus was adjusted to match the loudness in the test ear. Thwing found a maximum adaptation effect at the frequency of the adapting tone with continuously decreasing effects on either side. He suggested that the adaptation is proportional to the extent to which the excitation patterns of the test and adapting stimulus overlap. More data are needed for the evaluation of this hypothesis.

8 ABNORMALITIES OF LOUDNESS PERCEPTION IN IMPAIRED HEARING: LOUDNESS RECRUITMENT AND PATHOLOGICAL ADAPTATION

Hearing losses may be broadly categorized into two main types. The first type, conductive deafness, occurs when there is a defect, usually in the middle ear, which reduces the transmission of sound to the inner ear. For example, viscous fluid may build up in the middle ear as a result of infection or the stapes may be immobilized as a result of growth of bone over the oval window. Sometimes a conductive loss is produced by wax in the ear canal. In general, a conductive loss results in a more or less uniform hearing loss as a function of frequency; it can be regarded as resulting in a simple attenuation of the incoming sound. The difficulty experienced by the sufferer can be well predicted from the elevation in absolute threshold. A simple hearing aid is usually quite effective in such cases, and surgery can also be effective.

The second type of hearing loss is called sensorineural hearing loss, although it is also inaccurately known as 'nerve deafness'. Sensorineural hearing loss most commonly arises from a defect in the cochlea, and is then known as a cochlear loss. However, sensorineural hearing loss may also arise as a result of defects in the auditory nerve or higher centres in the auditory system. Hearing loss due to neural disturbances occurring at a higher point in the auditory pathway than the cochlea is known as retrocochlear loss. The particular difficulties experienced by the sufferer, and the types of symptoms exhibited, depend on which part of the system is affected. Often, the extent of the loss increases with frequency, especially in the elderly. However, the difficulty experienced by the sufferer is not always well predicted from the audiogram. Patients often have difficulty in understanding speech in noisy environments, and the condition is usually not completely alleviated by a hearing aid. Most sensorineural losses cannot be treated by surgery.

A   *Loudness recruitment*

One phenomenon which often occurs when there are defects in the cochlea is loudness recruitment. This refers to an unusually rapid growth of loudness as the sensation level of a tone is increased, and it might be observed as follows. Suppose that a patient has a hearing loss at 4000 Hz of 60 dB in one ear only. If a 4000 Hz tone is introduced into their normal ear at 100 dB SPL (which would also be about 100 dB above threshold for that ear), then the tone which sounds equally loud in their impaired ear will also have a level of about 100 dB SPL. Thus a tone which is only 40 dB above threshold in the impaired ear may sound as loud as a tone which is 100 dB above threshold in the normal ear; the ear with recruitment seems to 'catch up' with the normal ear in loudness. Notice that, although loudness recruitment is normally regarded as pathological, a phenomenon very much like it occurs in normal listeners for tones of very high and very low frequency. The loudness of these tones grows more rapidly per decibel than does the loudness for tones of middle frequencies (see section 3).

One method of detecting recruitment is based on the assumption that if loudness is increasing more rapidly than normal as the stimulus intensity is increased, then a smaller than normal intensity change will be required for a just-noticeable difference in loudness. Thus the difference limen (DL) for intensity should be abnormally small, particularly at low sensation levels, where the rate of growth of loudness is most rapid. This reasoning gives the basis for a number of clinical tests for recruitment, all of which assume that a smaller than normal DL will indicate the presence of recruitment. The most widely used of these is called the SISI (short increment sensitivity index) test (Jerger *et al.*, 1959).

Unfortunately the reasoning is not sound. We know from the results with normal subjects that loudness grows more rapidly with sound intensity for low-frequency tones than for middle-frequency tones, but the DL for intensity is not smaller for low-frequency tones. Similarly, in normal listeners the rate of growth of loudness with intensity is most rapid at low sound levels, but the intensity DL is largest at low sound levels. It appears that there is not necessarily a relationship between the rate of growth of loudness and the intensity DL. This has been directly confirmed by recent experiments (Zwislocki and Jordan, 1986; Viemeister and Bacon, 1988). The lack of relationship makes sense if we assume that the size of the DL is determined by variability in the loudness sensation, as well as its rate of growth. At low sound levels, or in the impaired ear, the variability may well be increased.

In spite of the difficulties of interpretation, a small size of the DL is sometimes associated with recruitment, especially for stimuli at low SLs. However, this applies only to modulated tones, or tones where the increment to be detected is superimposed on a steady background. Even in this case the test is not very reliable (Lamore and Rodenburg, 1980). Where the task is one of detecting a difference in intensity between two separate tone pulses, the intensity DL can be somewhat larger than normal in cases of recruitment. In cases where the hearing disorder is in the auditory nerve rather than in the cochlea (and recruitment is generally not seen), the intensity DL may be considerably larger than normal (Fastl and Schorn, 1981). An extensive review of the SISI test has been given by Buus *et al.* (1982a, b).

A second technique for measuring loudness recruitment is the alternate binaural loudness balance (ABLB) test, which can be applied when only one ear is affected. A tone of a given level in the normal ear is alternated with a variable tone of the same frequency in the impaired ear, and the level of the tone is adjusted to give a loudness match. This is repeated at a number of different levels, so that the rate of growth of loudness in the impaired ear can be compared with that in the normal ear. Hood (1972) has emphasized the importance of presenting the tones alternately at the two ears, rather than presenting sustained tones simultaneously at the two ears. The reason for this is that, for sustained tones, pathological adaptation (see below) may occur, so that the loudness decreases rapidly with increasing duration of the stimulus. Thus all tests designed to detect recruitment must involve either interrupted tones or abrupt changes in tonal intensity.

A third test for recruitment involves the measurement of loudness discomfort levels (LDLs). For most normal subjects, a tone becomes uncomfortably loud when its level reaches 100–110 dB SPL. For a patient with a nonrecruiting hearing loss (for example a conductive loss) the LDL may be much higher, whereas, if recruitment is present, the LDL will fall within the range for normal subjects. In general, if the range between the absolute threshold and the LDL is reduced compared to normal, this is indicative of loudness recruitment.

The phenomenon of loudness recruitment probably accounts for a statement which is often heard from patients with this type of hearing loss: "Don't shout; you're talking loud enough, but I can't understand what you are saying!" The patient may not be able to hear very faint sounds, but sounds of high intensity are just as loud as for a normal listener. However, sounds which are easily audible may not be easily intelligible.

The physiological causes of loudness recruitment are not entirely clear, but it occurs consistently in disorders of the cochlea, and is usually absent in conductive deafness and in retrocochlear deafness. It is probably connected with hair-cell damage, and in particular with damage to the outer hair cells. It is certainly the case that the outer hair cells are the most susceptible to damage (e.g. from intense auditory stimulation). However, there have been reports (Dix and Hood, 1973) of recruitment caused by brain stem disorders.

Evans (1975) has suggested that recruitment may be associated with the abnormally broad tuning curves which are commonly found when the functioning of the cochlea is impaired (see Chapter 1, section 5 and Chapter 3, section 10). If tuning curves are abnormally broad, with shallow slopes, then the rate at which activity spreads across the nerve fibre array, with increasing intensity, will be greater than normal. This could be the basis of loudness recruitment. One problem with this hypothesis is that is predicts 'over recruitment'; at very high sound levels the loudness in an impaired ear should actually exceed that in a normal ear. This does not usually happen. Furthermore, an experiment by Moore *et al.* (1985b) failed to support Evan's (1975) hypothesis. Moore and co-workers tested subjects with loudness recruitment in one ear only, so that loudness matches could be made between the normal and impaired ear. The tone in the impaired ear was presented in a bandstop noise which would have masked the edges of the excitation pattern of the tone. If Evans' hypothesis were correct, this noise should have reduced or abolished the loudness recruitment. In fact, the loudness of the tone in the impaired ear was almost unaffected by the bandstop noise. This indicates that abnormal spread of excitation is not the cause of loudness recruitment.

An alternative explanation for loudness recruitment is that it results from damage to or loss of the active process in the cochlea which enhances sensitivity for low input sound levels (see Chapter 1). This process is nonlinear, and it results in an amplification of the basilar membrane response to low level sounds, while leaving the response to high level sounds relatively unamplified. If the active process is lost, then the response to low level sounds is not amplified, and the absolute threshold is elevated. However, the response to high level sounds remains roughly the same as normal. This could explain loudness recruitment.

An equivalent explanation can be given in terms of neural responses. Assume, for simplicity, that loudness is coded is terms of which neurones are active at a given CF. Consider neural responses in a normal ear. At low sound levels, neurones with low thresholds would be active, whereas at high levels neurones with both low and high thresholds would be active (see section 6B). For an impaired ear, the thresholds of the high-threshold neurones may be almost unaffected, while the (normally) low-threshold neurones have elevated thresholds because of the loss of the active process. A high-level tone will excite both the (impaired) 'low-threshold' neurones and the high-threshold neurones, so that the loudness sensation is the same as normal. This hypothesis is attractive since it can explain why, in patients with impairments in one ear only, the loudness in the recruiting ear generally 'catches up with' and matches the loudness in the normal ear at high sound levels.

B Pathological adaptation

Abnormal metabolic processes in the cochlea or auditory nerve sometimes result in a very rapid decrease in neural responses, although the response to the onset of a sound may be normal or near normal. The psychological correlate of this is adaptation which is more extreme and more rapid than normal. This effect is usually greater in defects of the nerve fibres than of the cochlea itself, and so pathological adaptation is useful in the differential diagnosis of cochlear and retrocochlear defects (Jerger and Jerger, 1975).

There are several ways of studying this phenomenon, including the simultaneous dichotic loudness balance procedure which we described for normal adaptation. Since, however, pathological adaptation occurs at all sound levels, it can conveniently be studied with tones close to threshold. One way of doing this is to measure the difference in threshold for continuous and interrupted tones. For patients with conductive hearing loss, or for normal subjects, there is little difference between the two types of threshold. For a patient with a retrocochlear loss, the threshold for a continuous tone may be considerably higher than that for an interrupted tone. One very striking way of demonstrating this is first to determine the threshold for an interrupted tone. The sound level is then raised by 5 dB and the tone is presented continuously. After five or six seconds the sensation of tone will disappear completely, although for the normal listener the sensation would persist indefinitely. It is often necessary to raise the level of the tone by 20–30 dB before the sensation persists indefinitely for subjects with retrocochlear losses. It is easy to confirm that the effect is pathological adaptation rather than fatigue, by interrupting the tone at any time during the test; the original threshold is restored at once. These tests are known as tone decay tests (Jerger and Jerger, 1975).

It is clear that measures of recruitment and adaptation are of considerable use in the diagnosis of hearing disorders, and in identifying the site in the auditory pathway where the defect lies. Such measures also give us a valuable insight into the relationship between normal and abnormal functioning of the auditory system, and thus provide pointers for the direction of research in these areas. Studies of what can go wrong with the auditory system help us to understand how it normally works, and conversely a more complete knowledge of how the normal system functions is essential if we are to be able to work out exactly what has gone wrong in cases of hearing loss. A knowledge of the underlying processes involved in adaptation and fatigue is important in the interpretation of clinical data, and also indicates the need, as Hood (1972) puts it, "... for care in the design and execution of all audiological test procedures".

9   *GENERAL CONCLUSIONS*

In this chapter we have discussed a number of different aspects of the perception of loudness and the way it is coded in the auditory system. Absolute threshold curves show that we are most sensitive to middle frequencies (1000–5000 Hz). At least part of this sensitivity arises from the action of the outer and middle ear. Our absolute sensitivity is such that our ability to detect faint sounds would normally be limited by environmental noises, rather than by limits in the system itself. There is, however, considerable variability between different individuals, so that thresholds 20 dB on either side of the mean are still considered as 'normal'. Hearing losses with age are most marked at high frequencies. Noise exposure tends to produce the greatest hearing loss around 4000–6000 Hz.

Equal-loudness contours allow us to compare the loudnesses of sinusoids of different frequencies. In general, the shapes of equal-loudness contours are similar to absolute threshold curves at low levels, but become flatter at high levels. Thus, at high levels it is roughly true that tones of equal SPL sound equally loud regardless of frequency. The shapes of equal-loudness contours indicate that loudness grows more rapidly with increasing intensity for low frequencies and for very high frequencies than for middle frequencies. This means that the tonal balance of recorded sounds, such as speech or music, may be affected by the level at which the sounds are reproduced. Equal-loudness contours are used in the design of sound level meters, so that the readings obtained give a better indication of the perceived loudness than would readings based simply on physical intensity.

The techniques of loudness scaling – magnitude estimation and magnitude production – allow the construction of 'psychological' scales of loudness, the most common one being the sone scale suggested by S. S. Stevens (1957). Such scales are supposed to relate the perceived loudness of a given sound to its physical characteristics (such as intensity), and they have been utilized in models which allow the calculation of the loudness of any complex sound.

Absolute thresholds and the loudness of sounds both depend upon duration. Over a certain range of durations (about 15–150 ms) the ear appears to integrate sound energy for the purpose of detection. Thus, it is approximately true that threshold depends only on the total amount of energy in the stimulus, and not on how that energy is distributed over time. However, this does not hold at very long durations, probably because of the limited integration time of the ear. At very short durations 'energy splatter' in the signal may also reduce its detectability. There is some evidence that the integration time of the ear is shorter for high frequencies than for low. The loudness of short duration sounds may also depend upon their total energy, but the results are much less clear cut, and vary considerably according to the experimental technique used.

We are able to detect relatively small changes in sound level (0.5–2 dB) for a wide range of levels and for many types of stimuli. In general, discrimination performance, as measured by the Weber fraction ($\Delta I/I$), is independent of level for bands of noise, but improves at high levels for pure tones. Various psychoacoustic experiments indicate that, at high levels, information in neurones with CFs above and (to a lesser extent) below the frequency of the test tone contributes to intensity discrimination, but is not essential for it. In other words, spread of excitation is not essential for maintaining the wide dynamic range of the auditory system. Similarly, psychophysical experiments suggest that phase locking may play a role in intensity discrimination but it is not essential.

Recordings from single neurones in the auditory nerve indicate that the information contained in the firing rates of auditory neurones is more than sufficient to account for human intensity discrimination. Indeed, the information from only about 100 out of the 30 000 neurones would be sufficient. Thus, it appears that intensity discrimination is not limited by the information carried in the auditory nerve, but rather by the use made of that information at higher levels in the auditory system.

Exposure to auditory stimulation produces two types of changes in the responsiveness of the auditory system: the apparent magnitude of the stimulus may decrease, a process known as adaptation, and the absolute threshold measured after exposure may increase, a process known as fatigue. There are many problems associated with the measurement of these processes, and they are not always clearly separable.

Fatigue, as measured by temporary threshold shift (TTS), is generally small at low exposure intensities, but increases rapidly when the fatiguing stimulus is above about 90–100 dB SPL. This may indicate a division between fatigue that is physiological and transient in nature and fatigue that is more permanent and pathological in nature. TTS generally decreases with increasing recovery time, although a 'bounce' sometimes occurs about two minutes after cessation of the fatiguing stimulus. This may indicate that more than one process is involved in recovery. Recovery times vary considerably, but may be as long as 16 h or more following exposure to very intense sounds. Sound levels above 110–120 dB SPL may produce permanent hearing losses, particularly if the exposure is of long duration. Such sound levels are not uncommonly produced by rock and pop groups, and they may be easily obtained by many of the sets of headphones which are available on the domestic market.

Adaptation effects measured with the simultaneous dichotic loudness balance (SDLB) technique are generally quite rapid, the greatest adaptation occurring within one or two minutes of exposure. Adaptation measured in this way occurs at both high and low sound levels. In contrast, studies which avoid binaural interaction have shown that adaptation occurs only for low level tones (below 30 dB SL) and is strongest at high frequencies. The reasons for the discrepancies between the different methods remain to be explained.

In some cases of hearing loss, particularly when there is pathology of the cochlea, loudness recruitment may occur. Recruitment is an abnormally rapid growth of loudness with increase in intensity: the sufferer may have an elevated absolute threshold, but intense sounds are as loud as for a normal listener. One method of detecting recruitment is based on the assumption that it will be associated with an abnormally small intensity DL, but this assumption does not appear to be well founded. However, the detection of brief increments in sound level often is better than normal at low SLs. When only one ear is affected, recruitment can be detected by direct comparison with the normal ear, using a loudness balancing technique. When both ears are affected, recruitment may be revealed by a normal loudness discomfort level, but an elevated absolute threshold. Recruitment may be associated with hair-cell damage, particularly to the outer hair cells. It does not seem to be caused by an abnormal spread of excitation.

Pathological adaptation may occur when there are abnormal metabolic processes in the cochlea or auditory nerve, although the effect is usually greater in the latter case. The adaptation is more rapid and more extreme than normal, and is most easily measured for tones close to threshold; a continuous tone just above threshold may fade after a time and eventually become completely inaudible. However, the tone may easily be made audible once again by interrupting it.

Recruitment and pathological adaptation are useful measures in the differential diagnosis of cochlear and retrocochlear hearing loss and in addition they provide useful insights into the functioning of the auditory system. It is to be hoped that the future will see an increasing cooperation between clinical audiologists and otologists and the basic scientist. Theories about normal auditory functioning cannot be complete if they do not take into account the phenomena (such as recruitment) that are observed clinically, and clinical workers have much to gain from theories and data derived from studies of the normal human subject.

FURTHER READING

An extensive review of the perception of loudness may be found in:

Scharf, B. (1978). Loudness. In *Handbook of Perception*, Vol. 4 (eds E. C. Carterette and M. P. Friedman), Academic Press, New York.

A review and summary of the literature on loudness adaptation may be found in:

Scharf, B. (1981). Loudness adaptation. In *Hearing Research and Theory* (eds J. V. Tobias and E. D. Schubert), Academic Press, New York.

Demonstrations 4, 6, 7 and 8 of *Auditory Demonstrations* on CD are relevant to the contents of this chapter (see list of further reading for Chapter 1).

3

Frequency selectivity, masking and the critical band

1 INTRODUCTION

This chapter is concerned with the frequency selectivity of the auditory system. Frequency selectivity refers to our ability to resolve the sinusoidal components in a complex sound, and it plays a role in many aspects of auditory perception. However, it is often demonstrated and measured by studying masking. It is a matter of everyday experience that one sound may be obscured, or rendered inaudible, in the presence of other sounds. Thus music from a car radio may mask the sound of the car's engine, provided the music is somewhat more intense. Masking has been defined as:

(1) The *process* by which the threshold of audibility for one sound is raised by the presence of another (masking) sound. (2) The *amount* by which the threshold of audibility of a sound is raised by the presence of another (masking) sound. The unit customarily used is the decibel.   (American Standards Association, 1960)

It has been known for many years that a signal will most easily be masked by a sound having frequency components close to, or the same as, those of the signal (Mayer, 1894; Wegel and Lane, 1924). This led to the idea that our ability to separate the components of a complex sound depends, at least in part, on the frequency-resolving power of the basilar membrane. This idea will be elaborated later in this chapter. It also led to the idea that masking reflects the limits of frequency selectivity: if the selectivity of the ear is insufficient to separate the signal and the masker, then masking will occur. Thus, masking can be used to quantify frequency selectivity. Hence, much of this chapter will be devoted to studies of masking.

As well as having theoretical significance, a knowledge of the rules governing the masking of one sound by another can be very useful in practical situations. For example, one might want to know the extent to which noise from new machinery in a factory will interfere with the ability of workers to hold conversations or to detect warning signals. Masking is also used in the clinical assessment of hearing. For example, in a patient with one impaired and one normal ear, earphones may be used to present noise to the normal ear when testing the impaired ear, so as to prevent sound that 'leaks' across the head being heard in the normal ear.

An important physical parameter which affects masking is time. Most of this chapter will be devoted to simultaneous masking, in which the signal is presented at the same time as the masker. Later on we will discuss forward masking, in which the signal is masked by a preceding masker, and backward masking, in which the masker follows the signal.

2 THE CRITICAL BAND CONCEPT

A Fletcher's band-widening experiment and the power spectrum model

Fletcher (1940) carried out an experiment which has now become famous and which laid the foundation for the concept of the critical band. He measured the threshold of a sinusoidal signal as a function of the bandwidth of a bandpass noise masker. The noise was always centred at the signal frequency, and the noise power density was held constant. Thus, the total noise power increased as the bandwidth increased. This experiment has been repeated several times since then (Hamilton, 1957; Greenwood, 1961a; Spiegel, 1981; Schooneveldt and Moore, 1989). An example of the results, taken from Schooneveldt and Moore, is given in Fig. 3.1. The threshold of the signal increases at first as the noise bandwidth increases, but then flattens off, so that further increases in noise bandwidth do not change the signal threshold significantly.

To account for these results, Fletcher (1940) suggested that the peripheral auditory system behaves as if it contained a bank of bandpass filters, with continuously overlapping centre frequencies. These filters are now called the 'auditory filters'. Fletcher thought that the basilar membrane provided the basis for the auditory filters. Each location on the basilar membrane responds to a limited range of frequencies, so that each different point corresponds to a filter with a different centre frequency. Recent data are consistent with this point of view (Moore, 1986).

When trying to detect a signal in a noise background, the listener is assumed to make use of a filter with a centre frequency close to that of the signal. This filter will pass the signal but remove a great deal of the noise. Only the components in the noise which pass through the filter will have any effect in masking the signal. It is usually assumed that the threshold for the signal is

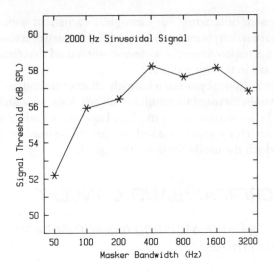

FIG. 3.1   The threshold of a 2000 Hz sinusoidal signal plotted as a function of the bandwidth of a noise masker centred at 2000 Hz. Notice that the threshold of the signal at first increases with increasing masker bandwidth and then remains constant. From Schooneveldt and Moore (1989).

determined by the amount of noise passing through the auditory filter; specifically, threshold is assumed to correspond to a certain signal-to-noise ratio at the output of the filter. This set of assumptions has come to be known as the 'power spectrum model' of masking (Patterson and Moore, 1986), since the stimuli are represented by their long-term power spectra, i.e. the relative phases of the components and the short-term fluctuations in the masker are ignored. We shall see later that the assumptions of this model do not always hold, but the model works well in many situations, and we will accept it for the moment.

In the band-widening experiment described above, increases in noise bandwidth result in more noise passing through the auditory filter, provided the noise bandwidth is less than the filter bandwidth. However, once the noise bandwidth exceeds the filter bandwidth, further increases in noise bandwidth will not increase the noise passing through the filter. Fletcher called the bandwidth at which the signal threshold ceased to increase the 'critical bandwidth'.

In analysing the results of his experiment, Fletcher made a simplifying assumption. He assumed that the shape of the auditory filter could be approximated as a simple rectangle, with a flat top and vertical edges. For such a filter all components within the passband of the filter are passed equally, and all components outside the passband are removed. The width of this passband is equal to the critical bandwidth described above. The term 'critical band' is often used to refer to this hypothetical rectangular filter.

Fletcher pointed out that the value of the critical bandwidth could be estimated indirectly, by measuring the threshold of a tone in broadband white noise, given the following hypotheses:

1. Only a narrow band of frequencies surrounding the tone – those falling within the critical band – contributes to the masking of the tone.
2. When the noise just masks the tone, the power of the tone divided by the power of the nöise inside the critical band is a constant, K.

As described in Chapter 1, noise power is usually specified in terms of the power in a band of frequencies 1 Hz wide (say from 1000 Hz to 1001 Hz). This is called the noise power density, and is denoted by the symbol N_o. For a white noise N_o is independent of frequency, so that the total noise power falling in a critical band W Hz wide is $N_o \times W$. According to Fletcher's second hypothesis,

$$P/(W \times N_o) = K$$

and

$$W = P/(K \times N_o).$$

By measuring P and N_o, and by estimating K, we can evaluate W.

The first hypothesis follows directly from Fletcher's experiment, although, as we shall see later, it is only an approximation. To estimate the value of the constant K, Fletcher measured the threshold for a tone in a band of noise whose width was less than the estimated critical bandwidth. In this case, K equals the ratio of the power of the tone to the power of the noise, since all of the noise passes through the auditory filter. Fletcher estimated K to equal 1, so that the value of W should be equal to P/N_o. The ratio P/N_o is now usually known as the critical ratio. Unfortunately, Fletcher's estimate of K has turned out not to be accurate. More recent experiments show that K is typically about 0.4 (Scharf, 1970). Thus, at most frequencies the critical ratio is about 0.4 times the value of the critical bandwidth estimated by more direct methods, such as the band-widening experiment. Also, K varies somewhat with centre frequency, so the critical ratio does not give a correct indication of how the critical bandwidth varies with centre frequency (Patterson and Moore, 1986). The difference between the critical ratio function (critical ratio as a function of frequency) and the generally accepted critical band function is illustrated in Fig. 3.2.

Since Fletcher first described the critical band concept, many different experiments have shown that listeners' responses to complex sounds differ

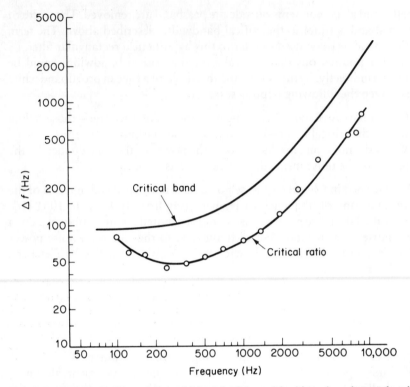

FIG. 3.2　A comparison of the width, Δf, of the critical band as determined by direct measures (upper curve) and as determined from the critical ratio. From Zwicker *et al.* (1957), by permission of the authors and *J. Acoust. Soc. Am.*

according to whether the stimuli are wider or narrower than the critical bandwidth. Further, these different experiments give remarkably similar estimates both of the absolute width of the critical band and of the way the critical bandwidth varies as a function of frequency. Thus the critical band phenomenon pervades and summarizes a great variety of data, and provides a valuable guide in the planning of experiments and the analysis of data. Some of the types of experiment in which critical band phenomena have been observed are described below.

B   The loudness of complex sounds

Consider a complex sound of fixed energy (or intensity) having a bandwidth of W. If W is less than the critical bandwidth, then the loudness of the sound is

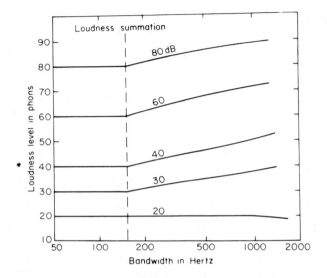

FIG. 3.3 The loudness level in phons of a band of noise centred at 1 kHz, measured as a function of the width of the band. For each of the curves, the overall sound level was constant, and its value, in dB SPL, is indicated in the figure. The dashed line shows that the bandwidth at which loudness begins to increase is roughly the same at all levels tested (except that no increase occurs at the lowest level). From Feldtkeller and Zwicker (1956) by permission of the authors and publisher.

more or less independent of W; the sound is judged to be about as loud as a pure tone of equal intensity lying at the centre frequency of the band. However, if W is increased beyond the critical bandwidth, the loudness of the complex begins to increase. This has been found to be the case for bands of noise (Zwicker *et al.*, 1957) and for complexes consisting of pure tones whose frequency separation is varied (Scharf, 1961, 1970) (see Fig. 3.3). The critical bandwidth for the data in Fig. 3.3 is about 160 Hz for a centre frequency of 1000 Hz. Thus, for a given amount of energy, a complex sound will be louder if the energy is spread over a number of critical bands, than if it is all contained within one critical band. This finding has been incorporated in the models described in Chapter 2, which allow the calculation of the loudness of almost any complex sound (see, for example, Zwicker and Scharf, 1965).

The increase in loudness with increasing bandwidth can be understood if we assume that when the bandwidth of a sound is sufficient to occupy more than one critical band, the loudness in adjacent, but nonoverlapping, bands is summed to give the total loudness. Consider the effect of taking two tones very close together in frequency, so as to occupy one critical band, and increasing their frequency separation so that two critical bands are occupied. The intensity in each band will now be half of what it was, since only one tone is present in each band. According to Steven's Power Law, $L = kI^{0.3}$ (see Chapter 2, section 4). Thus halving intensity is equivalent to a reduction in loudness to 0.81 of its original value. The total loudness in the two bands will be $2 \times 0.81 = 1.62$ times the original value. Thus increasing bandwidth beyond the critical band results in an increase in loudness. The argument can easily be extended to cover multicomponent complex tones and bands of noise (see Moore and Glasberg, 1986).

A corresponding explanation can be offered in terms of the neurophysiological data. When the two tones are very close in frequency they excite essentially the same set of neurones. If the two tones are separated in frequency, they excite essentially independent sets of neurones. Now at moderate and high intensities, the firing rates of individual neurones change relatively slowly as a function of intensity. Thus the decrease in neural firings as a result of halving the effective intensity exciting each set, is more than offset by the doubling of the number of neurones involved. If, then, loudness is related in some way to the total number of neural impulses evoked by the stimulus, it is clear that the loudness of the complex should be greater when the components are widely separated.

At low sensation levels (around 10–20 dB SL) the loudness of a complex sound is roughly independent of bandwidth. This also is easy to explain. At these low levels, neural firing rates change relatively rapidly with intensity, and so does loudness. The loudness of a single critical band changes almost in direct proportion to intensity, so that increasing the spread of energy from one to two critical bands, for example, produces two component bands each half as loud as the original sound (Scharf, 1970). The total loudness is equal to that of the original single band, so that loudness is independent of bandwidth. At very low sensation levels (below 10 dB), if we distribute the energy of a complex sound over a wide range of frequencies, then the energy in each critical band is insufficient to make the sound audible. Accordingly, near threshold, loudness must decrease as the bandwidth of a complex sound is increased from a subcritical value. As a consequence, if the intensity of a complex sound is increased slowly from a subthreshold value, the rate of growth of loudness is greater for a wideband sound than for a narrowband sound.

C   The threshold of complex sounds

When two tones with a small frequency separation are presented together, a sound may be heard even when either tone by itself is below threshold.

Gässler (1954) measured the threshold of multitone complexes consisting of evenly spaced sinusoids. The tones were presented both in quiet and in a special background noise, chosen to give the same masked threshold for each component in the signal. As the number of tones in a complex was increased, the threshold, specified in terms of total energy, remained constant until the overall spacing of the tones reached the critical bandwidth. Thereafter the threshold increased. The critical bandwidth for a centre frequency of 1000 Hz was estimated to be about 180 Hz. These results suggest that the energies of the individual components in a complex sound will sum, in the detection of that sound, provided the components lie within a critical band. When the components are distributed over more than one critical band, detection is less good.

Unfortunately, more recent data are not in complete agreement with those of Gässler. For example, Spiegel (1981) measured the threshold for a noise signal of variable bandwidth centred at 1000 Hz in a broadband background noise masker. The threshold for the signal as a function of bandwidth did not show a breakpoint corresponding to the critical bandwidth, but increased monotonically as the bandwidth increased beyond 50 Hz. Spiegel suggested that the ear is capable of integration over bandwidths much greater than the critical bandwidth.

D Two-tone masking

Zwicker (1954) measured the threshold for a narrow band of noise, of centre frequency f, in the presence of two tones, with frequencies on either side of f. He increased the frequency separation of the two tones, starting with a small separation, and found that threshold for the noise signal remained constant until the separation reached a critical value, after which it fell sharply. He took this critical value to be an estimate of the critical bandwidth. Unfortunately the interpretation of this experiment is complicated. One problem is that the lower of the two tones may interact with the noise band to produce combination products; these are frequency components not present in the stimulus applied to the ear, and they appear to result from a nonlinear process in the cochlea (see Chapter 1, section 5D and Chapter 5, section 5A). The listener may detect these combination products even though the signal itself is inaudible. When precautions are taken to mask the distortion products, then the threshold for the signal does not show an abrupt decrease, but decreases smoothly with increasing frequency separation between the two tones (Patterson and Henning, 1977; Glasberg *et al.*, 1984). Nevertheless, the results do clearly indicate the operation of a filtering mechanism in the ear. For an extensive review of results obtained using two-tone maskers, the reader is referred to Rabinowitz *et al.* (1980).

E   Sensitivity to phase

The sounds which we encounter in everyday life often change in frequency and amplitude from moment to moment. In the laboratory the perception of such sounds is often studied using either frequency-modulated or amplitude-modulated sine waves. Such waves consist of a carrier frequency (a sine wave) upon which some other signal is impressed. In amplitude modulation (AM) the carrier's amplitude is varied so as to follow the magnitude of a modulating sine wave, while the carrier frequency remains unchanged. In frequency modulation (FM) the carrier's instantaneous frequency is varied in proportion to the modulating signal's magnitude, but the amplitude remains constant. The two types of waveform are illustrated in Fig. 3.4. The expression describing an AM sinewave with carrier frequency f_c and modulating frequency g is

$$(1 + m \sin 2\pi gt) \sin 2\pi f_c t$$

where t is time, and m is a constant determining the amount of modulation; m is referred to as the modulation depth. When $m = 1$, the wave is said to be 100% modulated. The corresponding expression describing an FM sinewave is

$$\sin (2\pi f_c t + \beta \sin 2\pi gt)$$

In this case, β is usually referred to as the modulation index.

These complex waveforms can be analysed into a series of sinusoidal components. For an AM wave the results of the analysis are very simple: the spectrum contains just three frequency components with frequencies $f_c - g, f_c$ and $f_c + g$. For an FM wave the spectrum often contains many components, but if m is small, then the FM wave can also be considered as consisting of three components: $f_c - g, f_c$ and $f_c + g$. Under some conditions an AM wave and an FM wave may have components which are identical in frequency and amplitude, the only difference between them being in the relative phase of the components. If, then, the two types of wave are perceived differently, the difference is likely to arise from a sensitivity to the relative phase of the components.

Zwicker (1952) measured one aspect of the perception of such stimuli, namely the just-detectable amounts of amplitude or frequency modulation, for various rates of modulation. He found that for high rates of modulation, where the frequency components are widely spaced, the detectability of FM

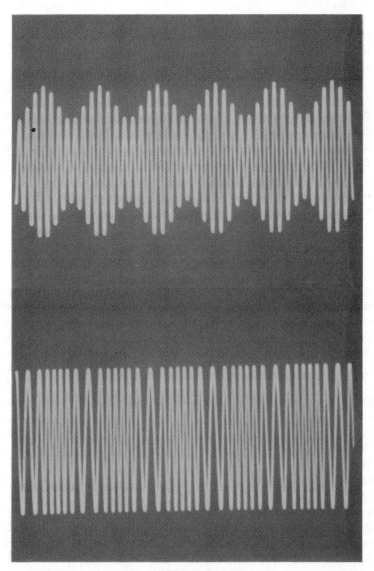

FIG. 3.4 Waveform of an amplitude-modulated wave (upper trace) and a frequency-modulated wave (lower trace).

and AM was equal when the components in each type of wave were of equal amplitude. However, when all three components fell within a critical band, AM was more easily detectable than FM. Thus it appears that we are only sensitive to the relative phase of the components, in the detection of modulation, when those components lie within a critical band. These results have been confirmed by Schorer (1986).

It is not at present clear whether this finding can be generalized to the perception of suprathreshold levels of modulation, or to other aspects of our sensitivity to phase. Indeed there is some evidence to the contrary. For example, it has been shown that subjects can detect phase changes between the components in complex sounds in which the components are separated by considerably more than a critical band (Raiford and Schubert, 1971; Lamore, 1975; Patterson, 1987a). Further work is needed to clarify the nature of these discrepancies, and to determine the applicability of the critical band concept to the phase sensitivity of the ear.

F   The discrimination of partials in complex tones

According to Ohm's (1843) Acoustical Law, the ear is able to hear pitches corresponding to the individual sinusoidal components in a complex periodic sound. In other words, we can 'hear out' the individual partials. Plomp (1964a) used a complex tone with 12 sinusoidal components to investigate the limits of this ability. The listener was presented with two comparison tones, one of which was of the same frequency as a partial in the complex; the other lay halfway between that frequency and the frequency of the adjacent higher or lower partial. The listener had to judge which of these two tones was a component of the complex. Plomp used two types of complex: a harmonic complex containing harmonics 1 to 12, where the frequencies of the components were integral multiples of that of the fundamental; and a nonharmonic complex, where the frequencies of the components were mistuned from simple frequency ratios. He found that for both kinds of complex only the first five to eight components could be 'heard out'. If it is assumed that a partial will only be distinguished when it is separated from its neighbour by at least one critical bandwidth, then the results can be used to estimate the critical bandwidth. Above 1000 Hz, the estimates obtained in this way coincide with other critical band measures. Below 1000 Hz the estimates are about two-thirds as large. When Plomp repeated the experiment using a two-tone complex, he found that the partials could be distinguished at smaller frequency separations than were found for multitone complexes.

Thus, while the results are roughly in line with other measures of critical bandwidth, there are discrepancies, especially at low frequencies. It is possible that the analysis of partials from a complex sound depends in part on factors other than pure frequency resolution. Some indication of this is given by the work of Soderquist (1970). He compared musicians and nonmusicians in a task very similar to that of Plomp, and found that the musicians were markedly superior. This result could mean that musicians have narrower critical bands, but this is unlikely if the critical band reflects a basic physiological process, as is generally assumed (Scharf, 1970). It seems more plausible that some other mechanism is involved in this task and that musicians, because of their greater experience, are able to make more efficient use of this mechanism. Haggard (1974) also reports comparisons of different measures of the critical bandwidth, and suggests that discrepancies at low frequencies may be explained by the intervention of mechanisms other than the critical band. This problem is discussed more fully later in this chapter.

G Interim summary

The examples given above show that the phenomenon of the critical band can be revealed in a great variety of different experiments. By and large, the results of the different experiments give reasonably consistent estimates of the value of the critical bandwidth; the critical band function shown in Fig. 3.2 was arrived at by combining the results from many different experiments. However, it is also clear that most of the experiments do not show a distinct breakpoint corresponding to the critical bandwidth. Rather, the pattern of results changes smoothly and continuously as a function of bandwidth.

The idea that there should be distinct breakpoints in the data goes back to Fletcher's approximation of the auditory filter as having the shape of a rectangle. Fletcher was well aware that the filter was not perfectly rectangular. He knew that a tone or narrow band of noise can mask another tone for frequency separations considerably exceeding the critical bandwidth. We are led to consider the critical band as resembling a filter with a rounded top and with sloping edges; the critical bandwidth then becomes some measure of the 'effective' bandwidth of this filter. We will now describe some attempts to measure the characteristics of the auditory filter, in other words, to derive the shape of the auditory filter.

3 ESTIMATING THE SHAPE OF THE AUDITORY FILTER

Most methods for estimating the shape of the auditory filter at a given centre frequency are based on the assumptions of the power spectrum model of masking. The threshold of a signal whose frequency is fixed is measured in the presence of a masker whose spectral content is varied. It is assumed, as a first approximation, that the signal is detected using the single auditory filter which is centred on the frequency of the signal, and that threshold corresponds to a constant signal-to-masker ratio at the output of that filter. The methods described below both use this same basic technique.

A   Psychophysical tuning curves

One method involves a procedure which is analogous in many ways to the determination of a neural tuning curve, and the resulting function is often called a psychophysical tuning curve (PTC). To determine a PTC the signal is fixed in level, usually at a very low level, say, 10 dB SL. The masker can be either a sinusoid or a narrow band of noise. When a sinusoid is used beats occur between the signal and masker, and these can provide a cue as to the presence of the signal. The effectiveness of this cue varies with the frequency separation of the signal and masker, since slow beats (which occur at small frequency separations) are more easily detected than rapid beats (see Chapter 4). This varying sensitivity to beats violates one of the assumptions of the power spectrum model of masking. This problem can be avoided by using a narrowband noise masker, since such a masker has inherent fluctuations in amplitude which prevent beats being detected. Thus noise is generally preferred (Patterson and Moore, 1986).

For each of several masker frequencies, the level of the masker needed just to mask the signal is determined. Because the signal is at a low level it is assumed that it will produce activity primarily in one auditory filter. It is assumed further that at threshold the masker produces a constant output from that filter, in order to mask the fixed signal. Thus the PTC will tell us the masker level required to produce a fixed output from the auditory filter as a function of frequency. Normally we determine a filter characteristic by plotting the output from the filter for an input varying in frequency and fixed in level (see Chapter 1, section 4 and Fig. 1.4). However, if the filter is linear the two methods will give the same result. Thus, if we assume linearity, the shape of the auditory filter can be obtained simply by inverting the PTC. Examples of some PTCs are given in Fig. 3.5.

The PTCs in Fig. 3.5 are very similar in general form to the neural tuning curves in Fig. 1.13. Remember that the neural tuning curves are obtained by determining the level of a tone required to produce a fixed output from a single neurone, as a function of the tone's frequency. The similarities in the procedures and the results encourage us to believe that the basic frequency selectivity of the auditory system is established at the level of the auditory

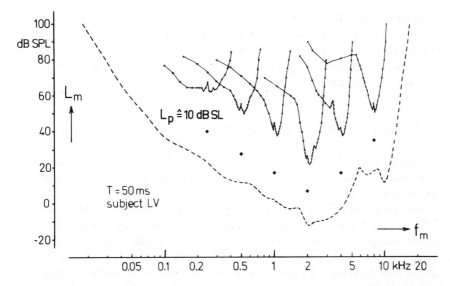

FIG. 3.5 Psychophysical tuning curves (PTCs) determined in simultaneous masking, using sinusoidal signals at 10 dB SL. For each curve, the solid diamond below it indicates the frequency and level of the signal. The masker was a sinusoid which had a fixed starting phase relationship to the brief, 50 ms, signal. The masker level, L_m, required for threshold is plotted as a function of masker frequency, f_m, on a logarithmic scale. The dashed line shows the absolute threshold for the signal. From Vogten (1974), by permission of the author.

nerve, and that the shape of the human auditory filter (or PTC) corresponds to the shape of the neural tuning curve. However, there is a need for caution in reaching this conclusion. In the determination of the neural tuning curve only one tone is present at a time, whereas for the PTC the masker and signal are presented simultaneously. This turns out to be an important point, and we will return to it later.

A second problem is that the neural tuning curve is derived from a single neurone, whereas the PTC inevitably involves activity over a group of neurones with slightly different CFs. Returning to the filter analogy, we have assumed in our analysis that only one auditory filter is involved, but it might be the case that the listener does not attend to just one filter. When the masker frequency is above the signal frequency the listener might do better to attend to a filter centred just below the signal frequency. If the filter has a relatively flat top, and sloping edges, this will considerably attenuate the masker at the filter output, while only slightly attenuating the signal. By using this off-centre filter the listener can improve performance. This is known as 'off-frequency listening', and there is now good evidence that humans do indeed listen 'off-frequency' when it is advantageous to do so. The result of off-frequency listening is that the PTC has a sharper tip than would be obtained if only one auditory filter were involved (Johnson-Davies and Patterson, 1979; O'Loughlin and Moore, 1981).

B   The notched noise method

Patterson (1976) has described an ingenious method of determining auditory filter shape which prevents off-frequency listening. The method is illustrated in Fig. 3.6. The signal is fixed in frequency, and the masker is a noise with a bandstop or notch centred at the signal frequency. The deviation of each edge of the noise from the centre frequency is denoted by Δf. The width of the notch is varied, and the threshold of the signal is determined as a function of notch width. Since the notch is symmetrically placed around the signal frequency, the method cannot reveal asymmetries in the auditory filter, and the analysis assumes that the filter is symmetric on a linear frequency scale. This assumption appears not unreasonable, at least for the top part of the filter and at moderate sound levels since PTCs are quite symmetric around the tips. For a signal symmetrically placed in a bandstop noise, the optimum signal-to-masker ratio at the output of the auditory filter is achieved with a filter centred at the signal frequency, as illustrated in Fig. 3.6. Using a filter not

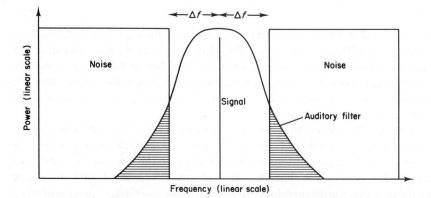

FIG. 3.6   Schematic illustration of the technique used by Patterson (1976) to determine the shape of the auditory filter. The threshold of the sinusoidal signal is measured as a function of the width of a spectral notch in the noise masker. The amount of noise passing through the auditory filter centred at the signal frequency is proportional to the shaded areas.

centred at the signal frequency reduces the amount of noise passing through the filter from one of the noise bands, but this is more than offset by the increase in noise from the other band.

As the width of the spectral notch is increased, less and less noise passes through the auditory filter. Thus the threshold of the signal drops. The amount of noise passing through the auditory filter is proportional to the area under the filter in the frequency range covered by the noise. This is shown as the shaded areas in Fig. 3.6. If we assume that threshold corresponds to a constant signal-to-masker ratio at the output of the filter, then the change in signal threshold with notch width tells us how the area under the filter varies with Δf. The area under a function between certain limits is obtained by integrating the value of the function over those limits. Hence by differentiating the function relating threshold to Δf, the height of the filter is obtained. In other words, the height of the filter for a given deviation, Δf, from the centre frequency is equal to the slope of the function relating signal threshold to notch width, at that value of Δf.

A typical auditory filter derived using this method is shown in Fig. 3.7. It has a rounded top and quite steep skirts. Unlike the simple rectangular filter, a filter with this shape cannot be completely specified with a single number, the critical bandwidth. However, some sort of summary statistic is useful, and one common measure is the bandwidth of the filter at which the response has

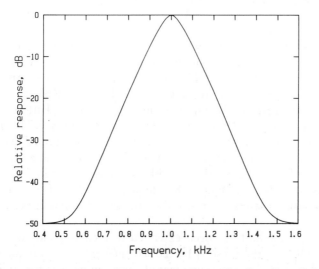

FIG. 3.7 A typical auditory filter shape determined using Patterson's method. The filter is centred at 1 kHz. The relative response of the filter (in dB) is plotted as a function of frequency.

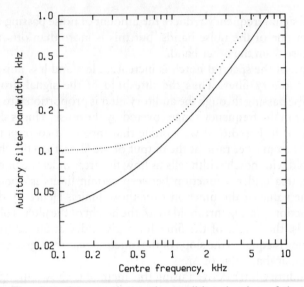

FIG. 3.8 The dotted curve shows the traditional value of the critical band-width as a function of frequency (Scharf, 1970). The solid curve shows the value of the ERB of the auditory filter as a function of frequency. The solid curve was obtained by combining the results of several experiments using Patterson's notched noise method of estimating the auditory filter shape. Adapted from Moore and Glasberg (1983a).

fallen by a factor of two in power, i.e. by 3 dB (see Chapter 1, section 4). The 3 dB bandwidths of the auditory filters derived using Patterson's method are typically between 10% and 15% of the centre frequency. An alternative measure is the equivalent rectangular bandwidth (ERB) (see Chapter 1, section 4). The ERBs of the auditory filters derived using Patterson's method are typically between 11% and 17% of the centre frequency. These values are quite close to the estimates of the critical bandwidth obtained in other ways, as described earlier. However, the values at low frequencies tend to be smaller than the traditional critical bandwidth estimates shown in Fig. 3.2 (Moore and Glasberg, 1983a). Figure 3.8 compares the ERB of the auditory filter estimated using Patterson's method with the traditional critical bandwidth function.

Patterson's method has been extended to include conditions where the spectral notch in the noise is placed asymmetrically about the signal frequency. This allows the measurement of any asymmetry in the auditory filter, but the analysis of the results is more difficult, and has to take off-frequency listening into account (Patterson and Nimmo-Smith, 1980). It is beyond the

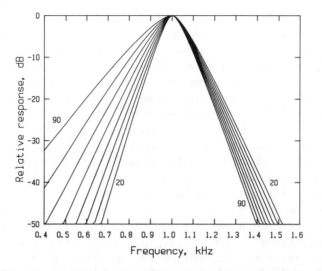

FIG. 3.9 The shape of the auditory filter centred at 1 kHz, plotted for input sound levels ranging from 20 to 90 dB SPL. The attenuation applied by the filter is plotted as a function of frequency. On the low frequency side, the filter becomes progressively less sharply tuned with increasing sound level. On the high frequency side, the sharpness of tuning increases slightly with increasing sound level. At moderate sound levels the filter is approximately symmetric on the linear frequency scale used. Adapted from Moore and Glasberg (1987).

scope of this book to give details of the method of analysis; the interested reader is referred to Patterson and Moore (1986) and Moore and Glasberg (1987). The results show that the auditory filter is reasonably symmetric at moderate sound levels, but becomes increasingly asymmetric at high levels, the low-frequency side becoming shallower than the high-frequency side. The shape of the auditory filter centred at 1 kHz is shown in Fig. 3.9 for a range of sound levels from 20 to 90 dB SPL.

C Some general observations on auditory filters

One question we may ask is whether the listener can only attend to one auditory filter at a time. The answer to this is obviously no, since many of the complex signals which we can perceive and recognize occupy more than one critical band; speech is a prime example of this. Indeed we shall see later that the perception of timbre seems to depend, at least in part, on the distribution of activity across different auditory filters. Furthermore, we shall see that the detection of a signal in a masker can sometimes depend on a *comparison* of the outputs of different auditory filters.

In spite of this, it is often possible to predict whether a complex sound will be detected in a given background noise by calculating the thresholds of the most prominent frequency components. If we know the shape of the auditory filter centred on each component, then we can calculate the amount of noise passing through the filter, and the signal-to-noise ratio at the output of the filter. If this ratio exceeds some criterion amount in any filter, then the signal will be detected. The criterion amount corresponds to a signal-to-noise ratio of about 1:2.5 or −4 dB; the signal will be detected if its level is not more than 4 dB below that of the noise at the output of the filter.

This model has practical applications, since it allows the prediction of appropriate levels for warning signals in factories and aircraft. In the past, when no theoretical model was available, the signals were often set at excessively high levels, to err on the side of 'safety'. The result was that when a signal 'went off' it was extremely aversive, and disrupted speech communication. The application of the auditory filter model has shown that sometimes signal levels can be reduced by 20 dB (a factor of 100 in power) and remain clearly audible (Patterson and Milroy, 1980).

Another question which arises is whether there is only a discrete number of critical bands, each one adjacent to its neighbours, or whether there is a continuous series of overlapping critical bands. For convenience, data relating to critical bands have often been presented as though the former were the case. For example, Scharf (1970) presented a table showing critical bandwidths for 24 successive critical bands, the upper cutoff frequency for each band being the same as the lower cutoff for the next highest band. While this method of presentation is convenient, it seems clear that critical bands are continuous rather than discrete; there has been no experimental evidence for any discontinuity or break between different critical bands. Thus we may talk about the critical band around any frequency in the audible range which we care to choose.

4　MASKING PATTERNS AND EXCITATION PATTERNS

So far we have discussed masking experiments in which the frequency of the signal is held constant, while the masker is varied. These experiments are most appropriate for estimating the shape of the auditory filter at a given centre frequency. However, many of the early experiments on masking did the opposite; the signal frequency was varied while the masker was held constant.

Wegel and Lane (1924) published the first systematic investigation of the masking of one pure tone by another. They determined the threshold of a signal with adjustable frequency in the presence of a masker with fixed frequency and intensity. The graph plotting masked threshold as a function of the frequency of the signal is known as a masking pattern, or sometimes as a masked audiogram. The results of Wegel and Lane were complicated by the occurrence of beats when the signal and masker were close together in frequency. To avoid this problem later experimenters (e.g. Egan and Hake, 1950; Greenwood, 1961a) have used a narrow band of noise as either the signal or the masker. Such a noise has 'built in' amplitude and frequency variations and does not produce regular beats when added to a tone.

The masking patterns obtained in these experiments show steep slopes on the low-frequency side, of between 80 and 240 dB/octave for pure-tone masking and 55–190 dB/octave for narrowband noise masking. The slopes on the high-frequency side are less steep and depend to some extent on the level of the masker. A typical set of results is shown in Fig. 3.10. Notice that on the high-frequency side the slopes of the curves tend to become shallower

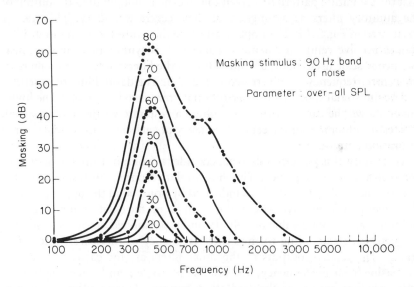

FIG. 3.10 Masking patterns (masked audiograms) for a narrow band of noise centred at 410 Hz. Each curve shows the elevation in threshold of a pure tone signal as a function of signal frequency. The overall noise level for each curve is indicated in the figure. Adapted from Egan and Hake (1950), by permission of the authors and *J. Acoust. Soc. Am.*

at high levels. Thus, if the level of a low-frequency masker is increased by, say, 10 dB, the masked threshold of a high-frequency signal is elevated by more than 10 dB; the amount of masking grows non-linearly on the high-frequency side. This has been called the 'upward spread of masking'.

The masking patterns do not reflect the use of a single auditory filter. Rather, for each signal frequency the listener uses a filter centred close to the signal frequency. Thus the auditory filter is shifted as the signal frequency is altered. One way of interpreting the masking pattern is as a crude indicator of the excitation pattern of the masker. The signal is detected when the excitation it produces is some constant proportion of the excitation produced by the masker in the frequency region of the signal. Thus the threshold of the signal as a function of frequency is proportional to the masker excitation level. The masking pattern should be parallel to the excitation pattern of the masker, but shifted vertically by a small amount. In practice, the situation is not so straightforward, since the shape of the masking pattern is influenced by factors such as off-frequency listening and the detection of combination tones produced by the interaction of the signal and the masker.

Moore and Glasberg (1983a) have described a way of deriving the shapes of excitation patterns using the concept of the auditory filter. They suggested that the excitation pattern of a given sound can be thought of as the output of the auditory filters as a function of their centre frequency. This idea is illustrated in Fig. 3.11. The upper portion of the figure shows auditory filter shapes for five centre frequencies. Each filter is symmetrical on the linear frequency scale used, but the bandwidths of the filters increase with increasing centre frequency, as illustrated in Fig. 3.8. The dashed line represents a 1 kHz sinusoidal signal whose excitation pattern is to be derived. The lower panel shows the output from each filter in response to the 1 kHz signal, plotted as a function of the centre frequency of each filter; this is the desired excitation pattern.

To see how this pattern is derived, consider the output from the filter with the lowest centre frequency. This has a relative output in response to the 1 kHz tone of about −40 dB, as indicated by point 'a' in the upper panel. In the lower panel, this gives rise to the point 'a' on the excitation pattern; the point has an ordinate value of −40 dB and is positioned on the abscissa at a frequency corresponding to the centre frequency of the lowest filter illustrated. The relative outputs of the other filters are indicated, in order of increasing centre frequency, by points 'b' to 'e', and each leads to a corresponding point on the excitation pattern. The complete excitation pattern was actually derived by calculating the filter outputs for filters spaced at 10 Hz intervals. In deriving the excitation pattern, excitation levels were expressed relative to the level at the tip of the pattern, which was arbitrarily labelled as 0 dB. To calculate the excitation pattern for a 1 kHz tone with a

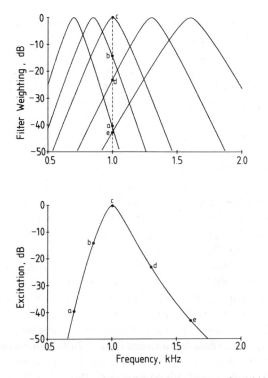

FIG. 3.11 An illustration of how the excitation pattern of a 1 kHz sinusoid can be derived by calculating the outputs of the auditory filters as a function of their centre frequency. The top half shows five auditory filters, centred at different frequencies, and the bottom half shows the calculated excitation pattern. See text for details. From Moore and Glasberg (1983a).

level of, say, 60 dB, the level at the tip would be labelled as 60 dB, and all other excitation levels would correspondingly be increased by 60 dB.

Note that, although the auditory filters were assumed to be symmetric on a linear frequency scale, the derived excitation pattern is asymmetric. This happens because the bandwidth of the auditory filter increases with increasing centre frequency. Note also, that the excitation pattern has the same general form as the masked audiograms shown in Fig. 3.10. This method of deriving excitation patterns is easily extended to the case where the auditory filters are asymmetric (Moore and Glasberg, 1987). Note, however, that whereas it is the lower side of the auditory filter which gets less steep with increasing level (see Fig. 3.9), it is the upper branch of the masked audiogram and the upper branch of the excitation pattern that become less steep with increasing level (see Fig. 3.10 and Fig. 2.7). This happens because the upper side of the excitation pattern is determined by the lower side of the auditory filter and vice versa.

5   THE NATURE OF THE CRITICAL BAND AND MECHANISMS OF MASKING

A   The origin of the auditory filter

The physiological basis of the critical band mechanism is still uncertain, although the frequency-resolving power of the basilar membrane is almost certainly involved. Indeed, there are many similarities between the frequency selectivity measured on the basilar membrane and frequency selectivity measured psychophysically (Moore, 1986). It appears that the critical bandwidth, or the ERB of the auditory filter, corresponds to a constant distance along the basilar membrane (Greenwood, 1961b; Moore, 1986); in humans each critical bandwidth corresponds to about 0.9 mm, regardless of the centre frequency. Further, the ERB of the auditory filter measured behaviourally in animals corresponds rather well with the ERB of tuning curves measured in single neurones of the auditory nerve in the same species. This is illustrated in Fig. 3.12 (data from Evans *et al.*, 1989). Behavioural ERBs were measured using bandstop noise (BSN) as described in section 3B, and using a different type of noise, comb-filtered noise (CFN).

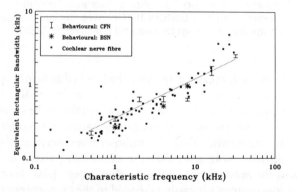

FIG. 3.12   A comparison of ERBs estimated from behavioural masking experiments and from neurophysiological measurements of the tuning curves of single neurones in the auditory nerve. All data were obtained from guinea pigs. There is a good correspondence between behavioural and neural data. From Evans *et al.* (1989).

Although this good correspondence between behavioural and neural ERBs suggests that the frequency selectivity of the auditory system is largely determined in the cochlea, it is possible that there is a sharpening process following the basilar membrane which results in an enhancement of frequency selectivity. This might be achieved by a process of lateral suppression or lateral inhibition. In such a process, weak inputs to one group of receptors (hair cells or neurones) would be suppressed by stronger inputs to adjacent receptors. This would result in a sharpening of the excitation pattern evoked by a stimulus. If the critical band mechanism depended on a neural inhibitory process, then we would expect that the process would take several milliseconds to become effective; work on lateral inhibition in other sensory systems, such as the visual system, has indicated a time constant of about 30 ms. Thus, the critical bandwidth measured with very brief signals should be greater than that measured with longer signals.

The data relevant to this issue are not entirely clear cut. Port (1963) found that measures of loudness summation for short duration stimuli (as short as 1 ms) gave the same value for the critical bandwidth as was found at long durations. Some other experimental results (e.g. Zwicker, 1965a,b; Srinivasan, 1971) have been taken to indicate a wider critical band at short durations. At the present time the reasons for the discrepancies are not entirely clear. Zwicker and Fastl (1972) in a review of this area concluded that the results which have been taken to indicate a wider critical band at short durations can, in fact, be explained in other ways, so that it is not necessary to assume a development of the critical band with time. Rather, the critical band mechanism may be viewed as a system of filters which are permanently and instantaneously present. This view has been supported by an experiment of Moore *et al.* (1987). They estimated the shape of the auditory filter using the notched noise method of Patterson (see section 3B). The signal was a brief (20 ms) tone presented at the start, the temporal centre, or the end of the 400 ms masker. The auditory filter shapes derived from the results did not change significantly with signal delay, suggesting that the selectivity of the auditory filter does not develop over time. On the other hand, measures of frequency selectivity obtained with tonal maskers do show a development of frequency selectivity with time (Bacon and Viemeister, 1985a; Bacon and Moore, 1986).

Overall, these results make it unlikely that any neural inhibitory process is involved in the formation of the critical band. It is possible, however, that some form of lateral suppression might operate at a very early stage in the processing of the auditory stimulus, for example, at the level of the hair cell (Sellick and Russell, 1979). Such a process could operate very fast. We will return to the question of lateral suppression in section 9.

B   The mechanism of masking – swamping or suppression?

There are now two common conceptions of the mechanism by which masking occurs. The first, which is most common among psychologists, is that masking involves the swamping of the neural activity evoked by the signal. If the masker produces a significant amount of activity in the channels (auditory filters or critical bands) which would normally respond to the signal, then the activity added by the signal may be undetectable. Consider, for example, the case of a tone together with a wideband white noise. When the tone is at its masked threshold, the level of the tone is about 4 dB less than the level of the noise in the critical band around the tone. This is the average discrepancy between critical bands and critical ratios; 4 dB corresponds to a power ratio of about 2.5 : 1. The combined excitation produced by the tone plus noise is about 1.5 dB higher in level than that produced by the noise alone. Thus one might argue that 1.5 dB represents the minimum increment in excitation necessary for detection of the tone. If the tone is much lower in level than the noise passing through the critical band, then it produces a negligible increment in excitation. For example, if the difference in levels is 20 dB, the increment in level is less than 0.05 dB. Thus the excitation produced by the tone is 'swamped' by that produced by the masker.

We should note that the task required of the subject may differ somewhat according to the manner of stimulus presentation. For a steady tone presented in a continuous background noise, the subject would have to detect that the excitation at some location (in one critical band) exceeded that at surrounding locations. Thus the subject would have to detect that there was a peak in the pattern of excitation (e.g. Greenwood, 1961a; Schubert, 1969). If, on the other hand, the tone was interrupted or presented intermittently, the subject could compare the level in the same critical band on successive occasions. This might make the task somewhat easier. Whichever of these two is appropriate, masking will only take place if the masker produces excitation in the channels (critical bands) which would otherwise respond to the signal.

An alternative view of masking, which is quite popular among neuro-physiologists (e.g. Delgutte, 1988), is that the masker suppresses the activity which the signal would evoke if presented alone. This is most easily explained by analogy with the 'two-tone suppression' observed in single neurones of the auditory nerve, which was described in Chapter 1, section 6F. The neural response to a tone at the CF of a neurone may be suppressed by a tone which does not itself produce excitatory activity in that neurone. The suppression may be sufficient to drive the firing rate of the neurone down to its spontaneous rate, and we might argue that this corresponds to the masking of the tone at CF. More generally, a masking sound might produce both excitation and suppression in the neurones responding to the signal, and masking might correspond to a mixture of swamping and suppression.

At the moment there seems to be no clear way of distinguishing between these two mechanisms of masking. However, there is general agreement that the threshold of a signal in simultaneous masking is quite well predicted by modelling the auditory system as a system of linear filters. Suppression is a markedly nonlinear process; the response to two simultaneous inputs is not the linear sum of the responses to each input separately. The fact that the linear model works so well encourages the belief that swamping is the major mechanism of simultaneous masking and that the effects of suppression are not revealed in simultaneous masking. A possible reason for this will be presented in section 9. We should not, however, rule out the possibility that suppression plays some role in simultaneous masking, and that it influences the results of other measures of the critical band. For example, suppression may well affect the loudness of complex sounds, and the way loudness changes with bandwidth.

C The neural code used for signal detection

So far we have discussed the basis of the auditory filter, and the mechanism by which the neural activity evoked by the signal might be 'masked'. We turn now to a consideration of what aspect of the neural activity evoked by the signal might be used for detection. The most common assumption is that the amount of activity is critical, and that neural firing rates are the important variable. However, an alternative possibility is that information in the temporal patterns of neural firing is used. The theoretical issues involved are in many ways similar to those which we discussed in relation to the intensity discrimination of signals in noise. Indeed, many researchers would consider that the detection of a signal in a masker is equivalent to the detection of an increment in intensity.

In response to a complex stimulus, the pattern of phase locking observed in a given neurone will depend upon which components in the stimulus are most effective in driving that neurone. For example, in response to two tones which are nonharmonically related, discharges may be phase locked to one tone, or the other, or both tones simultaneously. Which of these occurs is determined by the relative intensities of the two tones and their frequencies in relation to the response area of the neurone. When phase locking occurs to only one tone of a pair, each of which produces phase locking when presented alone, the temporal structure of the response may be indistinguishable from that which occurs when that tone is presented alone. Thus the dominant tone appears to 'capture' the response of the neurone. This effect appears to be partly mediated by suppression of the non-dominant tone, although in general it will arise from a mixture of swamping and suppression.

It is possible that the 'capture' effect underlies the masking of one tone by another. Clearly, the results we have described apply only to the responses of single auditory nerve fibres, and their application to the responses over an ensemble of nerve fibres is not entirely clear. However, recordings of the responses of many different nerve fibres within the same animal indicate that information about the relative levels of components in complex sounds is contained in the time patterns of neural impulses, even at sound levels sufficient to produce saturation in the majority of neurones (Kim and Molnar, 1979; Sachs and Young, 1980). In general, the temporal patterns of response are dominated by the most prominent frequency components in the complex stimulus, with the result that there may be little or no phase locking to weak components which are close in frequency to stronger ones. Thus it seems reasonable to suggest that a tone (with a frequency below about 5 kHz) will be masked when the subject cannot detect its effect on the time pattern of nerve impulses evoked by the stimulus as a whole.

This argument can easily be applied to the masking of a tone by wideband noise. A tone will evoke neural firings with a well-defined temporal pattern; the time intervals between successive nerve firings will be integral multiples of the period of the tone. A noise will evoke, in the same neurones, a much less regular pattern of neural firings. Thus we might argue that a tone will be detected when the nerve fibres responding to it show a certain degree of temporal regularity in their patterns of firing. If the temporal regularity is less than this amount the tone will be masked. Notice that the neurones involved in the detection of the tone will be those with CFs close to that of the tone. The action of the auditory filter will be important in reducing the contribution of the noise to the neural responses, and the neurones with CFs close to the tone frequency will be the ones showing the greatest degree of temporal regularity.

The idea that we use the temporal patterns of neural firing to analyse complex stimuli can provide an explanation for the discrepancies observed by Plomp (1964a) in human subjects' abilities to analyse partials from two-tone complexes and multitone complexes. As was mentioned earlier, Plomp found that a partial could only be 'heard out' from a multitone complex if that partial was separated from neighbouring partials by about one critical bandwidth. However, for a two-tone complex the partials could be identified for separations less than this. Figure 3.13 shows excitation patterns for a two-tone complex and a multitone complex. For a multitone complex, the excitation at CFs corresponding to the higher partials arises from the interaction of several partials of comparable effectiveness. Thus there is no CF where the temporal pattern of response is determined primarily by one partial. However, for a two-tone complex there are certain CFs where the

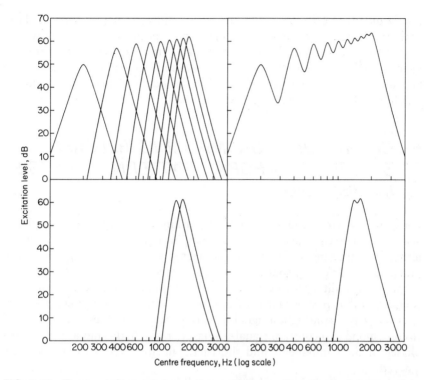

FIG. 3.13 The top left panel shows the excitation pattern for each harmonic in a complex tone containing the first nine harmonics of a 200 Hz fundamental. The top right panel shows the excitation pattern resulting from adding the nine harmonics together. The bottom left panel shows the excitation patterns for the seventh and eighth harmonics separately, and the bottom right panel shows the excitation pattern resulting from adding those two harmonics. For the two-tone complex, neurones with CFs below 1400 Hz would be phase locked primarily to the lower of the two harmonics, while neurones with CFs above 1600 Hz would be phase locked primarily to the upper of the two harmonics.

temporal pattern of response is dominated by one or the other of the component tones; this occurs at CFs just below and above the frequencies of the two tones. Thus the temporal patterns of firing in these neurones could signal the individual pitches of the component tones. This could explain why partials are more easily 'heard out' from a two-tone complex than a multitone complex.

It should be emphasized that the extent to which the auditory system is capable of analysing the time pattern of nerve firings is still a matter of debate (e.g. Whitfield, 1970). This is discussed more fully in Chapter 5, particularly in relation to the question of whether pitch perception involves the analysis of timing information. For the moment it is clear that neither masking nor the phenomena associated with the critical band involve simple processes, and that in seeking explanations of these we should be prepared to consider a number of possible underlying mechanisms.

6 CO-MODULATION MASKING RELEASE: SPECTRO-TEMPORAL PATTERN ANALYSIS IN HEARING

The power spectrum model of auditory masking assumes that the peripheral auditory system contains a bank of overlapping bandpass filters (the auditory filters). When trying to detect a sinusoidal signal of a given frequency in the presence of a masking sound, the observer is assumed to make use of the output of an auditory filter centred close to the signal frequency. In general, it is assumed that performance is based on the output of the single auditory filter which gives the highest signal-to-masker ratio, and threshold is assumed to correspond to a constant signal-to-masker ratio. In this model the relative phases of the components and short-term fluctuations of the masker are ignored.

As we have seen, this model works well in many situations. However, it clearly fails in others. In particular, there is good evidence that observers sometimes make comparisons *across* auditory filters, rather than listening through a single filter. Furthermore, temporal fluctuations of the masker can have important effects. This section reviews recent evidence for across-filter comparisons, emphasizing the importance of the temporal properties of the stimuli, and interpreting the results in terms of pattern analysis in the auditory system.

A Initial demonstrations of co-modulation masking release

Hall *et al.* (1984) were among the first to demonstrate that across-filter comparisons could enhance the detection of a sinusoidal signal in a fluctuating noise masker. The crucial feature for achieving this enhancement was that the fluctuations should be *coherent* or *correlated* across different frequency bands. In one of their experiments the threshold for a 1 kHz, 400 ms sinusoidal signal was measured as a function of the bandwidth of a noise

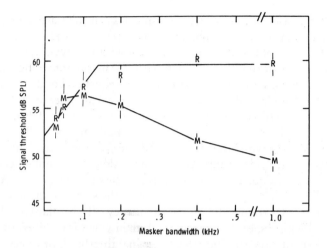

FIG. 3.14 The points labelled 'R' are thresholds for a 1 kHz signal centred in a band of random noise, plotted as a function of the bandwidth of the noise. The points labelled 'M' are the thresholds obtained when the noise was amplitude modulated at an irregular, low rate. For bandwidths of 0.2 kHz or more, the thresholds are lower in the modulated than in the random noise. This is called co-modulation masking release. From Hall *et al.* (1984), by permission of the authors and *J. Acoust. Soc. Am.*

masker, keeping the spectrum level constant. The masker was centred at 1 kHz. They used two types of masker. One was a random noise; this has irregular fluctuations in amplitude, and the fluctuations are independent in different frequency regions. The other was a random noise which was modulated in amplitude at an irregular, low rate; a noise lowpass filtered at 50 Hz was used as a modulator. The modulation resulted in fluctuations in the amplitude of the noise which were the same in different frequency regions. This across-frequency coherence was called 'co-modulation' by Hall *et al.* (1984). Figure 3.14 shows the results of this experiment.

For the random noise (denoted by R), the signal threshold increases as the masker bandwidth increases up to about 100–200 Hz, and then remains constant. This is exactly as expected from the traditional power spectrum model of masking (see section 2 and Fig. 3.1). The auditory filter at this centre frequency has a bandwidth of about 130 Hz. Hence, for noise bandwidths up to 130 Hz, increasing the bandwidth results in more noise passing through the filter. However, increasing the bandwidth beyond 130 Hz does not increase the noise passing through the filter, so threshold does not increase. The pattern for the modulated noise (denoted by M) is quite different. For noise bandwidths greater than 100 Hz, the signal threshold *decreases* as the bandwidth increases. This indicates that subjects can compare the outputs of different auditory filters to enhance signal detection. The fact that the decrease in threshold with increasing bandwidth only occurs with the modulated noise indicates that fluctuations in the masker are critical and that the fluctuations need to be correlated across frequency bands. Hence, this phenomenon has been called 'co-modulation masking release' (CMR). The amount of CMR in this experiment, defined as the difference in thresholds for random noise and modulated noise, was maximally about 10 dB.

A second way in which CMR can be demonstrated is by using narrow bands of noise, which have inherent relatively slow amplitude fluctuations. One band, the on-frequency band, is centred at the signal frequency. A second band, the flanking band, is centred away from the signal frequency, outside the critical band around the signal frequency. If the flanking band is uncorrelated with the on-frequency band, then when it is added to the on-frequency band it either has no effect on signal threshold, or it increases the signal threshold slightly. However, when the envelope of the flanking band is correlated with that of the on-frequency band (i.e. it has the same pattern of fluctuation over time), the flanking band can produce a release from masking, a CMR (Hall *et al.*, 1984; Schooneveldt and Moore, 1987). The release from masking can occur even if the signal and on-frequency band are presented to one ear and the flanking band is presented to the other ear (Cohen and Schubert, 1987; Schooneveldt and Moore, 1987). The magnitude of the CMR is usually defined as the difference in signal threshold for the condition with the uncorrelated flanking band and the condition with the correlated flanking band.

B   The role of within-channel cues

Schooneveldt and Moore (1987, 1989) have shown that modulation of a masker can produce a release from masking even when the masker's bandwidth is less than the auditory filter bandwidth. This release from masking cannot arise from comparisons of the outputs of different auditory filters, and hence it does not represent a CMR. Rather it results from a cue or cues available in the output of a single auditory filter. Schooneveldt and Moore called such cues 'within-channel cues'. One example of such a cue is a change in the pattern of envelope modulation which occurs when the signal is added to the masker; the envelope fluctuates less and the minima in the envelope tend to be less deep when the signal is present. This cue appears to be used in band-widening experiments such as illustrated in Fig. 3.14, but it can only be used when the signal duration is greater than about 100 ms (Schooneveldt and Moore, 1989).

Within-channel cues make it easy to overestimate the magnitude of CMR. However, the cues do not appear to be important for brief signals in band-widening experiments, or when the on-frequency and flanking bands are widely separated in frequency (Schooneveldt and Moore, 1987). They also do not occur when the on-frequency and flanking bands are presented to opposite ears. Hence, results for these conditions can be used to estimate the magnitude of the 'true' CMR.

C Factors influencing the magnitude of CMR

CMR measured in band-widening experiments (as in Fig. 3.14) occurs over a wide range of signal frequencies (500 to 4000 Hz), and does not vary greatly with signal frequency. CMR is largest when the modulation of the masker is at a low rate, and when the masker covers a wide frequency range. For signal durations of 100 ms or less, for which within-channel cues probably have little effect, CMR can be as large as 11 dB.

When CMR is measured using an on-frequency band and a flanking band, it generally falls in the range 1–6 dB when the flanking band is distant in frequency from the on-frequency band; this probably reflects a true CMR. The release from masking can be as large as 14 dB when the flanking band is close in frequency to the on-frequency band, but in this case within-channel cues probably influence the results. The true CMR appears to vary little with center frequency or with flanking-band frequency. CMR measured with a flanking band presented in the opposite ear to the signal-plus-masker also varies little with centre frequency or flanking-band frequency, and is typically 2–6 dB. Thus, across-filter comparisons can be made over a wide frequency range.

CMR measured with an on-frequency band and a flanking band tends to increase as the width of the bands of noise is decreased. This is probably a consequence of the fact that the rate of envelope fluctuations decreases as the bandwidth decreases; slow fluctuations lead to large CMR. CMR also increases if more than one flanking band is used.

D Models to explain CMR

Models proposed to explain CMR can be divided into two general categories. Those in the first category assume that the auditory system compares envelope modulation patterns at the outputs of auditory filters tuned to different centre frequencies. For a co-modulated masker without a signal, the modulation pattern is similar for all of the filters which are active. When a signal is added, the modulation pattern at the output of the auditory filter tuned to the signal frequency is altered. Thus, the presence of the signal is indicated by a *disparity* in the modulation pattern across different filters. The auditory system may be sensitive to this disparity.

A second category of model (Buus, 1985) assumes that the envelope fluctuations at the outputs of auditory filters tuned away from the signal frequency tell the listener the optimum times to listen for the signal, i.e. during the minima in the masker envelope. The signal-to-masker ratio is usually greatest during the masker minima, and the flanking band may help to indicate the exact times of the minima. This will be called the dip-listening model.

E   Experimental tests of the models

Richards (1987) tested the idea that the auditory system can detect disparities in envelope modulation patterns at the outputs of different auditory filters by requiring subjects to distinguish two stimuli. One stimulus consisted of two co-modulated bands of noise, i.e. two bands with the same envelope fluctuations. The other stimulus consisted of two bands with independent envelopes. Subjects were able to perform this task, indicating that across-filter disparities in modulation pattern can be detected.

Although disparities in modulation patterns across filters may be sufficient to produce a CMR, they do not appear to be necessary. This was demonstrated by Hall and Grose (1988). They used an on-frequency band and a flanking band as maskers, but the signal was a band of noise identical to the on-frequency band. Thus the addition of the signal to the on-frequency band merely resulted in a change of overall level, without changing the modulation pattern. They found a significant CMR. As well as indicating that a disparity in across-filter modulation patterns is not necessary to produce a CMR, the results also show that dip-listening is not necessary; for this particular signal, the signal-to-noise ratio is not greater at the masker minima than at the masker maxima. The results indicate that across-filter disparities in overall level are sufficient to produce a CMR. This finding is not consistent with either of the simple types of model of CMR described earlier.

In another experiment, Hall and Grose (1988) used a sinusoidal signal, but the level of the flanking band was varied randomly from one stimulus to the next. This would disrupt any cue related to across-filter differences in overall level. A substantial CMR was found, indicating that across-filter level differences are not necessary to produce a CMR. Presumably in this experiment the signal was detected either by dip-listening or by detecting across-filter disparities in modulation pattern.

Grose and Hall (1989) used as a masker a series of sinusoidal components which were sinusoidally amplitude modulated at a 10 Hz rate. The modulation was either in phase for all of the components (coherent modulation) or had a quasi-random phase for each component (incoherent modulation). The signal was a sinusoid coincident in frequency with the middle component of the masker. The difference in threshold for the two maskers gives a measure of CMR. They investigated the effect of presenting the signal as a series of brief tone pips which occurred either at minima or maxima in the envelope of the centre component of the masker. In the case of the masker with coherent modulation, the addition of the signal at either minima or maxima would have resulted in an across-filter envelope disparity. However, a CMR was found only in the former case. This supports the dip-listening model.

The results of these and other experiments suggest that CMR does not depend on any single cue or mechanism. Rather, it reflects the operation of flexible mechanisms which can exploit a variety of cues or combination of cues depending on the specific stimuli used.

F General implications of CMR

It seems likely that across-filter comparisons of temporal envelopes are a general feature of auditory pattern analysis, which may play an important role in extracting signals from noisy backgrounds, or separating competing sources of sound. As pointed out by Hall *et al.* (1984): "Many real-life auditory stimuli have intensity peaks and valleys as a function of time in which intensity trajectories are highly correlated across frequency. This is true of speech, of interfering noise such as 'cafeteria' noise, and of many other kinds of environmental stimuli". The experiments reviewed above suggest that we can exploit these coherent envelope fluctuations very effectively, and that substantial reductions in signal threshold can result. Other ways in which we separate competing sound sources will be discussed in Chapter 7.

7 PROFILE ANALYSIS

Green and his colleagues (Green, 1988) have carried out a series of experiments demonstrating that, even for stimuli without distinct envelope fluctuations, subjects are able to compare the outputs of different auditory filters to enhance the detection of a signal. They investigated the ability to detect an increment in the level of one component in a complex sound relative to the level of the other components; we will call the other components the 'background'. Usually the complex sound has been composed of a series of equal-amplitude sinusoidal components, uniformly spaced on a logarithmic frequency scale. To prevent subjects from performing the task by monitoring the magnitude of the output of the single auditory filter centred at the frequency of the incremented component, the overall level of the whole stimulus was varied randomly from one stimulus to the next, over a relatively large range (typically about 40 dB). This makes the magnitude of the output of any single filter an unreliable cue to the presence of the signal.

Subjects were able to detect changes in the relative level of the signal of only 1–2 dB. Such small thresholds could not be obtained by monitoring the magnitude of the output of a single auditory filter. Green and his colleagues have argued that subjects performed the task by detecting a change in the shape or profile of the spectrum of the sound; hence the name 'profile analysis'. In other words, subjects can compare the outputs of different auditory filters, and can detect when the output of one changes relative to that of others, even when the overall level is varied.

Green (1988) has given an extensive description of the main properties of profile analysis. Profile analysis is most effective when:

1. The background has a large spectral range. For example, for a 1000 Hz signal, the threshold is lower when the background extends from 200 to 5000 Hz than when it extends from 724 to 1380 Hz.
2. There are many rather than few components within the spectral range. Thus, increasing the number of components decreases the signal threshold. However, there is a limit to this effect. If some of the components fall close to the signal frequency, then they may have a masking effect on the signal. Thus, making the background too 'dense' (i.e. having many closely spaced components) can result in an increase in signal threshold.
3. The signal falls well within the frequency range of the background; threshold tends to rise when the signal is at the edge of the frequency range of the background.
4. The level of the signal component is similar to or slightly above the levels of the components in the background.
5. The background is composed of components with equal levels rather than levels which differ from component to component.

The first two aspects of profile analysis described above resemble CMR; recall that CMR is larger when the masker covers a wide frequency range or when several flanking bands are used. Indeed, profile analysis may be regarded as a special case of CMR, where the masker fluctuates randomly in level across stimuli but not within stimuli.

In one sense we should not find the phenomenon of profile analysis surprising. It has been known for many years that one of the main factors determining the timbre or quality of a sound is its spectral shape; this is discussed in more detail in Chapter 7. Our everyday experience tells us that we can recognise and distinguish familiar sounds, such as the different vowels, regardless of the levels of those sounds. When we do this, we are distinguishing different spectral shapes in the face of variations in overall level. This is functionally the same as profile analysis. The experiments on profile analysis can be regarded as a way of quantifying the limits of our ability to distinguish changes in spectral shape.

8 NONSIMULTANEOUS MASKING

'Simultaneous masking' is the term used to describe those situations where the masker is present throughout the presentation time of the signal. Time effects in masking have also been studied fairly intensively. Short signals, often called 'probes' are presented at various times in relation to the masker. Two basic types of nonsimultaneous masking can be distinguished: (1) backward masking, in which the probe precedes the masker (also known as pre-stimulatory masking); and (2) forward masking, in which the probe follows the masker (also known as post-stimulatory masking). Forward masking is just one of three conceptually distinct processes which may affect the threshold of a probe presented after another sound; the other two are adaptation and fatigue, which were discussed in Chapter 2. Forward masking is distinguished from adaptation and fatigue primarily by the fact that it occurs for maskers which are relatively short in duration (typically a few hundred milliseconds) and it is limited to signals which occur within a few hundred milliseconds after the cessation of the masker.

Although many studies of backward masking have been published, the phenomenon is poorly understood. The amount of backward masking obtained depends strongly on how much practice the subjects have received, and experiments in our laboratory suggest that highly practised subjects often show little or no backward masking. Thus, the larger masking effects found for unpractised subjects may reflect some sort of 'confusion' of the signal with the masker. In the paragraphs which follow, we will concentrate primarily on forward masking, which can be substantial even in highly practised subjects. The main properties of forward masking are as follows:

1. Forward masking is greater the nearer in time to the masker that the signal occurs. This is illustrated in the left panel of Fig. 3.15. When the delay D of the signal after the end of the masker is plotted on a logarithmic scale, the data fall roughly on a straight line. In other words, the amount of forward masking, in dB, is a linear function of $\log(D)$.
2. The rate of recovery from forward masking is greater for higher masker

levels. Thus, regardless of the initial amount of forward masking, the masking decays to zero after 100–200 ms.

3. Increments in masker level do not produce equal increments in amount of forward masking. For example, if the masker level is increased by 10 dB, the masked threshold may only increase by 3 dB. This contrasts with simultaneous masking, where, at least for wideband maskers, threshold usually corresponds to a constant signal-to-masker ratio. This effect can be quantified by plotting the signal threshold as a function of masker level. The resulting function is called a growth of masking function. Several such functions are shown in the right panel of Fig. 3.15. In simultaneous masking such functions would have slopes close to one. In forward masking the slopes are less than one, and the slopes decrease as the value of D increases (see Fig. 3.15).

4. The amount of forward masking increases with increasing masker duration for durations up to at least 20 ms. The results for greater masker durations vary somewhat across studies. Some studies show an effect of masker duration for durations up to 200 ms (e.g. Kidd and Feth, 1982),

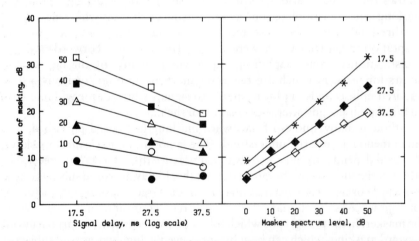

FIG. 3.15   The left panel shows the amount of forward masking of a brief 2 kHz signal, plotted as a function of the time delay of the signal after the end of the noise masker. Each curve shows results for a different noise spectrum level (10–50 dB). The results for each spectrum level fall on a straight line when the signal delay is plotted on a logarithmic scale, as here. The right panel shows the same thresholds plotted as a function of masker spectrum level. Each curve shows results for a different signal delay time (17.5, 27.5 or 37.5 ms). Note that the slopes of these growth of masking functions decrease with increasing signal delay. Adapted from Moore and Glasberg (1983b).

while others show little effect for durations beyond 50 ms (e.g. Fastl, 1976).

5. Forward masking is influenced by the relation between the frequencies of the signal and the masker (just as in the case of simultaneous masking). This is a point which will be discussed in more detail in the following section.

The basis of forward masking is still not clear. It could be explained in terms of a reduction in sensitivity of recently stimulated cells, or in terms of a persistence in the pattern of neural activity evoked by the masker. Both points of view can be found in the literature. Duifhuis (1973) has suggested that for small intervals between the signal and the masker (less than about 20 ms) the dominant component in both forward and backward masking results from a temporal overlap of cochlear responses. That is to say, the vibrations evoked by the first stimulus on the basilar membrane will not have completely died away before the second stimulus arrives. If this is the case, then backward and forward masking effects for short delay times should be more pronounced for low frequencies than for high (de Boer, 1969a, b). This should happen because the bandwidth of tuning on the basilar membrane is less at low frequencies than at high, and narrower filters 'ring' for longer times (see Chapter 1, section 4, and Fig. 1.5; see also, Chapter 4, section 3). A comparison of the results of different workers (Elliot, 1962; Gruber and Boerger, 1971; Patterson, 1971) reveals that this is indeed the case. Further, Duifhuis (1971) has demonstrated that for short time delays the masked threshold is affected by the relative phase of the masker and the signal, as would be expected if there were a temporal overlap of the patterns of vibration on the basilar membrane.

While at least part of the observed masking at short time delays may be explained in terms of temporal overlap of vibration patterns on the basilar membrane, it is clear that other processes must be involved. The 'ringing' on the basilar membrane would last for only a few milliseconds at medium to high frequencies, yet forward masking occurs for masker-signal intervals of at least 100 ms.

In summary, the empirical phenomena of forward masking are now fairly well known. The nature of the underlying processes is not fully understood. Contributions from a number of different sources may be important, these contributions being related to different levels in the auditory system. At the peripheral level, temporal overlap of patterns of vibration on the basilar membrane may be important, especially for small delay times between the signal and masker. Also at this level some sort of temporary fatigue may play a role in forward masking. At higher neural levels a persistence of the excitation pattern evoked by the masker may occur.

9   EVIDENCE FOR LATERAL SUPPRESSION FROM NONSIMULTANEOUS MASKING

The results from experiments on simultaneous masking can generally be explained quite well on the assumption that the peripheral auditory system contains a band of overlapping bandpass filters which are approximately linear. However, measurements from single neurones in the auditory nerve show significant nonlinearities. In particular, the response to a tone of a given frequency can sometimes be suppressed by a tone with a different frequency, giving the phenomenon known as two-tone suppression (see Chapter 1, section 6F and Fig. 1.18). For other complex signals, similar phenomena occur and are given the general name lateral suppression. This can be characterized in the following way. Strong activity at a given CF can suppress weaker activity at adjacent CFs. In this way, peaks in the excitation pattern are enhanced relative to adjacent dips. The question now arises as to why the effects of lateral suppression are not usually seen in experiments on simultaneous masking.

Houtgast (1972) has argued that simultaneous masking is not an appropriate tool for detecting the effects of lateral suppression. Its use is based upon the assumption that when the neural activity at a given CF is influenced by lateral suppression, the masked threshold for a test tone with frequency corresponding to that CF would also be affected. Houtgast argued that, in simultaneous masking, the masking stimulus and the test tone are processed simultaneously in the same channel. Thus any suppression in that channel will affect the neural activity caused by both the test tone and the masking noise. In other words, the signal-to-noise ratio in a given frequency region will be unaffected by lateral suppression, and thus the threshold of the test tone will remain unaltered.

Houtgast suggested that this difficulty could be overcome by presenting the masker and the test tone successively (i.e. by using a forward masking technique). If lateral suppression does occur, then its effects will be seen in the forward masking threshold curve provided: (1) in the chain of levels of neural processing the level at which the lateral suppression occurs is not later than the level at which most of the forward masking effect arises; (2) the suppression built up by the masker has decayed by the time that the test tone is presented (otherwise the problems described for simultaneous masking will be encountered).

Houtgast (1972) used a repeated-gap masking technique, in which the masker was presented with a continuous rhythm of 150 ms on, 50 ms off. Probe tones with a duration of 20 ms were presented in the gaps. In one experiment he used as maskers highpass and lowpass noises with sharp spectral cutoffs (96 dB/octave). He anticipated that lateral suppression would result in an enhancement of the neural representation of the spectral edges of the noise. Neurones with CFs well within the passband of the noise should have their responses suppressed by the activity at adjacent CFs. However, for neurones with a CF corresponding to a spectral edge in the noise, there should be a release from suppression, owing to the low activity in neurones with CFs outside the spectral range of the noise. This should be revealed as an increase in the threshold of the probe when its frequency coincided with the spectral edge of each noise band. The results showed the expected edge effects. No such effects were found in simultaneous masking. Thus, nonsimultaneous masking does reveal the type of effects which a suppression process would produce.

Houtgast (1972) also noted a very remarkable feature of the repeated-gap technique which had been reported earlier by Elfner and Caskey (1965): when the bursts of probe tone are just above the threshold, they sound like a continuous tone. Only at higher levels of the probe tone is the perception in accord with the physical time pattern, namely a series of tone bursts. Houtgast called the level of the probe tone, at which its character changed from pulsating to continuous, the pulsation threshold. He showed that the existence of such a pulsation threshold is a very general feature of alternating stimuli, and is not restricted to the alternation of two stimuli with a frequency component in common. However, the phenomenon does not occur when the masker contains no frequency component in the neighbourhood of the probe tone. He suggested the following interpretation of the phenomenon: "When a tone and a stimulus S are alternated (alternation cycle about 4 Hz), the tone is perceived as being continuous when the transition from S to tone causes no (perceptible) increase of nervous activity in any frequency region" (Houtgast, 1972). In terms of patterns of excitation this suggests that "the peak of the nervous activity pattern of the tone at pulsation threshold level just reaches the nervous activity pattern of S". Given this hypothesis, the pulsation threshold for a test tone as a function of frequency can be considered to map out the excitation pattern of the stimulus S. The pulsation threshold curve will thus reflect both the frequency-analysing properties of the cochlea and the effects of lateral suppression. We will discuss the pulsation threshold and its interpretation in Chapter 7. For the moment, we will accept it as providing a tool for mapping the representation of sounds in the auditory system. For convenience, we will refer to the measurement of the pulsation threshold as a nonsimultaneous masking technique.

Following the pioneering work of Houtgast, many workers have reported that there are systematic differences between the results obtained using simultaneous and nonsimultaneous masking techniques. One major difference is that nonsimultaneous masking reveals effects which can be directly attributed to suppression. A good demonstration of this involves a psycho-

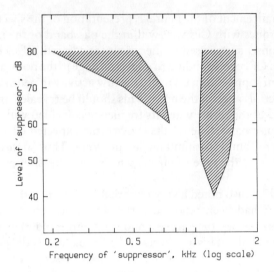

FIG. 3.16 Results of an experiment measuring pulsation thresholds for a 1 kHz 'signal' alternated with a two component 'masker'. One component was a 1 kHz tone which was fixed in level at 40 dB. The second component (the 'suppressor') was a tone which was varied both in frequency and in level. The shaded areas indicate combinations of frequency and level where the second tone reduced the pulsation threshold by 3 dB or more. Adapted from Houtgast (1974).

physical analogue of neural two-tone suppression. Houtgast (1973, 1974) measured the pulsation threshold for a 1 kHz 'signal' alternating with a 1 kHz 'masker'. He then added a second tone to the 'masker' and measured the pulsation threshold again. He found that sometimes the addition of this second tone produced a reduction in the pulsation threshold, and he attributed this to a suppression of the 1 kHz component in the 'masker' by the second component. If the 1 kHz component is suppressed, then there will be less activity in the frequency region around 1 kHz, producing a drop in the pulsation threshold. The second tone was most effective as a 'suppressor' when it was somewhat more intense than the 1 kHz component, and above it in frequency. A 'suppression' of about 20 dB could be produced by a 'suppressor' at 1.2 kHz. Houtgast mapped out the combinations of frequency and intensity over which the 'suppressor' produced a 'suppression' exceeding 3 dB. He found two regions, one above 1 kHz and one below, as illustrated in Fig. 3.16. The regions found were similar to the suppression areas which can be observed in single neurones of the auditory nerve (see Fig. 1.18). Similar results have been found using a forward masking technique (Shannon, 1976).

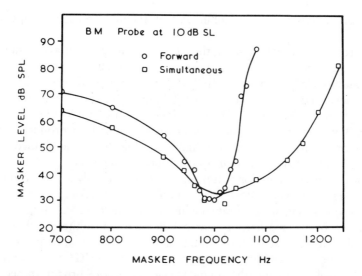

FIG. 3.17 Comparison of psychophysical tuning curves (PTCs) determined in simultaneous masking (squares) and forward masking (circles). The signal was a brief 1 kHz sinusoid with a level of 10 dB SL. From Moore (1978).

A second major difference between the two types of masking is that the frequency selectivity revealed in nonsimultaneous masking is greater than that revealed in simultaneous masking. A well-studied example of this is the psychophysical tuning curve (PTC), which was discussed in Section 3A. PTCs are obtained by determining the level of a masker required to mask a fixed signal as a function of masker frequency. We pointed out earlier the general resemblance in shape of the PTC and the neural tuning curve. PTCs determined in forward masking, or using the pulsation threshold method, are typically sharper than those obtained in simultaneous masking. An example is given in Fig. 3.17. The difference is particularly marked on the high-frequency side of the tuning curve. According to Houtgast (1974) this difference arises because the internal representation of the masker (its excitation pattern), is sharpened by a suppression process, with the greatest sharpening occurring on the low-frequency side. In simultaneous masking, the effects of suppression are not seen, since any reduction of the masker activity in the frequency region of the signal is accompanied by a similar reduction in signal evoked activity. In other words, the signal-to-masker ratio in the frequency region of the signal is unaffected by the suppression. In forward masking, on the other hand, the suppression does not affect the signal. For maskers with frequencies above that of the signal, the effect of suppression is to increase the masker level required to mask the signal. Thus the suppression is revealed as an increase in the high-frequency slope of the PTC.

According to this explanation, the PTC in simultaneous masking does not indicate the level of the masker required to produce a fixed amount of activity in the auditory filter centred at the signal frequency. Rather, it indicates the masker level required to produce a constant signal-to-masker ratio at the output of that filter. The PTC determined in nonsimultaneous masking would, however, indicate the masker level required to produce a fixed amount of activity at the output of that filter. Thus the nonsimultaneous PTC would provide a better analogue of the neural tuning curve.

Although this explanation is appealing, it is not the only way of accounting for the sharper PTC obtained in nonsimultaneous masking. An alternative explanation is that, in simultaneous masking, the low level signal may be suppressed by the masker, so that it falls below absolute threshold. The neural data indicate that tones falling outside of the region bounded by the neural tuning curve can produce suppression. Thus the PTC in simultaneous masking might map out the boundaries of the more broadly tuned suppression region (Delgutte, 1988). The signal in nonsimultaneous masking could not be suppressed in this way, so that, as for the other explanation, the nonsimultaneous PTC provides a better analogue of the tuning curve. A major difference between these two explanations is that the first assumes that suppression will sharpen the excitation pattern of a single sinusoidal component, whereas the second assumes only that one component may suppress another; suppression will not necessarily affect the internal representation of a single component. At present, there is no clear consensus as to which of these two views is correct. We should also remember that the shape of the PTC is likely to be influenced by off-frequency listening (see section 3), so that even in nonsimultaneous masking it will not correspond accurately to the neural tuning curve (O'Loughlin and Moore, 1981).

Several other methods of estimating frequency selectivity have indicated sharper tuning in nonsimultaneous masking. For example, auditory filter shapes estimated in forward masking using a notched-noise masker (as described in section 3B), have 3 dB bandwidths about 17% less and slopes about 50% greater than those estimated in simultaneous masking (Moore and Glasberg, 1981). This encourages us to believe that a general consequence of suppression is an enhancement of frequency selectivity.

We may conclude that results from nonsimultaneous masking do show clearly the types of effects which would be expected if a suppression mechanism were operating. The level at which the effects occur is uncertain, but the most common assumption has been that they arise at a very early stage in auditory processing, possibly at or close to the point of transduction of mechanical movements to neural impulses.

10 FREQUENCY SELECTIVITY IN IMPAIRED HEARING

There is now considerable evidence that frequency selectivity is impaired by damage to the cochlea. Chapter 1, section 5B reviewed some of the evidence that the tuning of the basilar membrane is physiologically vulnerable. Damage to the tuning can be reversed if the damaging agent (e.g. anoxia, noise exposure, drugs such as aspirin) is removed quickly enough. Otherwise, it is permanent. Evidence for vulnerability of tuning has also been obtained from studies of single neurones and from psychophysical studies.

Robertson and Manley (1974) showed that the normal, sharp tuning seen in auditory neurones can be altered by reducing the oxygen supply to the animal. Slowing the rate of ventilation makes the tuning curves less sharp, and at the same time decreases the sensitivity around the tip. These changes are reversible. Similar effects have been reported by Evans (1975), who also found that a reversible degradation in tuning could be produced by the ototoxic agents cyanide and frusemide. It appears that the normal sharp tuning of auditory nerve fibres depends upon a mechanism which is physiologically vulnerable, and that the loss of the sharp tuning is accompanied by an elevation in threshold. Evans and Harrison (1976) used the drug Kanamycin to produce selective damage to the outer hair cells of the cochlea. They found that the threshold and tuning properties of auditory nerve fibres are dependent on the integrity of the outer hair cells, even though the great majority of fibres innervate only inner hair cells.

There have been many psychophysical studies of frequency selectivity in the hearing impaired. Zwicker and Schorn (1978) measured psychophysical tuning curves (PTCs) in six different groups of subjects: normal hearing; conductive hearing loss; degenerative hearing loss (produced by ageing or progressive hereditary loss); noise-induced hearing loss; otosclerosis; and Ménière's disease. They found that the PTCs of the last four groups, where the hearing loss is assumed to involve a defect in the cochlea, were considerably flatter than those in the first two groups, where no defect of the cochlea is involved. This indicates a loss of frequency selectivity.

Florentine et al. (1980) used several of the methods which have been used to measure critical bandwidths in normally hearing subjects (section 2), and found that in patients with cochlear impairments all of the measures indicated a broadening of the critical band. Glasberg and Moore (1986) found that auditory filter shapes estimated using a notched noise masker were much broader than normal in cases of cochlear impairment. Some examples are given in Fig. 3.18. Pick et al. (1977) estimated auditory filter shapes in a different way, but came to essentially the same conclusion. Several studies have shown that there is a correlation between threshold elevation and filter

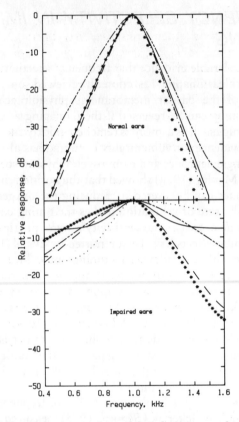

FIG. 3.18   Auditory filter shapes for a centre frequency of 1 kHz, estimated for five subjects each having one normal ear and one ear with a cochlear hearing loss. The relative response of each filter (in dB) is plotted as a function of frequency. The filter shapes for the normal ears are shown at the top, and those for the impaired ears at the bottom. Each line type represents results for one subject. Note that the filters for the impaired ears are broader than normal, particularly on the low frequency side. Data from Glasberg and Moore (1986).

bandwidth; higher absolute thresholds tended to be associated with broader filters.

It is worth considering the perceptual consequences of a loss in frequency selectivity. The first major consequence is a greater susceptibility to masking by interfering sounds. When we are trying to detect a signal in a noisy background we use the auditory filter(s) giving the best signal-to-noise ratio. In a normal ear, where the auditory filter is relatively narrow, all of the background noise except a narrow band around the signal frequency is attenuated at the filter output. In an impaired ear, where the filter is broader,

much more of the noise gets through the filter, so that the detectab
signal is reduced. Thus background noises severely disrupt the det
discrimination of sounds, including speech. This may partly account for the
great difficulties experienced by those with cochlear impairments in following speech in noisy situations such as in pubs or at parties.

A second, but related, difficulty is that of perceptually separating two or
more simultaneously presented sounds. Our ability to do this depends on
more than just frequency selectivity (see Chapter 7, section 3), but the
auditory filter mechanism undoubtedly plays a role. Thus, when the auditory
filter is broader than normal, it is much more difficult to hear out one voice
from a mixture of voices. Holding a conversation when two people are
talking at once can be very difficult for the hearing impaired person.

A third difficulty arises in the perceptual analysis of complex sounds, such
as speech or music. We will see in Chapter 7 that the perception of timbre
seems to depend upon the ear's frequency selectivity. When frequency
selectivity is impaired, the ability to detect differences in the spectral composition of sounds, and hence in timbre, is reduced. Thus it may be more
difficult for the impaired listener to tell the difference between different vowel
sounds, or to distinguish different musical instruments. We should note that
the provision of a hearing aid which simply amplifies sound will not
overcome any of the difficulties described in this section. Such an aid may help
to make sounds audible, but it does not correct the impaired frequency
selectivity.

11 GENERAL CONCLUSIONS

A great many of the phenomena discussed in this chapter can be understood
by considering the peripheral auditory system as containing a bank of
bandpass filters with continuously overlapping centre frequencies. The
basilar membrane appears to provide the initial basis of the filtering process.
The general properties of the frequency analysis carried out by the auditory
system are summarized in the critical band concept: listeners' responses to
complex stimuli differ depending on whether the components of the stimuli
fall within one critical bandwidth or are spread over a number of critical
bands. The critical band is revealed in experiments on masking, loudness,
absolute threshold, phase sensitivity, and the audibility of partials in complex
tones. We should remember, however, that the auditory filter does not have a
simple rectangular shape; rather it has a rounded top and sloping sides. The
value of the critical bandwidth should not be regarded as a complete
specification of the filter, but merely as a rough indication of its bandwidth.

The auditory filter can be thought of as a weighting function which
characterizes frequency selectivity at a particular centre frequency. Its band-

width for frequencies above 1 kHz is about 10–17% of the centre frequency. At moderate sound levels the auditory filter is roughly symmetric on a linear frequency scale. At high sound levels the low-frequency side of the filter becomes less steep than the high-frequency side.

The neural excitation pattern of a given sound represents the distribution of activity evoked by that sound as a function of the CF of the neurones stimulated. It resembles a blurred or smeared version of the magnitude spectrum of the sound. In psychophysical terms, the excitation pattern can be defined as the output of each auditory filter as a function of its centre frequency. Excitation patterns are usually asymmetric, being less steep on the high frequency side. The asymmetry increases with increasing sound level. The shapes of excitation patterns are similar to the masking patterns of narrowband maskers.

Simultaneous masking is usually explained in terms of two underlying processes. Masking may correspond to a 'swamping' of the neural activity of the signal, a suppression of that activity by the masker, or a mixture of the two. The neural code carrying information about the signal is uncertain. A common assumption is that the amount of neural activity in neurones with different CFs is important. An alternative assumption is that the time pattern of neural activity carries information, but this could only apply for stimulating frequencies below 4–5 kHz.

Although many phenomena in simultaneous masking can be explained by assuming that the listener monitors the single auditory filter which gives the highest signal-to-masker ratio, some experiments clearly show that listeners can compare the outputs of different auditory filters in order to enhance signal detection. If the masker is amplitude modulated in such a way that the modulation is coherent, or correlated, in different frequency bands, a reduction in signal threshold, known as co-modulation masking release (CMR), can occur. If the magnitude of the output from any single auditory filter is made an unreliable cue to the presence of the signal, by randomizing the overall sound level of each stimulus, then subjects can still detect the signal by comparing the outputs of different filters, a process called profile analysis.

The processes underlying the phenomena of forward and backward masking are poorly understood. A number of stages can be distinguished in these processes, which may be related to different levels of neural activity. Forward masking may depend on the persistence of responses on the basilar membrane (ringing), neural adaptation or fatigue, and the persistence of the neural activity evoked by the masker at some level of the auditory system.

Houtgast and others have shown that nonsimultaneous masking reveals suppression effects similar to the suppression observed in primary auditory neurones. This suppression is not revealed in simultaneous masking, possibly because suppression at a given CF does not affect the signal-to-masker ratio at that CF. One result of suppression is an enhancement in frequency selectivity, mainly on the high-frequency side of the tuning curve (the low-frequency side of the excitation pattern).

There is now a good deal of evidence that part of the ear's frequency selectivity is physiologically vulnerable. This has been shown both in neuro-physiological studies in animals, and in psychophysical studies in patients with hearing impairments of cochlear origin. The broadening of the auditory filter in hearing impaired people can produce several perceptual deficits which are not corrected by a conventional hearing aid.

12 APPENDIX: SIGNAL DETECTION THEORY

A Introduction

A great deal of Chapters 2 and 3 has been concerned with the measurement of thresholds. Classically, a threshold has been considered as that intensity of a stimulus above which it will be detected and below which it will not. It has been known for many years that this viewpoint is unsatisfactory; if the intensity of a stimulus is slowly increased from a very low value, there is no well defined point at which it suddenly becomes detectable. Rather there is a range of intensities over which the subject will sometimes report a signal and sometimes will not. Thus a plot of percentage correct detections against the intensity of the stimulus (such a plot is called a psychometric function) typically has the form shown in Fig. 3.19. A further problem is that a subject's

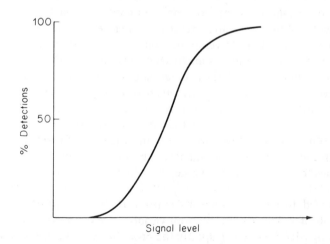

FIG. 3.19 A typical psychometric function showing how the percentage of times a signal is detected varies with signal level.

performance may be altered by changing the instructions, while at the same time the stimulus itself has remained unaltered. Thus it seems that factors not directly associated with the discriminability of the signal may influence the subject's performance. Signal detection theory provides a means of separating factors relating to criterion, motivation and bias from factors relating to purely sensory capabilities. It also enables us to account for the fact that responses may vary from trial to trial even when an identical stimulus is presented on each trial.

B   *The basic idea of signal detection theory*

The theory assumes that decisions are based upon the value of some internal variable x. The nature of x is not precisely specified. One might consider it to correspond to the 'sensory impression' evoked by the stimulus, or one might think of it in more physiological terms; x might correspond to the number of neural firings occurring in some particular channel during the presentation time of the stimulus. The important point is that such a variable exists and that its average value is monotonically related to the magnitude of the stimulus, i.e. increases in the magnitude of the stimulus will, on average, increase the value of x. The second important assumption of the theory is that the value of x will fluctuate from trial to trial, even though the same signal is presented. This variability may arise from two sources. The signal may actually be presented against a variable background, such as a noise, so that fluctuations in physical intensity occur. Alternatively, or in addition, the source of the variability may be neural; most neurones exhibit a pattern of random firings in the absence of external stimulation, so that the presence of a stimulus will be signalled as an increase in firing rate superimposed upon this pattern of random activity. Even in neurones with low spontaneous activity the response to a fixed stimulus may vary from trial to trial.

We see then that, although the average value of x will depend on whether a signal is present or absent, on any given trial the observer will never be absolutely sure that a signal has occurred, because of the inherent variability of x. Of course, if we make the signal sufficiently intense, the increase in x will be large compared with this variability, and thus the uncertainty becomes vanishingly small. But for faint signals the best that the observer can do is to make a guess on the basis of the value of x which occurred on that particular trial.

To proceed further, we have to make certain assumptions about the distribution of x. Since x is a random variable, we cannot predict its exact value on any trial, but we can specify the probability that x will fall within a specified range of values. One way of doing this is to plot a probability density

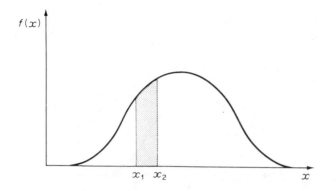

FIG. 3.20 A probability density function. The probability of x lying between the two values x_1 and x_2 is given by the shaded area under the curve. The total area under the curve is 1.

function, $f(x)$. The expression '$f(x)$' simply implies that f is a function of x. A probability density function, $f(x)$, is defined in such a way that the probability of x lying between x and $x + dx$ (where dx represents a small change in the value of x) is equal to $f(x)$ multiplied by dx. A probability density function is illustrated in Fig. 3.20. The quantity $f(x)dx$ can be seen to be equal to the area under the curve between the limits x and $x + dx$. More generally, the probability that x lies between two values, x_1 and x_2, is given by the area under the curve between these two points. Since, on any given trial, some value of x must occur, the total area under the curve is equal to 1.

Consider the situation where an observer is given a series of trials, on some of which a signal is present and on some of which it is absent. To describe this situation we need to specify two probability density functions; one describes the distribution of values of x when no signal is present (this is often denoted by $f(x)_N$, the suffix N referring to the 'noise', either external or neural, which gives rise to this distribution), and the other describes the distribution of values of x when a signal does occur (often denoted $f(x)_{SN}$). It is usually assumed that these two distributions are normal, or Gaussian, and that they have equal variances. There are some theoretical reasons for making this assumption, but normal distributions are also chosen because results are easier to handle in terms of the mathematics involved. The distributions are usually plotted with standard deviation units along the abscissa; in other words, they are scaled so as to have a standard deviation of unity. They will appear as in Fig. 3.21. For each of these two distributions the mean value of x corresponds to the peak in the distribution, and the separation between the two peaks, denoted by d' gives a measure of the separation of the two distributions, and thus of the discriminability of the signal.

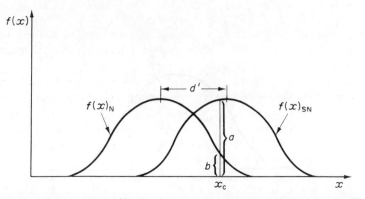

FIG. 3.21   The two distributions (probability density functions) which occur in response to 'noise' alone [$f(x)_N$], and 'noise' plus signal [$f(x)_{SN}$]. The separation between the means of the two curves, denoted by d', gives a measure of the discriminability of the signal. The criterion value is labelled x_c, and the ratio of the heights of the two curves at x_c, namely a/b, gives the likelihood ratio, β.

The theory assumes that the subject establishes a cutoff point corresponding to a particular value of x, which we denote x_c. If, on any given trial, the value of x which actually occurs is greater than x_c, the subject will report that a signal was present; otherwise they will report no signal. Just what value of x_c is chosen will depend upon the instructions to the subject, the probability of a signal, the system of rewards and punishments, previous experience and motivation. Since the exact nature of x is not specified, we cannot assign a number to x_c. To overcome this problem a new quantity is introduced – the likelihood ratio, β. This is defined as the ratio of the heights of the two distributions at x_c, i.e. as $f(x_c)_{SN}/f(x_c)_N$. In other words, the quantity β is equal to the likelihood ratio that a value of x of magnitude x_c arose from the presentation of a signal plus noise as opposed to noise alone. In Fig. 3.21 β is equal to a/b. In contrast to d' which gives a pure measure of the discriminability of the signal, β is related to the criterion of the subject and gives a measure of their degree of caution independent of any changes in sensory capability.

In a given experiment we can measure the proportion of times the subject responds yes when a signal is present, $P(H)$ (this is called the probability of a hit), and the proportion of times the subject responds yes when a signal is absent, $P(F)$ (this is called the probability of a false alarm). From these proportions, and given our assumption that the distributions are normal and of equal variance, it is easy to calculate the values of d' and β. A simple example of how this is done is given in Welford (1968: p. 33). In practice the situation is even easier than this, since tables exist giving the values of d' and β for any given values of $P(H)$ and $P(F)$.

The major advantage of signal detection theory, then, is that it enables us to separate changes in performance related to purely sensory factors from changes related to motivation or criterion. Notice that this can only be done by measuring the proportion of false alarms as well as the proportion of hits. Classical methods of determining thresholds, ignoring as they did the former measure, were not able to achieve this separation. We should note further that according to this theory there is no such thing as a sensory threshold; any given intensity of a signal presented to an observer will have associated with it a certain value of d', but there will be no particular value of the intensity which corresponds to threshold.

In practice, if we are interested in comparing the discriminability of different types of signals, we can measure the value of the signal needed to produce a particular value of d'. Alternatively, we can use a task which attempts to eliminate the effects of bias or criterion, so that threshold can be arbitrarily defined as corresponding to a particular percentage correct. One type of task which has proved useful in this respect is the two-alternative forced-choice (2AFC) task, in which there are two observation intervals, only one of which contains the signal. The theory assumes that for each observation interval a particular value of x occurs, and that the subject simply chooses the interval in which the largest value of x occurs. It turns out to be the case that results in a 2AFC task can be simply related to those in a 'single interval' task where the subject is simply required to say whether a signal was present or not on each trial; 76% correct in 2AFC corresponds to a d' of 1.

C Application of signal detection theory to models of masking

Although we do not need to specify the nature of x in order to apply this theory, many workers have considered what x might be. The question is equivalent to enquiring about the nature of the processes involved in masking – what features of a signal, or of its representation at a neural level, enable us to distinguish it from a masking stimulus. Some workers have considered that the masking of a tone by a noise can be explained purely in terms of the statistics of the stimuli; in other words, the variability of x arises primarily from the inherent variability of the stimuli rather than from any 'internal variability' in the sensory system of the listener. An example of this type of approach is given by the work of Jeffress (1964). He assumed that all stimuli are filtered, so that only a narrow band of frequencies in the noise contributes to the masking of the tone, i.e. he assumed a critical band mechanism. After this is a device which extracts the envelope of the filtered stimulus, and following this a criterion device. Jeffress showed that this model gave a good fit to much of the data obtained in detection experiments. Other workers (e.g. Swets *et al.*, 1962) have assumed that stimulus energy rather than the stimulus envelope is the feature on which decisions are based. Again, however, it is necessary to assume a critical band mechanism.

This class of models, in which variability in the signals rather than variability in the observer limits performance, may be considered as describing different types of 'ideal observer'. These models have never been intended as complete descriptions of the human observer, since it is clear that internal variability does play a significant role; human observers rarely, if ever, achieve the performance levels which would be predicted as 'ideal'. This does not mean, however, that the models are of no value. Rather, they provide "a class of normative models with which the observer's performance can be compared" (Tanner and Sorkin, 1972).

FURTHER READING

The following monograph has as its central theme the action of the ear as a frequency analyser. It is clearly written, and contains a discussion of several aspects of frequency selectivity which are beyond the scope of this book:

Plomp, R. (1976). *Aspects of Tone Sensation*. Academic Press, London and New York.

A very detailed review of the frequency selectivity of the ear, covering both physiological and psychological aspects, is the following collection of edited chapters:

Moore, B. C. J. (1986). *Frequency Selectivity in Hearing*. Academic Press, London.

A comprehensive review of profile analysis is:

Green, D. M. (1988). *Profile Analysis*. Oxford University Press, New York.

A comprehensible primer of signal detection theory may be found in:

McNicol, D. (1972). *A Primer of Signal Detection Theory*. Allen and Unwin, London.

Signal detection theory and its applications are covered in detail in:

Green, D. M. and Swets, J. A. (1974). *Signal Detection Theory and Psychophysics*. Kreiger, New York.

Demonstrations 1, 2, 3, 9, 10, 11, 32, 33 and 34 of *Auditory Demonstrations* on CD are relevant to the contents of this chapter (see list of further reading for Chapter 1).

4

The temporal resolution of the auditory system

1 INTRODUCTION

The temporal resolution of the auditory system refers to its ability to detect changes in stimuli over time, for example, to detect a brief gap between two stimuli or to detect that a sound is modulated in some way. This ability is also sometimes described as temporal acuity. Time is a very important dimension in hearing, since almost all sounds change over time. Furthermore, for sounds which convey information, such as speech and music, much of the information appears to be carried in the changes themselves, rather than in the parts of the sounds which are relatively stable. This point will be expanded in Chapters 7 and 8. It is important to distinguish between temporal resolution (or acuity) and temporal integration (or summation). The latter refers to the ability of the auditory system to add up information over time to enhance the detection or discrimination of stimuli, and it has been described already in this book in connection with absolute thresholds and loudness (Chapter 3, Section 5).

A major difficulty in measuring the temporal resolution of the auditory system is that changes in the time pattern of a sound are generally associated with changes in its magnitude spectrum. Thus, the detection of a change in time pattern can sometimes depend not on temporal resolution per se, but on the detection of the spectral change. As an example, consider the task of distinguishing a single brief click from a pair of clicks separated by a short time interval. Assume that the energy of the single click is the same as that of the pair of clicks, so that the two sounds are similar in loudness. At first sight, this task appears to give a direct measure of temporal resolution. The results show that subjects can distinguish the single click from the click pair when the gap between the two clicks in a pair is only a few tens of microseconds (Leshowitz, 1971). This appears to indicate remarkably fine temporal resolution.

The interpretation is not, however, so straightforward. The magnitude

137

spectrum of a pair of clicks is different from the magnitude spectrum of a single click; at some frequencies the single click has more energy and at others it has less energy. Subjects are able to detect these spectral differences, either by monitoring the energy within single critical bands, or by detecting the differences in spectral shape of the two sounds (as occurs in profile analysis; see Chapter 3). The spectral differences in this case are most easily detected at high frequencies. When a noise is added to mask frequencies above 10 kHz, the threshold value of the gap increases dramatically. Thus, the results of this experiment cannot be taken as a direct measure of temporal resolution.

There have been two general approaches to getting around this problem. One is to use signals whose magnitude spectrum is not changed when the time pattern is altered. For example, the magnitude spectrum of white noise remains flat if the noise is interrupted, i.e. if a gap is introduced into the noise. The second approach uses stimuli whose spectra are altered by the change in time pattern, but extra background sounds are added to mask the spectral changes. We will consider both of these approaches.

2   TEMPORAL RESOLUTION MEASURED BY THE DISCRIMINATON OF STIMULI WITH IDENTICAL MAGNITUDE SPECTRA: BROADBAND SOUNDS

A   The detection of gaps in broadband noise

As mentioned above, the long-term magnitude spectrum of broadband white noise remains the same if the noise is briefly interrupted. Thus, the threshold for detecting a gap in a broadband noise provides a simple and convenient measure of temporal resolution. Usually a two-alternative forced-choice (2AFC) procedure is used: the subject is presented with two successive bursts of noise and either the first or the second burst (at random) is interrupted to produce the gap. The task of the subject is to indicate which burst contained the gap. Results obtained using this task show that the gap threshold is typically 2–3 ms (Plomp, 1964b; Penner, 1977). The threshold increases at very low sound levels, when the level of the noise approaches the absolute threshold, but is relatively invariant with level for moderate to high levels.

B   The discrimination of time-reversed signals

The long-term magnitude spectrum of a sound is not changed when that sound is time reversed (played backwards in time). Thus, if a time reversed sound can be discriminated from the original, this must reflect a sensitivity to the difference in time pattern of the two sounds. This was exploited by Ronken (1970), who used as stimuli pairs of clicks differing in amplitude. One click, labelled A, had an amplitude greater than that of the other click, labelled B. Typically the amplitude of A was twice that of B. Subjects were required to distinguish click pairs differing in the order of A and B: either AB or BA. The ability to do this was measured as a function of the time interval or gap between A and B. Ronken found that subjects could distinguish the click pairs for gaps down to 2–3 ms. Thus the limit to temporal resolution found in this task is similar to that found for the detection of a gap in broadband noise. It should be noted that, in this task, subjects do not hear the individual clicks within a click pair. Rather, each click pair is heard as a single sound with its own characteristic quality. For example, the two click pairs AB and BA might sound like 'tick' and 'tock'.

Ronken's experiment has been repeated several times, mostly with similar results. However, Resnick and Feth (1975) showed that the interclick interval required for threshold varied systematically as a function both of overall sound level and of the relative level of the clicks within a pair; the thresholds ranged from 0.5 to 1.8 ms. Also, one study has shown much greater temporal acuity. Henning and Gaskell (1981), using very brief clicks ($20\,\mu$s), found that the order of the click pairs could be discriminated for click pair durations down to 0.25 ms. The reasons for the discrepancies between the different results are unclear.

C   Temporal modulation transfer functions

The experiments described above each give a single number to describe temporal resolution. A more general approach is to measure the threshold for detecting changes in the amplitude of a sound as a function of the rapidity of the changes. In the simplest case, white noise is sinusoidally amplitude modulated, and the threshold for detecting the modulation is determined as a function of modulation rate. The function relating threshold to modulation rate is known as a temporal modulation transfer function (TMTF). Modulation of white noise does not change its long-term magnitude spectrum. An example of the results is shown in Fig. 4.1, adapted from Bacon and Viemeister (1985b). For low modulation rates, performance is limited by the amplitude resolution of the ear, rather than by temporal resolution. Thus, the threshold is independent of modulation rate for rates up to about 16 Hz. As the rate increases beyond 16 Hz, temporal resolution starts to have an effect; the threshold increases, and for rates above about 1000 Hz the modulation cannot be detected at all. Thus, we become progressively less sensitive to amplitude modulation as the rate of modulation increases. The shapes of

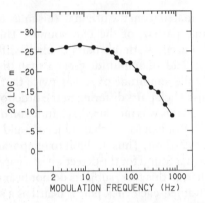

FIG. 4.1 A temporal modulation transfer function (TMTF). A broadband white noise was sinusoidally amplitude modulated, and the threshold amount of modulation required for detection is plotted as a function of modulation rate. The amount of modulation is specified as 20 log (m), where m is the modulation depth (see Chapter 3, Section 2E). The higher the sensitivity to modulation, the more negative is this quantity. Adapted from Bacon and Viemeister (1985b) by permission of the authors.

TMTFs do not vary much with overall sound level, but the ability to detect the modulation does worsen at low sound levels.

Measurements of the TMTF were initially motivated by the possibility that temporal resolution could be modelled as a linear system (e.g. Viemeister, 1979). In a linear system, the response to any complex stimulus can be predicted by summing the responses to the individual sinusoidal components of that stimulus (see Chapter 1, Section 3). If the detection of modulation could be modelled as a linear system, then the detectablity of any form of amplitude modulation (e.g. square-wave modulation) could be predicted from the TMTF. Although this approach has had only limited success, TMTFs have formed the basis for some models of temporal resolution which are discussed in Section 5.

3   *TEMPORAL RESOLUTION MEASURED BY THE DISCRIMINATON OF STIMULI WITH IDENTICAL MAGNITUDE SPECTRA: EFFECTS OF CENTRE FREQUENCY*

All the experiments described in Section 2 used broadband stimuli. Thus they provide no information regarding the question of whether the temporal resolution of the ear varies with centre frequency. It has often been suggested

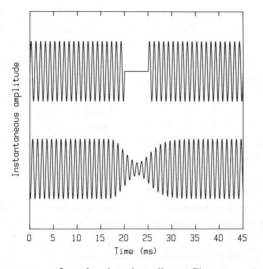

FIG. 4.2 The response of a simulated auditory filter to a 1 kHz sinusoid containing a 5 ms gap. The upper trace shows the input to the filter, and the lower trace shows the output. The filter was centred at 1 kHz and its characteristics were chosen to simulate those of a human auditory filter with the same centre frequency. Only the portions of the waveforms immediately before and after the gap are shown. Note that the gap is partially filled in by the ringing in the filter.

that, in theory, temporal resolution should be poorer at low frequencies than at high. This idea is based on the assumption that temporal resolution might be limited by the response time of the auditory filters. For example, if a stimulus is turned off and on again to form a temporal gap, ringing in the auditory filters might partially fill in the gap, so that the output of the auditory filters would show only a small dip. This is illustrated in Fig. 4.2 which shows the response of a simulated auditory filter to a sinusoid containing a brief gap. The narrower the bandwidth of a filter, the longer is its response time. The auditory filters have narrower bandwidths at low frequencies than at high. Thus, if the responses of the auditory filters limit temporal resolution, resolution should be worse at low frequencies than at high. The experiments described in the rest of this section provide an initial test of this idea.

A   Time-reversed sinusoids

Green (1973) used time-reversed stimuli like those of Ronken (1970) to measure temporal resolution, but instead of clicks he used brief pulses of a sinusoid. Each stimulus consisted of a brief pulse of a sinusoid in which the level of the first half of the pulse was 10 dB different from that of the second half. Subjects were required to distinguish two signals, differing in whether the half with the high level was first or second. Green measured performance as a function of the total duration of the stimuli. The threshold, corresponding to 75% correct discrimination, was similar for centre frequencies of 2 and 4 kHz, and was between 1 and 2 ms. However, the threshold was slightly higher for a centre frequency of 1 kHz, being between 2 and 4 ms. Thus, these data suggest that the response time of the auditory filters was not important above 2 kHz, but may have played a role below that.

It is interesting that performance in this task was actually a non-monotonic function of duration. Performance was good for durations in the range 2–6 ms, worsened for durations around 16 ms, and then improved again as the duration was increased beyond 16 ms. For the very short durations, subjects listened for a difference in quality between the two sounds – rather like the 'tick' and 'tock' described earlier for Ronken's stimuli. At durations around 16 ms, the tonal quality of the bursts became more prominent, and the quality differences were harder to hear. At much longer durations the soft and loud segments could be separately heard, in a distinct order. It appears, therefore, that performance in this task was determined by two separate mechanisms.

B   The discrimination of Huffman sequences

Patterson and Green (1970) and Green (1973) have studied the discrimination of a class of signals which have the same long-term magnitude spectrum, but which differ in their short-term spectra. These sounds are called Huffman sequences. Essentially, they are brief broadband sounds, like clicks, except that the energy in a certain frequency region is delayed relative to that in other regions. The amount of the delay, the centre frequency of the delayed frequency region, and the width of the delayed frequency region can all be varied. If subjects can distinguish a pair of Huffman sequences differing, for example, in the amount of delay in a given frequency region, this implies that they are sensitive to the difference in time pattern. Green (1973) measured the ability of subjects to detect differences in the amount of delay in three frequency regions: 650 Hz, 1900 Hz and 4200 Hz. He found similar results for all three centre frequencies: subjects could detect differences in delay time of about 2 ms regardless of the centre frequency of the delayed region. Thus the results of this task provide no support for the idea that the response of the auditory filter limits temporal resolution for centre frequencies of 650 Hz and above.

4 DETECTION OF TEMPORAL GAPS IN NARROWBAND SOUNDS

In this section we consider the detection of temporal gaps in narrowband sounds. For such sounds, the introduction of a gap results in spectral splatter; energy is spread outside the nominal bandwidth of the sound. To prevent the splatter being detected, the sounds are presented in a background sound, usually a noise, designed to mask the splatter. Unfortunately, the noise used to mask the splatter also has effects within the frequency band of interest, making the gap harder to detect. Thus the level and spectrum of the noise have to be carefully chosen so as to be sure that the splatter is masked while minimizing within-band masking effects.

A Detection of gaps in narrowband noise

Several researchers have measured thresholds for detecting gaps in narrowband noises (e.g. Fitzgibbons and Wightman, 1982; Shailer and Moore, 1983; Buus and Florentine, 1985). An example of the results, taken from Shailer and Moore (1983) is shown in Fig. 4.3. The stimulus containing the gap was a noise with bandwidth one-half of the centre frequency, and a continuous background noise with a notch of the same width was used to mask splatter. The gap thresholds are large (about 22 ms) at the lowest centre

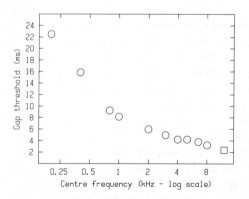

FIG. 4.3 Gap thresholds for noise bands plotted as a function of centre frequency. The bandwidth of the noise was 0.5 times the centre frequency. The square at the right hand side shows the gap threshold for wideband noise. Adapted from Shailer and Moore (1983).

frequency used (200 Hz) and decrease monotically with increasing centre frequency. The gap thresholds for the highest centre frequency (8 kHz) are similar to those found with broadband noise (about 3 ms). This suggests that the results obtained with broadband noise reflect the use of information from the higher-frequency regions of the spectrum.

In contrast to the results with Huffman sequences, these results show a very large effect of centre frequency, which is consistent with the idea that the response time of the auditory filter affects gap thresholds at low frequencies. To test this idea, Shailer and Moore (1983) measured auditory filter shapes in the same subjects as used for the gap detection task. This was done using the notched noise method described in Chapter 3, section 3B. Recall that the response time of a filter is inversely related to its bandwidth. Shailer and Moore found that, for centre frequencies up to 1 kHz, the gap thresholds were approximately equal to the reciprocals of the auditory filter bandwidths. For centre frequencies above this, the gap thresholds were larger than the reciprocals of the filter bandwidths. This suggests that temporal resolution in this task is limited by the response time of the auditory filter for centre frequencies up to 1 kHz, but above that some other process limits performance.

One problem in interpreting these experiments is that the bandwidth of the stimuli used increased with increasing centre frequency; the bandwidth was always one half of the centre frequency. Noise bands have inherent fluctuations in amplitude, and the rapidity of these fluctuations increases with increasing bandwidth. It has been suggested that gap thresholds for noise bands may be partly limited by the inherent fluctuations in the noise (Shailer and Moore, 1983, 1985; Green, 1985). Randomly occurring dips in the noise may be 'confused' with the gap to be detected. The confusion would be maximal for dips comparable in duration to the gap. In practice, this means that noise with a narrow bandwidth, and hence slow fluctuations, would create the greatest confusion and give the largest gap thresholds. The data are consistent with this view: gap thresholds for narrowband noises increase with decreasing noise bandwidth (Shailer and Moore, 1983, 1985). Furthermore, gap thresholds measured with very narrow noise bands show little effect of centre frequency (Shailer and Moore, 1985; de Filippo and Snell, 1986).

It appears that gap thresholds for noise bands depend both upon the inherent fluctuations in the noise and on the effects of the auditory filters (Shailer and Moore, 1983, 1985; Moore and Glasberg, 1988a). This is illustrated in Fig. 4.4. Each panel of the figure shows a sample of noise containing a gap (upper trace) and the output of a simulated auditory filter in response to that stimulus (lower trace). The filter is always centred on the passband of the noise.

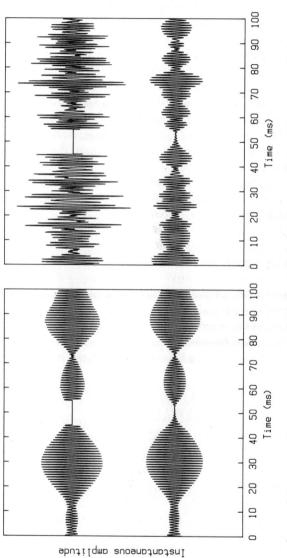

FIG. 4.4 In each panel, the upper trace shows a sample of narrowband noise containing a 10 ms gap, and the lower trace shows the output of a simulated auditory filter in response to that noise. The noises and the filter are centred at 1 kHz. In the left panel, the noise bandwidth is 50 Hz, which is less than the filter bandwidth of 130 Hz. In the right panel the noise bandwidth is 500 Hz.

When the noise bandwidth is less than the auditory filter bandwidth (left panel), the temporal pattern of the fluctuation in the noise is hardly changed by the filter. Ringing in the filter has the effect of partially filling in the gap, but does not fill the gap completely. The gap threshold then depends primarily on the confusability of the gap with the inherent fluctuations of the noise itself, and does not change with centre frequency. When the noise bandwidth is greater than the auditory filter bandwidth (right panel), the fluctuations at the output of the filter are slower than those at the input. For a gap to be reliably detected, it has to be longer than a typical dip in the output of the filter. Thus, the filter bandwidth rather than the stimulus bandwidth is the factor limiting the gap threshold. This explains why gap thresholds decrease with increasing centre frequency for noise bandwidths greater than the auditory filter bandwidth (as shown in Fig. 4.3).

Gap thresholds for narrowband noises tend to decrease with increasing sound level for levels up to about 30 dB above absolute threshold, but to remain roughly constant after that.

B   Detection of gaps in sinusoids

Shailer and Moore (1987) studied the ability of subjects to detect temporal gaps in sinusoids. The sinusoids were presented in a continuous noise with a spectral notch at the frequency of the sinusoids. The results were strongly affected by the phase at which the sinusoid was turned off and on to produce the gap. The three phase conditions used are illustrated in Fig. 4.5. For all

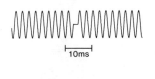

FIG. 4.5 The three phase conditions used by Shailer and Moore (1987) to measure gap thresholds for sinusoids. For each condition, the stimulus shown is a 400 Hz sinusoid with a 1.9 ms gap. The three conditions are: standard phase (top), reversed phase (middle), and preserved phase (bottom).

conditions, the portion of the sinusoid preceding the gap ended with a positive-going zero-crossing. In other words, the sinusoid was turned off as the waveform was about to change from negative to positive values. The three conditions differed in the phase at which the sinusoid was turned on at the end of the gap: for the 'standard' phase condition (top trace), the sinusoid started at a positive-going zero-crossing; for the 'reversed' phase condition (middle trace), the sinusoid started at a negative-going zero-crossing; and for the 'preserved' phase condition (bottom trace) the sinusoid started at the phase it would have had if it had continued without interruption. Thus, for the preserved-phase condition it was as if the gap had been 'cut out' from a continuous sinusoid.

Examples of psychometric functions for the three conditions are shown in Fig. 4.6. The frequency of the sinusoid was 400 Hz. A two-alternative forced-choice task was used, so chance performance corresponds to 50% correct. For the preserved-phase condition, performance improves monotonically with increasing gap duration, as might be expected. However, for the other

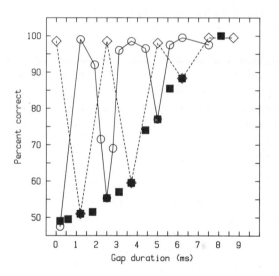

FIG. 4.6 An example of the results of Shailer and Moore (1987), showing data for one subject for a signal frequency of 400 Hz. Psychometric functions for gap detection are plotted for the standard phase (circles), reversed phase (diamonds) and preserved phase (filled squares) conditions. When the gap is an integer multiple of the signal period, P (=2.5 ms), the standard phase condition is identical to the preserved phase condition. Similarly, when the gap is $(n + 0.5)P$, where n is an integer, the reversed phase condition is identical to the preserved phase condition. Adapted from Shailer and Moore (1987).

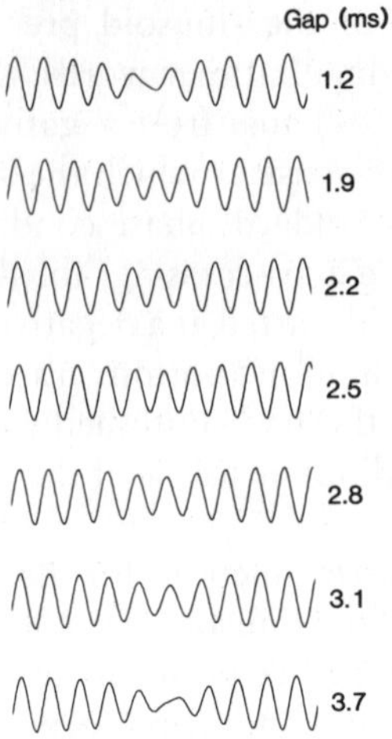

Gap (ms)

FIG. 4.7 The output of a simulated auditory filter centred at 400 Hz in response to 400 Hz sinusoids containing gaps ranging in duration from 1.2 to 3.7 ms, for the standard phase condition.

two conditions the psychometric functions are distinctly nonmonotonic. For the standard-phase condition, the gap is difficult to detect when its value is an integer multiple of the period (P) of the signal, i.e., 2.5 ms and 5 ms. Conversely, the gap is easy to detect when its value is $(n + 0.5)P$, where $n = 0$ or 1. The psychometric function for the reversed phase condition shows poor performance when the gap duration is $(n + 0.5)P$, where $n = 0$ or 1, and good performance when the gap duration is nP.

Shailer and Moore (1987) explained these results in terms of ringing in the auditory filter. Their argument is illustrated in Fig. 4.7, which shows responses of a simulated auditory filter with a centre frequency of 400 Hz to a series of stimuli from the standard-phase condition, with gap durations ranging from 1.2 to 3.7 ms. When the sinusoid is turned off at the start of the gap, the filter continues to respond or ring for a certain time. If the gap duration is 2.5 ms, corresponding to one whole period of the sinusoid, the sinusoid following the gap is in phase with the ringing response. In this case the output of the filter shows only a small dip, and we would expect gap detection to be difficult. This is exactly what is observed. For a gap duration of 1.2 ms or 3.7 ms, the sinusoid following the gap is out of phase with the ringing response. Now the output of the filter passes through zero before returning to its steady-state value. The resulting dip in the filter output is larger, and is much easier to detect. This explains why the psychometric function is nonmonotonic for the standard-phase condition. Similar arguments explain the nonmonotonicities for the reversed-phase condition. For the preserved phase condition, the sinusoid following the gap is always in phase with the ringing response of the auditory filter. Thus, the dip in the output of the auditory filter increases monotonically with increasing gap duration, and the psychometric function is monotonic.

The results for the preserved-phase condition can be used to estimate the gap threshold corresponding to 75% correct. For the data shown in Fig. 4.4, the gap threshold is about 4.5 ms. Shailer and Moore (1987) found that the gap threshold was roughly constant at about 5 ms for centre frequencies of 400, 1000 and 2000 Hz. Data for one subject indicated that the gap threshold increased somewhat, to 7 ms, for a centre frequency of 200 Hz. Overall, then, while the auditory filter seems to play a role in determining the form of the results for the standard- and reversed-phase conditions, gap thresholds estimated from the preserved-phase condition do not show a strong effect of centre frequency. This appears puzzling, since we might have expected that ringing in the auditory filter would lead to larger gap thresholds at low centre frequencies. We will return to this point later.

5 MODELLING TEMPORAL RESOLUTION

In the previous sections we considered the role of the auditory filter in limiting temporal resolution. While there is evidence that the auditory filter does play a role in some measures of temporal resolution, its influence is seen mainly at low frequencies, below about 1 kHz. The response of the auditory filter at high frequencies is too fast for it to be a limiting factor in most tasks involving temporal resolution. This has led to the idea that there is a process at levels of the auditory system higher than the auditory nerve which is 'sluggish' in some way, thereby limiting temporal resolution. Models of temporal resolution are especially concerned with this process. The models assume that the internal representation of stimuli is 'smoothed' over time, so that rapid temporal changes are lost but slower ones are preserved. Although this smoothing process almost certainly operates on neural activity, the most widely used models are based on smoothing a simple transformation of the stimulus, rather than its neural representation. This is done for simplicity and mathematical convenience, even though it is not very realistic.

A   Models based on a lowpass filter

A popular model of temporal resolution (e.g. Rodenburg, 1977; Viemeister, 1979) is illustrated in Fig. 4.8. There is an initial stage of bandpass filtering,

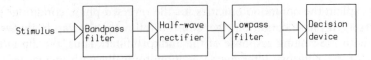

FIG. 4.8   A block diagram of a model of temporal resolution. See text for details.

reflecting the action of the auditory filters. For simplicity, only one filter is shown; in reality there would be an array of parallel channels, each like that shown in the figure. The filter is followed by some sort of nonlinear device; the figure shows a half-wave rectifier. This passes portions of the waveform of one polarity (say, the positive parts), but does not pass portions of the opposite polarity. This resembles the way that neural spikes tend to occur for a particular polarity of the stimulating waveform (see Chapter 1, section 6E). The output of the rectifier is always positive, even though the waveform passing through the filter has positive and negative portions of roughly equal magnitude. The output of the rectifier is fed through a lowpass filter. This has the effect of 'smoothing' the output of the rectifier. In effect, the output of the lowpass filter resembles the amplitude envelope of the output of the bandpass filter. However, rapid envelope fluctuations are reduced in magnitude, while slower ones are preserved. The output of the lowpass filter is fed to the final stage of the model, a decision device. This model has been considered most often in the context of the TMTF. Indeed, it has sometimes been assumed that the shape of the TMTF for broadband noise is largely determined by the lowpass filter stage of the model in Fig. 4.8 (Rodenburg, 1977).

   A variation on this type of model is illustrated in Fig. 4.9. As before, the initial stages are a bandpass filter and a nonlinear device. However, the nonlinear device in this case has a square-law characteristic: the instantaneous value of the output is proportional to the square of the instantaneous value of the input. This gives a quantity which is always positive and which is related to the instantaneous power at the output of the bandpass filter. The next stage is a temporal integrator which sums the energy occurring within a certain time interval or 'window'. The window is assumed to slide in time, so that the output of the temporal integrator is like a running average of the input. This has the effect of smoothing rapid fluctuations while preserving

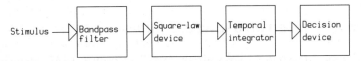

FIG. 4.9   A variation of the type of model shown in Fig. 4.8.

slower ones. The temporal integrator is equivalent to the lowpass filter in Fig. 4.8, except that the smoothing is applied to a power-like quantity rather than an amplitude-like quantity. Finally, as before, the output of the temporal integrator is fed to a decision device.

B The nature of the decision device

The nature of the decision device, or the rule used by the decision device, may vary with the task being considered. To account for TMTFs, several different decision rules have been suggested. Rodenburg (1977) suggested that the threshold for detecting amplitude modulation of a given rate depends on the magnitude of the output of the lowpass filter; the decision device in this case is simply a threshold device. Modulation would be detected if the output of the lowpass filter exceeded a certain magnitude. In a 2AFC task, the subject would simply choose the observation interval for which the output from the lowpass filter was higher. Viemeister (1979) suggested that decisions are based on the variance of the output of the lowpass filter; this variance would be greater for a modulated waveform than for an unmodulated waveform. Finally, Green and Forrest (1988) have suggested that the output of the lowpass filter is repeatedly sampled during an observation interval, and decisions are based on the ratio of the highest sample value to the lowest sample value; this ratio would tend to be greater for modulated than for unmodulated waveforms. Note that the ratio would be greater than one for an unmodulated noise, because of the inherent fluctuations in the noise. At present, there seems to be no obvious way of deciding among these decision rules.

For other types of task, a different decision rule might be used. Consider, for example, the task of detecting a gap in a sinusoidal stimulus. Figure 4.10 shows the output of the different stages of the model in Fig. 4.9 for sinusoidal input signals with a 5 ms gap (the model in Fig. 4.8 would give similar results). Inputs with centre frequencies of 400, 1000 and 2000 Hz are shown. After passing through a simulated auditory filter centred at the signal frequency, each gap is partially filled in, so the output of the filter shows a dip rather than a silent gap (just as in Fig. 4.7). For the 400 Hz signal, the dip in the output of the filter is shallow, but lasts for a relatively long time. For the 2000 Hz signal, the dip is deep but lasts for only a short time. After passing through the sliding temporal integrator (or lowpass filter), the fine structure of the signal is lost, and the gap is filled in even more. It is usually assumed that the gap will be detected if the dip in the output of the temporal integrator exceeds a certain threshold value, which is typically about 2 dB. Notice that the dip is similar for the three centre frequencies used. This explains why Shailer and Moore

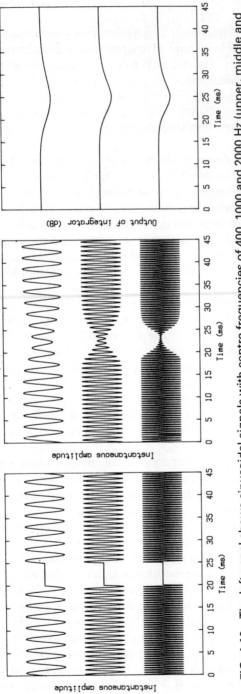

FIG. 4.10 The left panel shows sinusoidal signals with centre frequencies of 400, 1000 and 2000 Hz (upper, middle and lower traces, respectively), each containing a 5 ms gap. The middle panel shows the outputs of simulated auditory filters centred at the frequency of each signal. The right panel shows the results of passing the outputs of the simulated filters through the remaining stages of the model shown in Fig. 4.9, namely a square law device and a sliding temporal integrator. See text for details.

(1987) found that gap thresholds for sinusoids were almost independent of centre frequency (see section 4B). To explain the fact that performance is not perfect in this task, it has to be assumed that there is some inherent variability in one or more stages of the model. For example, the decision stage of the model might itself have an internal noise which limits resolution.

In summary, the rule used by the decision device may vary depending on the task required. Although it is easy to suggest plausible rules, it is difficult to demonstrate that a particular rule is actually being used.

C The characteristic of the lowpass filter

Although all the stages of the model can affect performance in tasks requiring temporal resolution, it is often felt that the stage which is most directly related to temporal resolution is the lowpass filter or temporal integrator. Thus, it would be desirable to be able to determine the characteristics of this stage independently of the other stages.

Consider first the model illustrated in Fig. 4.8. As mentioned above, it has sometimes been suggested that the TMTF for broadband noise is largely determined by the lowpass filter stage of the model. If this were true, then the TMTF would define the shape of the lowpass filter, and thus the characteristics of the model could be completely determined by empirical data. In practice there are problems. The shape of the TMTF predicted by the model is actually affected by the characteristics of the initial bandpass filter, by the type of nonlinearity assumed (square-law device or rectifier), by the characteristics of the lowpass filter and by the decision rule used (Viemeister, 1979; Green and Forrest, 1988). Thus there is no simple way to define the shape of the lowpass filter independently of the other stages of the model. Furthermore, to account for TMTFs for broadband noise, it has to be assumed that the initial bandpass filter is broader than the auditory filter (Viemeister, 1979). This would imply that the outputs of several different auditory filters could be combined at some level in the auditory system, so as to enhance temporal resolution.

Consider now the model illustrated in Fig. 4.9, in which the lowpass filter is implemented as a sliding temporal integrator. In the simplest form of this model, all the power within the window is weighted equally to determine the output. The window in this case is often described as 'rectangular' and the window is completely defined by its duration. However, it is more realistic to assume that power occurring more recently in time (close to the end of the window) is more important than power occurring earlier (close to the start of the window). This can be modelled by considering the window as a weighting function, having a particular mathematical form, such as an exponential

(Munson, 1947; Zwislocki, 1969). The output of the temporal integrator then becomes a weighted sum of the input power, with recently occurring power receiving the greatest weight. This weighting function can be considered as a temporal domain analogue of the auditory filter. The auditory filter shape was once approximated as a rectangle, and was later shown to be more accurately characterized as a weighting function with a rounded top and sloping skirts (see Chapter 3). Similarly, the temporal integrator can be approximated by a rectangular window, but is more accurately characterized as a nonrectangular weighting function. The form of this weighting function is sometimes referred to as the 'shape' of the temporal window. The task of determining this shape is equivalent to the task of determining the shape of the lowpass filter in the model of Fig. 4.8.

Some recent experiments (Moore *et al.*, 1988; Plack and Moore, 1989) have been devoted to determining the shape of the hypothetical temporal window. It is beyond the scope of this book to go into the details of the experiments. Briefly, the results confirm that the temporal window is not rectangular, and that power at times close to the end of the window is weighted more than power at times close to the start of the window. The shape of the temporal window is almost invariant with centre frequency, but the effects of the auditory filter can produce an apparent broadening of the window at low centre frequencies; a broader temporal window is associated with poorer temporal resolution. Finally, the results show that the temporal window broadens somewhat as the sound level decreases.

To summarize the essential features of this class of model, the stimulus is assumed to be bandpass filtered, passed through a nonlinear device, and lowpass filtered (or, equivalently, passed through a sliding temporal integrator). Temporal resolution depends upon four factors: the shape and bandwidth of the initial bandpass filter; the type of nonlinearity assumed; the cutoff frequency and slope of the lowpass filter (or the shape of the weighting function describing the temporal window); and the nature and sensitivity of the decision device following the lowpass filter.

D   Models incorporating compressive nonlinearities

The models described above assume that a simple transformation of the stimulus magnitude is integrated over time. However, it seems more realistic to assume that neural activity is integrated (Divenyi and Shannon, 1983; Shannon, 1986). Unfortunately, it is much more difficult to construct a model based on this assumption, since we do not know the level in the auditory system at which the integration takes place, and since it would be necessary to include a variety of complex phenomena such as neural saturation and adaptation. An intermediate step is to model one or more of the basic properties of the transformation from stimulus magnitude to neural activity. One such property is the fact that the number of neural spikes evoked by a stimulus is not directly proportional to the stimulus intensity. Rather it is a nonlinear, compressive function of stimulus intensity; the number of spikes grows more slowly than the stimulus intensity. One way of modelling this is by a power function. The number of spikes, N, is assumed to be proportional to the stimulus intensity, I, raised to a power, n, where $n < 1$. For example, if $n = 0.3$, then a tenfold increase in power would lead to a doubling of the number of neural spikes (see, for example, Chapter 3, section 2B).

Several workers have suggested models of temporal resolution in which there is a compressive nonlinearity prior to the temporal integrator (Penner, 1980; Penner and Shiffrin, 1980; Shannon, 1986). In these models, temporal resolution is determined by the type of nonlinearity assumed, as well as by the temporal integrator and the sensitivity to changes in the output of the integrator. These models are complex, and it is beyond the scope of this book to describe them in detail. However, they do appear to be successful in accounting for certain aspects of forward and backward masking.

E   Comparison of the models

The models described above all have in common some type of smoothing device, which removes rapid fluctuations but preserves slower ones. The models described in section A achieve the smoothing by a sequence of stages including: a bandpass filter (the auditory filter); a nonlinear device (rectifier or square-law device); and a lowpass filter (or temporal integrator). For the model illustrated in Fig. 4.8, the lowpass filter essentially extracts the amplitude envelope of the output of the bandpass filter, and the smoothing is applied to that envelope. For the model illustrated in Fig. 4.9, the smoothing is applied to the power at the output of the auditory filter. Thus, the models are conceptually similar, except that one operates in terms of amplitude, and the other operates in terms of power. At present, there appear to be no strong reasons for preferring one approach over the other. The models outlined in section D include a compressive nonlinearity before the temporal integrator. They are perhaps more realistic physiologically, but they are more complex, and are less easy to implement.

One limitation of all the models is that they are restricted to accounting for the type of task which requires resolution within a particular frequency channel. However, certain types of tasks clearly require comparisons *across* different frequency channels. For example, the discrimination of Huffman sequences involves comparing the time of arrival of energy in different frequency bands (see section 3B). At present, we do not have good models to account for performance on this type of task. It is noteworthy, however, that the discrimination of Huffman sequences is one of the few tasks which shows no variation of temporal resolution with centre frequency.

6   GENERAL CONCLUSIONS

The temporal resolution of the auditory system can be measured with many different types of signals and in a variety of tasks. In all cases, it is important to ensure that cues in the long-term magnitude spectrum of the stimuli are not being used to perform the task.

For broadband noises, the threshold for detecting a temporal gap is typically 2–3 ms, except at very low levels, where the threshold increases. For pairs of clicks differing in amplitude, the threshold value of the gap between the clicks required to distinguish their order is also about 2–3 ms, although some experiments have given smaller thresholds. The threshold for detecting sinusoidal amplitude modulation of broadband noise varies with the modulation frequency; the threshold is low at low modulation frequencies and increases with increasing modulation frequency. The function describing modulation thresholds as a function of modulation rate is known as a temporal modulation transfer function (TMTF).

Narrowband sounds allow the measurement of temporal resolution at different centre frequencies. We might expect temporal resolution to be poorer at low centre frequencies because of ringing in the auditory filters; the filters at low centre frequencies have narrow bandwidths and they therefore have a long response time. Some experiments show the expected effect, while others do not.

Thresholds for the discrimination of time reversed sinusoids and Huffman sequences (section 3) are typically in the range 2–3 ms, and vary only slightly with centre frequency. Thresholds for detecting gaps in narrowband noises are large (up to 22 ms) at low centre frequencies, but decrease to about 3 ms at high centre frequencies. The results for these noises seem to be strongly influenced both by the action of the auditory filter and by the inherent fluctuations in the noises. Randomly occuring dips in the noises may be confused with the gap to be detected. The detection of a gap in a sinusoid is strongly affected by the phase at which the sinusoid is turned off and on to produce the gap. The psychometric functions for some conditions show distinct nonmonotonicities which can be explained in terms of ringing in the auditory filter. Gap thresholds for sinusoids do not vary markedly with centre frequency, but may worsen slightly at very low centre frequencies. Overall, the results for different types of narrowband signals suggest that the auditory filter may affect temporal resolution at low frequencies, but it has little effect for centre frequencies above about 1 kHz.

Models to account for temporal resolution all assume that there is a process which smooths the internal representation of auditory stimuli, but they differ in the way that the smoothing is implemented. The models have a number of stages including: a bandpass filter (the auditory filter); a nonlinear device (a rectifier or square-law device); a smoothing device (lowpass filter or temporal integrator); and a decision device. Temporal resolution can be affected by all of the stages of the models. Some models additionally assume a compressive nonlinearity before the temporal integrator. All of these models are successful in accounting for certain aspects of the data, but none is completely general. In particular, they do not account for performance in tasks which require a comparison of the timing of events in different frequency channels.

Other aspects of temporal resolution are discussed later. Specifically, Chapter 6, section 12 discusses temporal resolution in binaural processing, and Chapter 7, section 4C discusses judgements of the temporal order of sounds.

FURTHER READING

The following book is the proceedings of a conference on temporal resolution. The chapters by Green and by Buus and Florentine are of particular relevance to this chapter.

Michelsen, A. (1985). *Time Resolution in Auditory Systems*. Springer-Verlag, Berlin.

5
Pitch perception

1 INTRODUCTION

In this chapter we will consider the perception of the pitch of both pure and complex tones. Pitch may be defined as "that attribute of auditory sensation in terms of which sounds may be ordered on a musical scale" (American Standards Association, 1960). In other words, variations in pitch give rise to a sense of melody. Pitch is related to the repetition rate of the waveform of a sound; for a pure tone this corresponds to the frequency and for a periodic complex tone to the fundamental frequency. There are, however, exceptions to this simple rule, as we shall see later. Since pitch is a subjective attribute, it cannot be measured directly. Assigning a pitch value to a sound is generally understood to mean specifying the frequency of a pure tone having the same subjective pitch as the sound.

2 THEORIES OF PITCH PERCEPTION

For many years there have been two different theories of pitch perception. One, the 'place' theory of hearing has two distinct postulates. The first is that the stimulus undergoes some sort of spectral analysis in the inner ear, so that different frequencies (or frequency components in a complex stimulus) excite different places along the basilar membrane, and hence neurones with different CFs (this is called tonotopic organization; see Chapter 1, section 6B). The second is that the pitch of a stimulus is related to the pattern of excitation produced by that stimulus; for a pure tone the pitch is generally assumed to correspond to the position of maximum excitation. The first of these two postulates is now well established, and has been confirmed in a number of independent ways, including direct observation of the movement of the basilar membrane (see Chapter 1). The second is still a matter of dispute.

An alternative to the place theory, which will be called the 'temporal' theory, suggests that the pitch of a stimulus is related to the time pattern of the neural impulses evoked by that stimulus. Nerve firings tend to occur at a particular phase of the stimulating waveform, and thus the intervals between successive neural impulses approximate integral multiples of the period of the stimulating waveform (this is called phase locking; see Chapter 1, section 6E). The temporal theory could not work at very high frequencies, since phase locking does not occur for frequencies above about 5 kHz. However, this is not a serious problem, since the tones produced by musical instruments, the human voice and most everyday sound sources all have fundamental frequencies below this range.

A difficulty for the place theory arises when we consider complex tones. These produce patterns of excitation along the basilar membrane which do not show a single well-defined maximum; rather there is a distribution of excitation with many maxima. The largest maximum may not be at the CF corresponding to the fundamental component. However, the perceived pitch, in general, still corresponds to this component. We shall discuss later how the place theory may be modified to account for this.

3 THE PERCEPTION OF THE PITCH OF PURE TONES

In this section we shall discuss theories which attempt to explain how we perceive and discriminate the frequency of pure tones. The main topics which we shall discuss are: the size of the frequency difference limen (the smallest detectable change in frequency, abbreviated DL); changes in the size of the DL with frequency; and the perception of musical intervals as a function of frequency. It is important to distinguish between frequency selectivity and frequency discrimination. The former refers to the ability to resolve the frequency components of a complex sound, as discussed in Chapter 3. The latter refers to the ability to detect changes in frequency over time. As explained below, for place theories, frequency selectivity and frequency discrimination are closely connected; frequency discrimination depends upon the filtering which takes place in the cochlea. For temporal theories, frequency selectivity and frequency discrimination are not necessarily closely connected.

A The frequency discrimination of pure tones

There have been two common ways of measuring frequency discrimination. One measure involves the presentation of two successive steady tones with slightly different frequencies. The subject is asked to judge whether the first or the second has the higher pitch. The order of the tones is varied randomly from trial to trial, and the frequency DL is usually taken as that frequency separation between the pulses for which the subject achieves 75% correct responses. This measure will be called the DLF. A second measure uses tones which are frequency modulated (FM) at a low rate (typically 2–4 Hz). The amount of modulation required for detection of the modulation is determined. This measure will be called the FMDL.

Early studies of frequency discrimination mainly measured FMDLs (e.g. Shower and Biddulph, 1931; Zwicker, 1956). Recent studies have concentrated more on the measurement of DLFs. A summary of the results of some of these studies is given in Fig. 5.1, taken from Wier *et al.* (1977). Expressed in Hz, the DLF is smallest at low frequencies, and increases monotonically with increasing frequency. Expressed as a proportion of centre frequency, the DLF tends to be smallest for middle frequencies, and larger for very high and very low frequencies. Wier *et al.* (1977) found that the data describing the DLF as a function of frequency fell on a straight line when plotted as log(DLF) against √(frequency); the axes are scaled in this way in Fig. 5.1. The

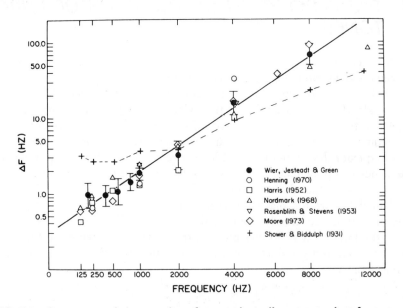

FIG. 5.1 Summary of the results of several studies measuring frequency discrimination thresholds. The thresholds, ΔF, are plotted in Hz as a function of frequency. All of the studies measured DLFs except that of Shower and Biddulph; they measured FMDLs. From Wier *et al.* (1977), by permission of the authors and *J. Acoust. Soc. Am.*

theoretical significance of this is not clear. FMDLs, shown as the dashed line in Fig. 5.1, tend to vary less with frequency than DLFs. Both DLFs and FMDLs tend to get somewhat smaller as the sound level increases.

A basic problem for any theory of hearing is to account for the remarkably small size of the frequency DLs; for a frequency of 1 kHz and at a moderate sound level (60–70 dB SPL), the DLF is about 2 Hz. Zwicker (1970) has attempted to account for frequency discrimination in terms of changes in the excitation pattern evoked by the stimulus when the frequency is altered. This is a place model. Zwicker inferred the shapes of the excitation patterns from masked audiograms such as those shown in Fig. 3.10 (see Chapter 3 for details). In his original formulation of the model, Zwicker intended it to apply only to FMDLs; others have tried to apply the model to account for DLFs.

According to Zwicker's model, a change in frequency will be detected whenever the excitation level at some point on the pattern changes by more than a certain threshold value. Zwicker suggested that this value was about 1 dB. The change in excitation level is always greatest on the steeply sloping low-frequency side of the excitation pattern (see Fig. 5.2). Thus, in this model, the detection of a change in frequency is functionally equivalent to the detection of a change in level on the low-frequency side of the excitation

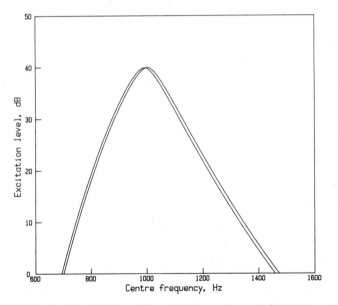

FIG. 5.2 Schematic representation of the patterns of excitation evoked by two tones of slightly different frequency; the frequencies of the tones are 995 and 1005 Hz and their level is 40 dB. The greatest difference in excitation level for the two patterns occurs on the steeply sloping low-frequency side.

pattern. Maiwald (1967) has shown that the steepness of the low-frequency side is roughly constant when expressed in units of the critical bandwidth rather than in terms of linear frequency. The slope has a value of 27 dB/bark (a bark is a unit of one critical bandwidth). Thus Zwicker's model predicts that the frequency DL at any given frequency should be a constant fraction (1/27) of the critical bandwidth at that frequency; a change in frequency of 1/27 bark should give a change in excitation level of 1 dB. FMDLs do conform fairly well to the predictions of the model. However, DLFs vary more with frequency than predicted by the model; at low frequencies DLFs are smaller than predicted, while at high frequencies they are slightly larger than predicted (Moore and Glasberg, 1986).

Henning (1966) has pointed out a problem with the measurement of frequency DLs at high frequencies; the frequency changes may be accompanied by correlated loudness changes. These occur because the response of headphones on real ears is generally very irregular at high frequencies, and there is also a loss of absolute sensitivity of the observer at high frequencies (see the right-hand half of Fig. 2.1). These loudness changes may provide observers with usable cues in the detection of frequency changes. To prevent subjects from using these cues, Henning (1966) measured DLFs for tones whose level was varied randomly from one stimulus to the next. The random variation in level produced changes in loudness which were large compared with those produced by the frequency changes. Henning found that DLFs at high frequencies (4 kHz and above) were markedly increased by the random variation in level, whereas those at low frequencies were not.

Although Henning's experiment was carried out primarily to assess the importance of loudness cues in frequency discrimination, his data also provide a test of Zwicker's model. If the detection of frequency changes were based on the detection of changes in excitation level on the low-frequency side of the excitation pattern, then the introduction of random variations in level should markedly impair frequency discrimination; the small change in excitation level produced by a given frequency change would now be superimposed on much larger random changes in level. This predicted impairment of frequency discrimination was found only at high frequencies. Thus, Henning's data are consistent with Zwicker's model for high frequencies but not for low frequencies. However, Emmerich *et al.* (1989) repeated Henning's experiment and found that random variations in level did result in larger DLFs at low frequencies (0.5–4.0 kHz). Although these data appear to support Zwicker's model, Emmerich and co-workers argued that this was not necessarily true. They presented evidence that the impairment produced by the randomization of level could be attributed to slight changes in the pitches of the sinusoidal signals with changes in level (see section C for a description of such changes).

Moore and Glasberg (1989) also measured DLFs for tones whose level was randomized from one stimulus to the next, but they randomized the level over a relatively small range (6 dB instead of 20 dB as used by Henning and Emmerich *et al.*) to minimize changes of pitch with level. The 6 dB range was still large relative to the changes in excitation level produced by small frequency changes. They found only a very small effect of the randomization of level; the DLFs were, on average, only 15% greater than those measured with the level fixed. The DLFs measured with the level randomized were smaller than predicted by Zwicker's model for frequencies from 0.5 to 4.0 kHz. At 6.5 kHz (the highest frequency tested), the data were not inconsistent with the model.

An alternative way of testing Zwicker's model is to use a stimulus which has energy distributed over a range of frequencies and whose magnitude spectrum has a certain slope. The slope of the excitation pattern of such a stimulus cannot be steeper than the slope of the physical spectrum. This approach was adopted by Moore (1972, 1973a). He measured DLFs for tone pulses of various durations. For a short duration tone pulse, the frequency spectrum contains energy at frequencies other than the nominal frequency of the tone pulse (see Chapter 1, section 2B). The shorter the tone pulse is made, the wider the range of frequencies over which the energy is spread. Below some critical duration the slope of the spectral envelope will be less than the slope of the excitation pattern evoked by a long duration pure tone. Thus, if Zwicker's model is correct, this physical slope will limit performance at short durations. The results showed that at short durations observers did better than predicted for all frequencies up to 5 kHz. At about this frequency the DLs showed a sharp increase in value (see Fig. 5.3).

In summary, Zwicker's model predicts that frequency DLs should vary with frequency in the same way as the critical bandwidth. It also predicts that random variations in level should markedly increase frequency DLs. The results for DLFs are not consistent with these predictions. DLFs vary more with frequency than the critical bandwidth, and the effect of randomizing level is smaller than predicted, except at high frequencies. Furthermore, DLFs for short duration tones are smaller than predicted by Zwicker's model, except above 5 kHz. Other data, reviewed in Moore and Glasberg (1986), also suggest that Zwicker's model does not adequately account for DLFs. The results for FMDLs reviewed here are generally not inconsistent with Zwicker's model, although other data suggest that it may not be entirely adequate even for these (Feth, 1972; Coninx, 1978).

Although we have concentrated on Zwicker's model, other place models (e.g. Corliss, 1967; Henning, 1967; Siebert, 1968, 1970) also have difficulty in accounting for DLFs. All place models predict that frequency discrimination should be related to frequency selectivity; the sharper the tuning of

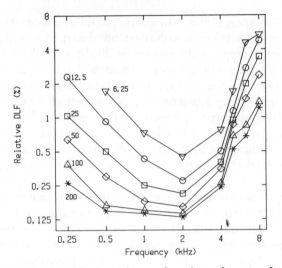

FIG. 5.3 Values of the DLF plotted as a function of centre frequency and expressed as a percentage of centre frequency (log scale). The number by each curve is the duration of the tone pulses in ms. Notice the sharp increase in the size of the DLFs which occurs around 5 kHz.

peripheral filtering mechanisms, the smaller should be the frequency DL. Thus, all place models predicted that the frequency DL should vary with frequency in the same way as the critical bandwidth. The failure of this prediction suggests that some other mechanism is involved.

The results are consistent with the idea that DLFs are determined by temporal information (phase locking) for frequencies up to about 4–5 kHz, and by place information above that. The precision of phase locking decreases with increasing frequency above 1–2 kHz, and it is completely absent above about 5 kHz. This can explain why DLFs increase markedly above this frequency. One difficulty with the temporal theory is that so far there has been no evidence of a physiological mechanism which would carry out the time measurements involved with sufficient accuracy. The DL size at 1 kHz requires that a time interval of 1 ms be measured with an accuracy of about 2 μs. When we consider that there is a certain 'jitter' in the initiation of nerve impulses, which, according to de Boer (1969a), has a standard deviation of about 100 μs for a 1 kHz tone, the problem becomes even more acute; the mechanism must also be required to 'average' over time and over different auditory nerve fibres. However, Goldstein and Srulovicz (1977) have shown that it is possible to predict the dependence of the frequency DL on frequency and duration by assuming that the auditory system processes the time intervals between successive nerve impulses, ignoring higher-order temporal dependencies.

The two mechanisms we have been discussing are not, of course, mutually exclusive; it is likely that place information is available over almost all of the auditory range but that temporal mechanisms allow better frequency discrimination for frequencies up to about 4–5 kHz

B   The perception of musical intervals

If a tone evokes a pitch, then a sequence of tones with appropriate frequencies should evoke the percept of a melody. One way of measuring this aspect of pitch perception is to require subjects to make judgements about the musical relationship of a sequence of two or more pure tones. For example, two tones which are separated in frequency by an interval of one octave (i.e., one has twice the frequency of the other) sound similar. They are judged to have the same name on the musical scale (for example, C or D).

If subjects are presented with a pure tone of a given frequency, f_1, and are asked to adjust the frequency, f_2 of a second tone so that it appears to be an octave higher in pitch, they will generally adjust f_2 to be roughly twice f_1. However, when f_1 lies above 2.5 kHz, so that f_2 would lie above 5 kHz, octave matches become very erratic. It appears that the musical interval of an octave is only clearly perceived when both tones are below 5 kHz.

Other aspects of the perception of pitch also change above 5 kHz. For example, a sequence of pure tones above 5 kHz does not produce a clear sense of melody. This has been confirmed by experiments involving musical transposition. For example, Attneave and Olson (1971) asked subjects to reproduce sequences of tones (e.g. the NBC chimes) at different points along the frequency scale. Their results showed an abrupt breakpoint at about 5 kHz, above which transposition behaviour was erratic.

In summary, it appears that only pure tones below 5 kHz have a pitch in the sense that a sequence of tones can evoke a sense of musical interval or melody. A sequence of pure tones above 5 kHz does not evoke a clear sense of melody, although differences in frequency can be heard. This is consistent with the idea that the pitch of pure tones is determined by different mechanisms above and below 5 kHz, specifically, by temporal mechanisms at low frequencies and place mechanisms at high frequencies.

C   The variation of pitch with level

The pitch of a pure tone is primarily determined by its frequency. However, sound level also plays a small role. On average, the pitch of tones below about 2000 Hz decreases with increasing level, while the pitch of tones above about 4000 Hz increases with increasing sound level. The early data of Stevens

(1935) showed rather large effects of sound level on pitch, but more recent data generally show much smaller effects (e.g. Verschuure and van Meeteren, 1975). For tones between 1 and 2 kHz, changes in pitch with level are generally less than 1%. For tones of lower and higher frequencies, the changes can be larger (up to 5%). There are also considerable individual differences both in the size of the pitch shifts with level, and in the direction of the shifts.

It has sometimes been argued that pitch shifts with level are inconsistent with the temporal theory of pitch; neural interspike intervals are hardly affected by changes in sound level over a wide range. However, changes in pitch with level could be explained by the place theory, if shifts in level were accompanied by shifts in the position of maximum excitation on the basilar membrane. On closer examination, these arguments turn out to be rather weak. Although the temporal theory assumes that pitch depends on the temporal pattern of nerve spikes, it also assumes that the temporal information has to be 'decoded' at some level in the auditory system. In other words, the time intervals between neural spikes have to be measured. It is quite possible that the mechanism which does this is affected by which neurones are active and by the spike rates in those neurones; these in turn depend on sound level.

The argument favouring the place mechanism is also weak. Chapter 2, section 7B, presented evidence from studies of auditory fatigue (temporary threshold shift) that the peak in the pattern of excitation evoked by low-frequency tones (around 1 kHz) shifts towards the base of the cochlea with increasing sound level. The base is tuned to higher frequencies, so the basalward shift should correspond to hearing an increase in pitch. At high sound levels the basalward shift corresponds to a shift in frequency of one-half octave or more. Thus the place theory predicts that the pitch of a 1 kHz tone should increase with increasing sound level, and the shift should correspond to half an octave or more at high sound levels. In fact, the pitch tends to decrease with increasing sound level, and the shift in pitch is always much less than half an octave.

At present there is no generally accepted explanation for the shifts in pitch with level. Given this, it seems that the existence of these pitch shifts cannot be used to draw any strong conclusions about theories of pitch.

D   General conclusions on the pitch perception of pure tones

Several lines of evidence suggest that place mechanisms are not adequate to explain the frequency discrimination of pure tones. Contrary to the predictions of place theories, the DLF does not vary with frequency in the same way as the critical bandwidth. Also, the DLF for short-duration tones is smaller than predicted by place theories except for frequencies above 5 kHz. This suggests that the DLF is determined by temporal mechanisms at low frequencies and by place mechanisms at high frequencies. The perception of sequences of pure tones also changes above 4–5 kHz. It seems that a sequence of tones only evokes a sense of musical interval or melody when the tones lie below 4–5 kHz, in the frequency range where temporal mechanisms probably operate.

4 THE PITCH PERCEPTION OF COMPLEX TONES

As was stated earlier in this chapter, the classical place theory has difficulty in accounting for the perception of complex tones. For such tones the pitch does not, in general, correspond to the position of maximum excitation on the basilar membrane. A striking illustration of this is provided by the 'phenomenon of the missing fundamental'. Consider, as an example, a sound consisting of short impulses (clicks) occurring 200 times per second. This sound has a low pitch, which is very close to the pitch of a 200 Hz pure tone, and a sharp timbre. It contains harmonics with frequencies 200, 400, 600, 800 . . . etc. Hz. However, it is possible to filter the sound so as to remove the 200 Hz component, and it is found that the pitch does not alter; the only result is a slight change in the timbre of the note. Indeed, we can eliminate all except a small group of midfrequency harmonics, say 1800, 2000 and 2200 Hz, and the low pitch still remains, although the timbre is now markedly different.

Schouten (1940) called this low pitch associated with a group of high harmonics the residue. He pointed out that the residue is distinguishable, subjectively, from a fundamental component which is physically presented or from a fundamental which may be generated (at high sound pressure levels) by nonlinear distortion in the ear. Thus it seems that the perception of a residue pitch does not require activity at the point on the basilar membrane which would respond maximally to a pure tone of similar pitch. This is confirmed by a demonstration of Licklider (1956) which showed that the low pitch of the residue persists even when the low-frequency channels are masked with low-frequency noise. Thus it seems that low pitches may be perceived via those neural channels that normally respond to the high or middle frequency components of a signal. Several other names have been used to describe residue pitch, including 'periodicity pitch', 'virtual pitch' and 'low pitch'. We shall use the term residue pitch. We shall see later that even when the fundamental component of a complex tone is present, the pitch of the tone is usually determined by harmonics other than the fundamental. Thus the perception of a residue pitch should not be regarded as unusual. Rather, residue pitches are what we normally hear when we listen to complex tones.

Several models have been proposed to account for residue pitch. These models may be divided into two broad classes. The first class (which we will call 'pattern recognition' models) assumes that the pitch of a complex tone is derived from neural signals corresponding to more primary sensations, such as the pitches of the individual partials. The second class of model assumes that pitch is based on time interval measurement. In particular, it has been suggested that the pitch of a complex tone is related to the time interval between corresponding points in the fine structure of the signal close to adjacent envelope maxima (Schouten *et al.*, 1962). If nerve firings tend to occur at these points (i.e. phase locking occurs), then this time interval will be present in the time pattern of neural impulses. Let us examine each class of model in more detail.

A   Pattern recognition models

Pattern recognition models propose that the perception of the pitch of a complex tone involves two stages. The first stage is a frequency analysis which determines the frequencies of some of the individual sinusoidal components of the complex tone. The second stage is a pattern recognizer which determines the pitch of the complex from the frequencies of the resolved components. Early models of this type were rather vague about the exact way in which the pattern recognizer might work, but a common idea was that it tried to find a fundamental frequency whose harmonics matched the frequencies of the resolved components of the stimulus as closely as possible (Thurlow, 1963; Whitfield, 1967, 1970).

These theories were inadequate in the sense that they did not state exactly what components of a complex stimulus are important in determining the pitch of the complex as a whole. For example, Whitfield (1970) said that "pitch is related to some weighted average of all the components", and that "the way in which this average is taken is complex". To see why this point is important consider the experiments of Schouten *et al.* (1962). They investigated the pitch of amplitude modulated sine waves, which have just three sinusoidal components. If a 'carrier' of frequency f_c is amplitude modulated by a modulator with frequency g, then the modulated wave contains components with frequencies $f_c - g$, f_c, and $f_c + g$ (see Chapter 3, section 2E). For example, a 2000 Hz carrier modulated 200 times per second contains components at 1800, 2000 and 2200 Hz, and has a pitch which is similar to that of a 200 Hz sine wave.

Consider now the effect of shifting the carrier frequency to, say, 2040 Hz. The complex now contains components at 1840, 2040 and 2240 Hz. This stimulus would be very unlikely to occur naturally; how will the pattern recognizer choose the appropriate matching pattern? One possibility is that pitch is determined on the basis of the spacing between adjacent partials, in which case the pitch would be unaltered. On the other hand, the partials correspond to the 46th, 51st and 56th harmonics of a 40 Hz fundamental, and so an appropriate matching stimulus would have the same pitch as a 40 Hz sinusoid. In fact, the perceived pitch, in this particular case, corresponds roughly to that of a 204 Hz sinusoid. In addition, there is an ambiguity of pitch, so that matches around 185 Hz and 227 Hz are also found.

A model to account for this effect has been proposed by Walliser (1968, 1969a–c). His model does not specify the mechanisms by which the pitch of a complex tone will be perceived, but provides a rule for determining the residue pitch of complex tones. There are two parts to the rule: (1) The pitch corresponding to the frequency difference between neighbouring partials (i.e. the envelope repetition rate) is approximately determined. This may be inferred from the pitch differences between adjacent partials (for high repetition rates where partials are well separated), or it may be determined from 'the roughness sensation' (for low repetition rates where the partials are closely spaced). The 'roughness sensation' seems to be related to fluctuations in the envelope of the stimulus. (2) A subjective subharmonic of the lowest present partial is found, such that the pitch of this subharmonic lies as close as possible to the pitch determined in (1). A subharmonic has a frequency which is obtained by dividing the original frequency by an integer.

To illustrate the working of the rule consider again the example discussed above, of a complex tone with components at 1840, 2040 and 2240 Hz. The envelope repetition rate, which is the same as the spacing between adjacent partials, is 200 Hz. The lowest partial is 1840 Hz, and the subharmonic of this which lies closest to 200 Hz is 204.4 Hz (1840 divided by 9). This corresponds closely to the perceived pitch.

Terhardt (1972a,b) has modified and elaborated this model, suggesting that a residue pitch will always be a subharmonic of a dominant partial rather than simply the lowest partial. By dominant he meant "partials which are resolvable", i.e. which can be heard out from the complex as a whole. Terhardt suggested that these dominant partials lie in the frequency region between 500 and 1500 Hz. According to this model, then, a residue pitch will only be heard when at least one partial can be resolved from the complex. When the partials are too close together in frequency, they will no longer be resolvable, and no residue pitch should be heard.

Terhardt (1974) has extended this model still further to include a learning phase. Since speech frequently contains harmonic complex tones (see Chapter 8), we are repeatedly exposed to such tones from the earliest moments in life. Terhardt suggested that as a result of this exposure we learn to associate a given frequency component with the subharmonics of that component; these will occur together in harmonic complex sounds. After the learning phase is completed, stimulation by a single pure tone produces pitch cues corresponding to subharmonics of that tone. When a harmonic complex tone is presented, the pitch cues corresponding to these subharmonics coincide at certain values. The largest number of coincidences occurs at the fundamental frequency and this determines the overall pitch of the sound. This is illustrated in Table 5.1, for a complex tone consisting of three components: 800, 1000 and 1200 Hz.

Table 5.1.   Frequencies of the subharmonics of the components in a harmonic complex tone.

Frequency of component Hz			Value of integer divisor
800	1000	1200	
400	500	600	2
266.7	333.3	400	3
200	250	300	4
160	*200*	240	5
133.3	166.7	*200*	6

It may be seen that the greatest number of coincidences in the subharmonics occurs at 200 Hz, which corresponds to the perceived pitch. For nonharmonic complex tones, such as those used by Schouten *et al.* (1962), there are no exact coincidences, but the frequency at which there are several near coincidences predicts the perceived pitch quite well. Notice that this model requires that more than one partial can be analysed from the complex tone in order for a residue pitch to be perceived.

An alternative model, although one still dependent on the resolution of individual frequency components in a complex tone, has been presented by Goldstein (1973). In this model the pitch of a complex tone is derived by a central processor which receives information only on the frequencies, and not on the amplitudes or phases, of individual components. The processor presumes that all stimuli are periodic and that the spectra comprise successive harmonics (which is the usual situation for naturally occurring sounds). The processor finds the harmonic series which provides the 'best fit' to the series of components actually presented. For example, if we present components at

1840, 2040 and 2240 Hz (as in the experiment by Schouten and co-workers described above), then a harmonic complex tone with a fundamental of 204 Hz would provide a good 'match'; this would have components at 1836, 2040 and 2244 Hz. The perceived pitch is in fact close to that of a 204 Hz sinusoid. According to this model, errors in estimating the fundamental occur mainly through errors in estimating the appropriate harmonic number. In the above example the presented components were assumed by the processor to be the 9th, 10th and 11th harmonics of a 204 Hz fundamental. However, a reasonable fit could also be found by assuming the components to be the 8th, 9th and 10th harmonics of a 226.7 Hz fundamental, or the 10th, 11th and 12th harmonics of a 185.5 Hz fundamental. Thus the model predicts the ambiguities of pitch which are actually observed for this stimulus; pitch matches tend to lie in three groups around 186, 204 and 227 Hz. The extent to which such multimodal pitch matches occur is predicted to depend upon the accuracy with which the frequencies in the stimulus are represented at the input to the central processor.

All of the models which we have described in this section depend on the spectral resolution of individual components in the stimulus. It is predicted that no residue pitch will be heard if no frequency components can be resolved or 'heard out' from the complex. We will discuss the experimental evidence relating to this in section 5A. The mechanism by which individual partials would be analysed from a complex tone has not generally been specified, although Terhardt (1972a,b) has suggested that this could operate via an extended place principle, and that the basic determinant of the pitch of a complex sound is the spatial pattern of activity on the basilar membrane. This is not a necessary assumption for these models. Indeed Goldstein (1973) was careful to state that

> ... the concept that the optimum processor operates on signals representing the constituent frequencies of complex-tone stimuli does not necessarily imply the use of tonotopic or place information per se as the measure of frequency. For example, temporal periods of pure tones are not ruled out as the measure of frequency.

As we saw in section 3, there is quite good evidence that temporal mechanisms play a part in our perception of pure tones, at least for frequencies up to 5 kHz. Thus, it is likely that the analysis of partials from a complex tone, and the determination of their pitches, relies at least in part on temporal mechanisms. Given this assumption, these models could still hold, but the basic data on which they operated would be the temporal patterns of firing in different groups of auditory neurones. We shall discuss later some of the experimental evidence which is relevant to these models. Let us now turn to the second main type of model – the 'temporal' models.

B Temporal models

Consider again the example of a pulse train of repetition rate 200/s, containing harmonics at 200, 400, 600 ... Hz. The lower harmonics in this sound are analysed into effectively separate locations on the basilar membrane, and the timing of the neural firings derived from these locations relates to the frequencies of those harmonics rather than to the repetition rate of the complex as a whole. However, the patterns of vibration on the basilar membrane corresponding to the higher harmonics overlap to some extent, so that the waveform on the basilar membrane results from the interference of a number of harmonics, and shows a periodicity the same as that of the input waveform. The timing of neural impulses derived from such a region is related to the repetition rate of the original input waveform. This is illustrated in Fig. 5.4 (see also Fig. 1.10).

These considerations lead to a theory whose development is mainly due to Schouten (1940, 1970). We summarize below the major points of his theory.

1. The ear analyses a complex sound into a number of components each of which is separately perceptible.
2. Some of these components correspond with individual partials present in the input waveform. These components have a pure tone quality.
3. One or more components may be perceived which do not correspond with any individual sinusoidal oscillation, but which are a collective manifestation of some of those oscillations which are not or are scarcely individually perceptible. These components (residues) have an impure, sharp tone quality.
4. The ear ascribes a pitch to a residue by virtue of the periodicity of the total waveform of the harmonics which are responsible for this residue.
5. The pitch ascribed to a complex sound is the pitch of that component to which the attention, by virtue either of its loudness or of its contrast with former sounds, is most strongly drawn.

In general, the residue is the most prominent component in a complex sound, and thus the pitch of the whole sound will be given by the pitch of the residue. We see, then, how a low pitch may be signalled through those neural channels which normally respond to the high or middle frequency components of a complex sound.

Notice a major difference between this model and the pattern recognition models, such as Terhardt's model. The pattern recognition models require that one or more partials in the complex sound should be resolvable from the complex in order for a low residue pitch to be heard, whereas Schouten's model requires that at least two partials are interacting in order for the

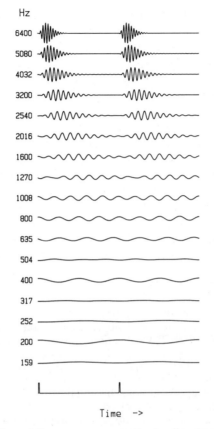

FIG. 5.4 A simulation of the responses on the basilar membrane to periodic impulses of rate 200 pulses per second. Each number on the left represents the frequency which would maximally excite a given point on the basilar membrane. The waveform which would be observed at that point, as a function of time, is plotted opposite that number. This figure can be compared with Fig. 1.10, which represents the envelope of responses to the same stimulus.

residue to be heard. And according to Schouten's model, a residue pitch may still be heard when none of the individual partials is separately perceptible.

Consider how Schouten's model deals with the complex tone which we discussed earlier in relation to the pattern recognition models; this contained components of 1840, 2040 and 2240 Hz. If we compare the waveform of this signal and the waveform of a signal containing components at 1800, 2000 and 2200 Hz, we see that, while the envelope repetition rates are the same, the time interval between corresponding peaks in the fine structure of the

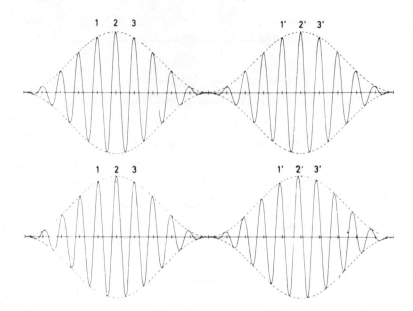

FIG. 5.5 Waveforms for two amplitude-modulated sine waves. In the upper waveform the carrier frequency (2000 Hz) is an exact multiple of the modulation frequency (200 Hz). Thus the time intervals between corresponding peaks in the fine structure, 1-1', 2-2', 3-3', are 5 ms, the period of the modulation frequency. In the lower waveform the carrier frequency is shifted slightly upwards. Thus, 10 complete cycles of the carrier occur in slightly less than 5 ms, and the time intervals between corresponding points on the waveform, 1-1', 2-2', 3-3', are slightly shorter than 5 ms. The lower waveform has a slightly higher pitch than that of the upper. From Plomp (1968), by permission of the author.

waveform is slightly different (see Fig. 5.5). Since these signals contain only a narrow range of frequency components, the waveforms on the basilar membrane would not be greatly different from those of the physically presented signals; the basilar membrane would not separate the individual components to any great extent. Thus, if nerve firings tend to occur at peaks in the fine structure of the waveform close to envelope maxima, the timing of the nerve impulses will convey slightly different pitches for the two stimuli. These differences in the time pattern of neural impulses have been observed by Javel (1980).

Nerve spikes can occur at any of the prominent peaks in the waveform, labelled 1, 2, 3 and 1', 2', 3'. Thus the time intervals between successive nerve spikes fall into several groups, corresponding to the intervals 1–1', 1–2', 1–3', 2–1', etc. This can account for the fact that the pitches of these stimuli are ambiguous. For the signal containing components at 1840, 2040 and 2240 Hz, one of these time intervals would correspond to a pitch of about 204 Hz, which is what is normally reported.

We see that it is necessary to refine Schouten's original theory, particularly with respect to point 4. The pitch of the residue is determined by the time interval between peaks in the fine structure of the waveform (on the basilar membrane) close to adjacent envelope maxima. If more than one possible time interval is present, the pitch corresponds, in general, to the interval which is most prominent, although sometimes ambiguity of pitch may occur. If we consider the representation of the signal on a neural level, in terms of the time pattern of nerve firings, then, just as was the case for pure tones, the time intervals between nerve firings rather than the overall rate of firing will be important. If the system were simply counting the number of impulses per second, then the pitch shifts observed by Schouten and co-workers would not have occurred.

5 EXPERIMENTAL EVIDENCE RELEVANT TO THE PATTERN RECOGNITION AND TEMPORAL MODELS

A The 'existence region' of the tonal residue

According to the pattern recognition theories, a residue pitch should only be heard when at least one of the sinusoidal components of the stimulus can be heard out. Thus a residue pitch should not be heard for stimuli containing only very high unresolvable harmonics. Ritsma (1962) investigated the audibility of residue pitches, for amplitude-modulated sinusoids containing three components, as a function of the modulation rate and the harmonic number (carrier frequency divided by modulation rate). Later (Ritsma, 1963) he extended the results to complexes with a greater number of components. He found that the tonal character of the residue pitch existed only within a limited frequency region, referred to as the 'existence region'. When the harmonic number was too high (above about 20), only a kind of high buzz of undefinable pitch was heard. He found, further, that some harmonics below 5 kHz had to be present for a residue pitch to be heard, and that the modulation rate had to be below about 800 Hz. Other workers (Plomp, 1967; Moore, 1973b) have found, using complex tones with a greater number of components, that residue pitches can be perceived for repetition rates up to about 1400 Hz.

Consider the implications of these results for the pattern recognition models. In Chapter 3 we discussed Plomp's (1964a) experiments which showed that for a partial within a multi-tone complex only the first 5–8 harmonics are separately perceptible, although the limit was somewhat higher for two-tone complexes. Since Ritsma (1962) found a tonal residue for complexes which only contained harmonics around the 20th, it would seem that under some conditions a residue pitch can be heard when none of the individual components is separately perceptible. We can describe these results in terms of the critical band concept; roughly speaking, components separated by a critical bandwidth or more will not interact, and will be separately perceptible, whereas components within a critical bandwidth will interact and will not produce separate pitches. Ritsma's results seem to indicate that a residue pitch can be heard when the components do not fall in separate critical bands and so should not be separately perceptible. However, this interpretation has been questioned. It is likely that Ritsma's results were influenced by the presence of combination tones in the frequency region below the lowest components in the complex tones, as has since been pointed out by Ritsma himself (1970).

A combination tone may be defined as a perceived tone not present in the sensations produced by the constituent components of the stimulus when they are presented singly. Certain combination tones, which were briefly mentioned in Chapter 1 (section 5D), have pitches corresponding to frequencies $f_1 - K(f_2 - f_1)$, where f_1 and f_2 are the frequencies of the tones which are physically presented and K is an integer. They correspond to lower partials of the complex which is physically presented. For example, if two tones with frequencies 1800 Hz and 2000 Hz are presented, the combination tone for $K = 1$ will have a frequency of 1600 Hz ([2 × 1800] − 2000). Combination tones of this type, and particularly those with a pitch corresponding to frequency $2f_1 - f_2$, have been shown to be audible even at moderate intensities (Plomp, 1965; Goldstein, 1967). Smoorenburg (1970) suggested that these combination tones, rather than the physically presented partials, are dominant in determining the pitch of a complex tone containing only high harmonics. Thus, in Ritsma's experiments, the effective harmonic number would have been lower than the nominal harmonic number.

Moore (1973b) carried out a series of experiments in an attempt to determine more clearly whether a residue pitch can be heard when no individual components are resolvable. He first determined that the lowest partial in a multitone complex was more easily audible than any of the other partials. In fact, it was about as easily audible as a partial in a two-tone complex. He then determined the audibility of the lowest partial in a multitone complex as a function of the frequency separation of the partials. A condition was included where a band of noise was present in the frequency region below the lowest partial. This band would have masked any combination tones present. The functions relating audibility to separation were then compared with the frequency separation of the harmonics for which a complex tone produced a well defined residue pitch, using the same set of subjects. Again a 'noise' condition was included, so that combination tones in the frequency region below the lowest presented partial could not influence the results. Moore found that, for high harmonic numbers, there was a range of conditions over which a residue pitch could be heard when none of the individual partials would have been separately perceptible.

Moore and Rosen (1979) investigated subjects' abilities to identify simple melodies which were 'played' by varying the repetition rate of pulse trains. The pulse trains were filtered so as to contain only high, unresolvable harmonics, and a low frequency noise was present to mask combinations tones. In order to determine whether these stimuli evoked a sense of musical interval, performance was compared with that obtained when the tunes were played as a pattern of sinusoidal frequencies in which the pitch changes were clearly audible, but the musical intervals had been distorted; the musical scale was either 'compressed' or 'expanded'. This preserves the pitch contour but makes the musical intervals sound 'wrong'. Moore and Rosen found that performance was superior for the highpass filtered pulse trains, and concluded that stimuli containing only high, unresolvable harmonics can evoke a sense of musical interval, and hence of pitch. The pattern recognition models cannot account for this. We should note, however, that the pitch of highpass filtered pulse trains is much less clear than that heard when lower harmonics are present.

B   The principle of dominance

According to pattern recognition theories, the lower resolvable harmonics are the most important for determining pitch. For temporal theories the higher, unresolved harmonics are the most important, since interference of harmonics is essential for the extraction of residue pitch. Ritsma (1967a) carried out an experiment to determine which components in a complex sound are most important in determining its pitch. He presented complex tones in which the frequencies of a small group of harmonics were multiples of a fundamental which was slightly higher or lower than the fundamental of the remainder. The subject's pitch judgements were used to determine whether the pitch of the complex as a whole was affected by the shift in the group of harmonics. Ritsma found that:

> For fundamental frequencies in the range 100 Hz to 400 Hz, and for sensation levels up to at least 50 dB above threshold of the entire signal, the frequency band consisting of the third, fourth and fifth harmonics tends to dominate the pitch

sensation as long as its amplitude exceeds a minimum absolute level of about 10 dB above threshold.

Thus Ritsma introduced the concept of dominance:

> ... if pitch information is available along a large part of the basilar membrane the ear uses only the information from a narrow band. This band is positioned at 3–5 times the pitch value. Its precise position depends somewhat on the subject. (Ritsma, 1970)

This finding has been broadly confirmed in other ways (Ritsma, 1967b; Bilsen and Ritsma, 1967), although the data of Moore et al. (1984, 1985c) show that there are large individual differences in which harmonics are dominant, and for some subjects the first two harmonics play an important role. Other data also show that the dominant region is not fixed in terms of harmonic number, but also depends somewhat on absolute frequency (Plomp, 1967; Patterson and Wightman, 1976). For high fundamental frequencies (above about 1000 Hz), the fundamental is usually the dominant component, while for very low fundamental frequencies, around 50 Hz, harmonics above the fifth may be dominant (Moore and Glasberg, 1988b).

On the whole, these results support the pattern recognition theories. The 3rd, 4th and 5th harmonics are relatively well resolved on the basilar membrane, and are usually separately perceptible. On the other hand, the overlap of vibration patterns on the basilar membrane would also be sufficient to provide temporal information about the periodicity of the input waveform. Thus, in the dominant region, both spectral and temporal analyses would appear to be possible. It is should also be noted that for very low fundamental frequencies, around 50 Hz, the dominant region appears to lie above the 5th harmonic. For centre frequencies above 250 Hz, the critical bandwidth is greater than 50 Hz, so that individual components in the dominant region would not be resolvable (Moore and Glasberg, 1988b).

C Evidence for the role of central mechanisms in the perception of complex tones

Houtsma and Goldstein (1972) conducted perhaps the first experiment which demonstrates that a residue pitch may be heard when there is no possibility of an interaction of components in the cochlea. They investigated the perception of stimuli which comprised just two harmonics with successive harmonic numbers, e.g. the fourth and fifth harmonics of a (missing) fundamental. On each trial, subjects were presented with two successive two-tone complexes with different (missing) fundamentals, and were required to identify the musical interval corresponding to the fundamentals. Harmonic numbers were randomized from note to note, so that the subjects could not use cues associated with the pitches of individual harmonics in order to extract the musical interval. They found that performance was good for low harmonic numbers, but fell to chance level for harmonic numbers above about 10–12. They found further that subjects were able to identify melodies when the stimuli were presented dichotically (one harmonic to each ear). At high sound levels, monaural performance was superior to dichotic, whereas at low levels (20 dB SL) there was no difference between the two conditions. Houtsma and Goldstein suggested that the differences at high levels resulted from the influence of combination tones, which would lower the effective harmonic number. They considered that if an allowance were made for the effect of combination tones, then there would be essentially no difference between the monaural and dichotic conditions.

These results cannot be explained in terms of Schouten's model, or indeed in terms of any model which requires an interaction of components on the basilar membrane. They imply that "the pitch of these complex tones is mediated by a central processor operating on neural signals derived from those effective stimulus harmonics which are tonotopically resolved" (Houtsma and Goldstein, 1972). In other words, these experiments clearly indicate that the pitch of a complex tone can be mediated by some sort of pattern recognition process. However, it is not yet entirely clear that the findings apply to the pitches of complex tones in general. The pitch of a two-tone complex is not very clear; indeed, many observers do not hear a single low pitch, but rather perceive the component tones individually (Smoorenburg, 1970). Residue pitches are generally much more distinct when greater numbers of harmonics are present. It does seem to be the case that two-tone complexes only produce a residue pitch for harmonic numbers below about 10, whereas the limit is somewhat higher for multitone complexes (Ritsma, 1962; Moore, 1973b; see section 5A). Thus some factor other than our ability to analyse individual components from complex tones affects the upper limit of the existence region.

Houtgast (1976) has reported an even more extreme example of hearing a residue pitch in the absence of interaction of components. He showed that, if a context was provided to focus the attention of the subject on pitches in a particular range, a single harmonic was capable of evoking the perception of a low residue pitch. He set up his experiment as follows. Subjects were presented with two successive harmonic complex signals which differed in fundamental frequency by 3%. On each trial the subject had to say whether the pitch of the second signal was higher or lower than that of the first. The signals did not have any harmonics in common, so that subjects could not simply listen to the pitches of the individual harmonics in order to perform the task. The first signal always contained six harmonics and had a clear unambiguous pitch. The second signal initially had three harmonics, but after a certain number of trials this number was reduced to two, and finally to one. In the absence of any background noise performance was very poor, and was at chance level (50%) for the one-component signal. Thus a single sinusoidal component in quiet does not lead to the percept of a residue pitch. However, when the experiment was conducted with a background noise, performance improved considerably; a score of 80% was obtained for the one-component signal. It appears that a single sinusoidal component has the potential to evoke subharmonic pitches. When the sensory information is made ambiguous, by the presence of a background noise, these potential pitches are more likely to be perceived. If the subject's attention is focused in a particular pitch range, then the subharmonic pitch in this range may be the dominant percept.

Yet another demonstration that interaction of components is not essential for the perception of a residue pitch is provided by an experiment of Hall and Peters (1981). They investigated the pitch associated with stimuli consisting of three harmonics which were presented successively in time rather than simultaneously. Each sinusoidal component lasted 40 ms, and there was a 10 ms pause between components. They found that, in the absence of a background noise, only pitches corresponding to the individual components were heard. However, when a background noise was present, pitches corresponding to the missing fundamental were heard. This result resembles that of Houtgast (1976), except that it was not necessary to provide a prior context to direct the subject's attention. It appears that noise enhances a synthetic mode of pitch perception, in which information is combined over different frequency regions and over time to produce a residue pitch. In quiet, an analytic mode of perception is more likely, so that the individual components are heard separately.

We may conclude, then, that the pitch of a complex tone can be derived from neural signals corresponding to individual partials in the complex, at least for stimuli with low harmonics and containing only a small number of harmonics. It is still not established whether the information about these partials is coded in terms of place or in terms of the temporal patterns of neural firing. Houtsma and Goldstein (1972) concluded that "all the constraints could conceivably be met by mechanisms based on either time or place information". But it is noteworthy that residue pitches are only observed when harmonics (or combination tones) are present with frequencies below about 5 kHz (Ritsma, 1962, 1963; Moore, 1973b). We saw earlier in this chapter that it is likely that temporal mechanisms are important in the perception of pure tones for frequencies up to about 5 kHz, but that above this only place mechanisms could operate. Thus, residue pitches are only heard when harmonics are present in the frequency region where temporal information is available.

D Pitches based upon purely timing information

A number of workers have investigated pitches evoked by stimuli which contain no spectral peaks, and which therefore would not produce a well-defined maximum on the basilar membrane. Such pitches presumably cannot arise on the basis of place information, and so provide evidence for the operation of temporal mechanisms.

Miller and Taylor (1948) presented random white noise that was turned on and off abruptly and periodically, at various rates, by an electronic switch. Provided care is taken to eliminate switching transients (clicks), the interrupted noise has a flat long-term magnitude spectrum. They reported that the noise had a pitch-like quality for interruption rates between 100 and 250 Hz. Pollack (1969) has shown that some subjects are able to adjust sinusoids to have the same pitch as the interrupted noise for interruption rates up to 2000 Hz. They adjust the frequency of the sinusoid to be roughly equal to the interruption rate of the noise.

Burns and Viemeister (1976, 1981) showed that noise that was sinusoidally amplitude modulated had a pitch corresponding to the modulation rate. As for interrupted noise, the long-term magnitude spectrum of white noise remains flat after modulation. They found that the pitch could be heard for modulation rates up to 800–1000 Hz, and that subjects could recognize musical intervals and melodies played by varying the modulation rate.

These experiments support the idea of a temporal pitch mechanism in the auditory system. However, the pitch of interrupted noise or of modulated noise is not very clear. This could be because it is only the envelope which is periodic. The fine structure of the waveform differs from one envelope period to the next. Many subjects do not report a pitch sensation at all, although most can hear that something pitch-like changes when the interruption rate is changed. This phenomenon, that a pitch is heard more clearly if it is varied, seems to be quite a general one, and is often marked for residue pitches.

A number of experiments have been reported showing pitch sensations as a result of the binaural interaction of noise stimuli. Huggins and Cramer (1958) fed white noise from the same noise generator to both ears, via headphones. The noise to one ear went through an allpass filter, which passed all audible frequency components without change of amplitude, but produced a phase change in a small frequency region. A faint pitch was heard corresponding to the frequency region of the phase transition, although the stimulus presented to each ear alone was white noise, and produced no pitch sensation. The effect was only heard when the phase change was in the frequency range below about 1 kHz. A phase shift of a narrow band of the noise results in that band being heard in a different position in space from the rest of the noise (see Chapter 6). This spatial separation presumably produces the pitch-like character associated with that narrow band.

Fourcin (1970) used two noise sources, which we shall denote n_1 and n_2. n_1 was fed via headphones to the two ears, producing a sound image localized in the middle of the head. n_2 was also fed to both ears, but the input to one ear was delayed by a certain time, T, producing a second sound image localized to one side (see Chapter 6). Sometimes the observer simply heard two separate sound images, neither of which had a pitch. At other times, however, a faint pitch was heard, whose position was not well defined, but which was generally heard in the middle of the head. When the observed pitches were matched to pure tones (of frequency f), the matches could be described by a function of the form $1/T = 4f/3$.

Bilsen and Goldstein (1974) reported that a pitch may be perceived when just one noise source is used, presented binaurally, but with a delay at one ear. For delays shorter than about 2 ms a single noise image is reported, whose perceived position depends on the delay. For longer time delays the image remains at the side of the head and becomes more diffuse, and, in addition, "a faint but distinct pitch image corresponding to $1/T$ appears in the middle of the head". As for the pitches reported by Fourcin, the effect only occurs at low frequencies; the highest pitches reported by Bilsen and Goldstein correspond to frequencies of about 500 Hz.

The exact mechanism which gives rise to these pitches remains to be elucidated. In all three of the experiments producing pitches by binaural interaction, the stimuli presented to each ear separately conveyed no spectral information. Therefore, timing information must be used in the creation of a central pattern of neural activity from which the pitch is extracted. In other words, information about the relative phases of components in the two ears must be preserved up to the point in the auditory system where binaural interaction occurs. We shall see in Chapter 6 that we are only able to use phase differences between the two ears in the localization of sounds for frequencies up to about 1500 Hz, and it seems that pitches perceived by binaural interaction are limited to this region. The necessity for binaural interaction means that there is no good reason to regard 1500 Hz as a limit for temporal coding in general.

A feature of all these pitches is that they are very faint, and indeed many observers do not hear them at all. They may arise from the operation of a mechanism which is not normally involved in pitch extraction, but is primarily concerned with the localization of sound, and the extraction of signals from noise. Indeed, one of the models put forward to explain the pitches of these stimuli, and to account for the factor of 4/3 which was found in Fourcin's experiments (Bilsen and Goldstein, 1974), is based on Durlach's equalization and cancellation model, which is a model designed to account for the detection of signals in noise under binaural listening conditions (see Chapter 6). Nordmark (1970) has pointed out there are many similarities in the systems involved in pitch and localization, especially when periodic stimuli are used. The relationship of the faint pitches heard with noise stimuli to the much clearer pitches observed in situations where spectral information is available is not, at the moment, clear.

6   A SCHEMATIC MODEL FOR THE PITCH PERCEPTION OF COMPLEX TONES

It is now quite clear that the perception of a particular pitch does not depend on a high level of activity at a particular place on the basilar membrane, or in a particular group of peripheral neurones. The pitch of complex tones is, in general, mediated by harmonics higher than the fundamental, so that similar pitches may arise from quite different distributions of neural activity. For stimuli containing a wide range of harmonics, the low harmonics, up to the 5th, tend to dominate the pitch percept. These harmonics lie in the range where it is possible to resolve and hear them out as separate entities. This supports the pattern recognition models of pitch perception. However, it is possible to hear a residue pitch when the harmonics are too high to be resolved. This cannot be explained by the pattern recognition models, but can be explained by the temporal models. The temporal models, on the other hand, cannot account for the fact that it is possible to hear a residue pitch when there is no possibility of the components of the complex tone interacting in the peripheral auditory system.

It seems that none of the theories presented so far can account for all of the experimental data. We next present a schematic model which incorporates features of both the temporal models and the pattern recognition models, and which can account, in a qualitative way, for all of the data. Since this model was proposed, in the first and second editions of this book (1977, 1982), several similar models have been presented, some of which are more quantitative (e.g. van Noorden, 1982; Patterson, 1987b; Meddis and Hewitt, 1988). The model is illustrated in Fig. 5.6. The first stage in the model is a bank of bandpass filters with continuously overlapping centre frequencies. These are the auditory filters or critical bands. The outputs of the filters in response to a complex tone have the form shown in Fig. 5.4. The filters responding to low harmonics have outputs which are approximately sinusoidal in form; the individual harmonics are resolved. The filters responding to

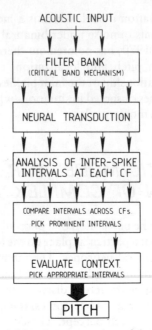

ACOUSTIC INPUT

FILTER BANK
(CRITICAL BAND MECHANISM)

NEURAL TRANSDUCTION

ANALYSIS OF INTER-SPIKE
INTERVALS AT EACH CF

COMPARE INTERVALS ACROSS CFs.
PICK PROMINENT INTERVALS

EVALUATE CONTEXT.
PICK APPROPRIATE INTERVALS

PITCH

FIG. 5.6   A schematic model for the perception of the pitch of complex tones. The model depends upon both place and timing information.

higher harmonics have outputs corresponding to the interaction of several harmonics. The waveform is complex, but has a repetition rate corresponding to that of the input.

The next stage in the model is the transduction of the filter outputs to neural impulses. The temporal pattern of firing in a given neurone reflects the temporal structure of the waveform driving that neurone. Say, for example, that the input has a fundamental frequency of 200 Hz. The fourth harmonic, at 800 Hz, is well resolved in the filter bank, and hence the neurones with CFs close to 800 Hz respond as if the input were an 800 Hz sinusoid. The time intervals between successive nerve impulses are multiples of the period of that tone, i.e. 1.25, 2.5, 3.75, 5.0 . . . ms (see Fig. 1.17). Neurones with higher CFs, say around 2000 Hz, are driven by a more complex waveform. The temporal structure of the response is correspondingly complex. Each peak in the fine structure of the waveform is capable of evoking a spike, so that many different time intervals occur between successive spikes. The interval corresponding to the fundamental, 5 ms, is present, but other intervals, such as 4.0, 4.5, 5.5 and 6.0 ms, also occur (Evans, 1978; Javel, 1980).

The next stage in the model is a device which analyses, separately for each CF, the interspike intervals which are present. The range of intervals which can be analysed is probably limited, and varies with CF. At a given CF the device probably operates over a range from about 0.5/CF to 15/CF seconds. This range is appropriate for the time intervals which would occur most often.

The next stage is a device which compares the time intervals present in the different channels, and searches for common time intervals. The device may also integrate information over time. In general the time interval which is found most often corresponds to the period of the fundamental component. Finally the time intervals which are most prominently represented across channels are fed to a decision mechanism which selects one interval from among those passed to it. This device incorporates memory and attention processes, and may be influenced by immediately preceding stimuli, context, conditions of presentation, and so on. The perceived pitch corresponds to the reciprocal of the final interval selected.

Consider how this model deals with a complex tone composed of a few low harmonics, say the 3rd, 4th and 5th harmonics of a 200 Hz (missing) fundamental. In those neurones responding primarily to the 600 Hz component, an analysis of time intervals between successive nerve firings would reveal intervals of 1.67, 3.33, 5.0, 6.67 . . . ms, each of which is an integral multiple of the period of that component. Similarly the intervals in the 800 Hz 'channel' are 1.25, 2.5, 3.75, 5.0 . . . ms, while those in the 1000 Hz 'channel' are 1, 2, 3, 4, 5 . . . ms. The only time interval which is in common across all of the channels is 5 ms; this corresponds to the pitch of the missing fundamental. Thus this stimulus will evoke a clear, unambiguous pitch.

Consider next what happens when a small group of high harmonics is presented, say the 12th, 13th and 14th harmonics of 200 Hz. These harmonics are not resolved in the filter bank, and so essentially only one channel of timing information is available. Furthermore, the time interval information is ambiguous, many values closely spaced around 5 ms being present. Thus, while a pitch corresponding to the missing fundamental may be perceived, that pitch is weak and ambiguous, as is observed psychophysically. This can explain why lower harmonics tend to dominate in the perception of pitch; the temporal information they provide is far less ambiguous, provided that information is combined across channels. The pitch associated with high harmonics can be made more clear by increasing the number of harmonics, since the ambiguities can be reduced by comparing across channels. This also is observed psychophysically.

If a small group of very high harmonics is presented, then they may fail to evoke a sense of musical pitch. This can be explained in terms of the limited range of time intervals which can be analysed at each CF. For harmonics above about the 15th, the time interval corresponding to the fundamental falls outside the range which can be analysed in the channel responding to those harmonics. This is one factor contributing to the limited existence region of the tonal residue (section 5A). The other factor is the absolute upper limit for phase locking. When the harmonics lie above 5 kHz the fine structure of the waveform at the filter output is no longer preserved in the temporal patterning of neural impulses. Thus the later stages of analysis of interspike intervals do not reveal the regularities necessary to determine the fundamental.

The way in which this model determines the pitch for a group of low harmonics resembles that proposed by Terhardt (1974). In his model each partial gives rise to potential pitches corresponding to subharmonics of that partial, and the perceived pitch is that for which the number of coincidences is greatest. In our model these subharmonic pitches correspond to the interspike intervals evoked by a given partial. For example, a 1 kHz tone evokes intervals of 1, 2, 3, 4, 5 ... ms, and these correspond to pitches of 1000, 500, 333.3, 250, 200 ... Hz. The differences between the models are as follows: Terhardt's model requires a learning phase in which the associations between partials and subharmonics are learned, whereas in our model the subharmonics occur automatically in the temporal patterns of neural firing. Secondly, Terhardt's model cannot explain the pitch produced by high, unresolved harmonics, whereas in our model they arise as part of the same process as is used for lower harmonics.

The way that our model deals with the pitch of nonharmonic complex tones depends on the spacing of the components relative to their centre frequency. If the components are widely spaced, and therefore resolvable, the pitch of the complex is determined in a similar way to that proposed by Terhardt. Say, for example, that components at 840, 1040 and 1240 Hz are presented. The time intervals in the 840 Hz channel will be 1.19, 2.38, 3.57, 4.76, 5.95 ... ms, all of which are integral multiples of the period, 1.19 ms. Similarly, the intervals in the 1040 Hz channel are 0.96, 1.92, 2.88, 3.85, 4.8, 5.76 ... ms, and those in the 1240 Hz channel are 0.81, 1.61, 2.42, 3.22, 4.03, 4.84 ... ms. In this case there is no time interval which is exactly the same in all channels, but there is a near coincidence at 4.8 ms, the intervals in the three channels being 4.76, 4.8 and 4.84 ms. The perceived pitch thus corresponds to the reciprocal of 4.8 ms, i.e. 208 Hz. When the components are closely spaced, and therefore unresolvable, then the pitch is derived from the time interval which is most prominently represented in the pattern of neural impulses evoked by the complex. In this case our model works in the same way as the temporal model outlined in section 4B. The perceived pitch corresponds to the time interval between peaks in the fine structure of the waveform (at the output of the auditory filter) close to adjacent envelope maxima. The pitch is ambiguous since several 'candidate' time intervals may be present.

In our model, just as in the other models we have discussed, combination tones may play a role in determining the pitch percept. Their role may be particularly important when the stimulus itself contains only closely spaced components. The combination tones act like lower partials, and are more resolvable than the partials physically present in the stimulus.

The pitches of stimuli without spectral peaks, such as periodically interrupted noise, are explained by the model as arising from the time interval information present primarily in the channels with high CFs, where the filter bandwidths are wider. When a filter has a wide bandwidth, the temporal structure of the input tends to be preserved at the output (see Chapter 1, section 4 and Fig. 1.5, and Chapter 4). Thus the temporal patterns of firing reflect the interruption of the noise. However, the time intervals between successive nerve impulses are much less regular than for a periodic sound, since the exact waveform of the noise varies randomly from moment to moment; the only regularity is in the timing of the envelope, not the fine structure. Thus the pitch of interrupted noise is weak.

The simple model we have presented does not account for the pitches which arise from a combination of the information at the two ears. However, it can easily be extended to do this by making the following reasonable assumptions. There is a separate filter bank, transduction mechanism and interval analyser for each ear. There is also a device determining interaural time intervals for spikes in channels with corresponding CFs (see Chapter 6). The results of the separate interval analysis for each ear, and of the interaural interval analysis, are fed to a common central interval comparator and decision mechanism.

In summary, the model we have presented can account for the major features of the pitch perception of complex tones, including the dominant region, the existence region of the residue, the pitch of nonharmonic complexes, and pitches produced by binaural interaction. Furthermore, it is consistent with the evidence presented earlier in this chapter that the pitch of pure tones is determined primarily by temporal mechanisms for frequencies up to 5 kHz. Notice, however, that both place and temporal analysis play a crucial role in the model; neither alone is sufficient.

7 THE PERCEPTION OF PITCH IN MUSIC

Since this topic could easily occupy a book of its own, we limit ourselves to discussing certain selected aspects related to the rest of this chapter. Other relevant material will be found in Chapter 7.

A   Octaves, musical intervals and musical scales

It has been known for very many years that tones which are separated by an octave (i.e. where the frequencies are in the ratio 2:1) have an essential similarity, and indeed are given the same name (C, D, etc.) in the traditional musical scale. It is also the case that other musical intervals correspond to simple ratios between the frequencies of the tones. For example, a fifth corresponds to a frequency ratio of 3:2; a major third to 5:4; and a minor third to 6:5. When musical notes in these simple ratios are sounded simultaneously, the sound is pleasant, or consonant, whereas departures from simple, integral ratios, as in certain progressive modern music, tend to result in a less pleasant or even a dissonant sound. This does not always hold for pure tones, a pair of which tend to be judged as consonant as soon as their frequency separation exceeds a critical bandwidth (Plomp and Levelt, 1965). However, complex tones blend harmoniously and tend to produce chords only when their fundamental frequencies are in simple ratios. In this situation several of their harmonics will coincide, whereas for nonsimple ratios the harmonics will differ in frequency, and produce beating sensations. Thus at least part of the dissonance may be explained in terms of this beating, or interference, of harmonics on the basilar membrane when the harmonics are close together, but not identical, in frequency. This cannot account for the whole of the effect, however; a pronounced dissonance from two mistuned pure tones may be heard when the tones are presented one to each ear. It is of interest, then, to consider why we prefer certain frequency ratios, for both the simultaneous and successive presentation of tones; why octaves sound so similar; and why some sounds are consonant and others dissonant.

One type of theory suggests that we learn about octave relationships and about other musical intervals by exposure to harmonic complex sounds (usually speech sounds) from the earliest moments in life. For example, the first two harmonics in a periodic sound have a frequency ratio 2:1, the 2nd and 3rd have a ratio 3:2, the 3rd and 4th 4:3, etc. Thus by exposure to these sounds we learn to associate harmonics with particular frequency ratios. We discussed earlier in this chapter Terhardt's (1974) suggestion that such a learning process could account for the perception of residue pitch. If judgements of similarity and of consonance or dissonance also depend upon familiarity, then a learning process will also account for our perception of musical intervals (Terhardt, 1974).

An alternative theory suggests that we prefer pairs of tones for which there is a similarity in the time patterns of neural discharge. This view was put forward as early as 1898 by Meyer, and has since been supported by Boomsliter and Creel (1961), among others. If it is the case that the pitch of a complex tone results from an analysis and correlation of the temporal patterns of firing in different groups of auditory neurones, then such an analysis would also reveal similarities between different tones when they are in simple frequency ratios. It is certainly the case that both our sense of musical pitch and our ability to make octave matches largely disappear above 5 kHz, the frequency at which neural synchrony no longer appears to operate (see section 3B). Furthermore, the highest note (fundamental) for instruments in the orchestra lies just below 5 kHz. One could argue from this that our lack of musical pitch at high frequencies is a result of a lack of exposure to tones at these frequencies. However, notes produced by musical instruments do contain harmonics above 5 kHz, so that if the learning of associations between harmonics were the only factor involved, there would be no reason for the change at 5 kHz.

It is of interest that the musical scale in general use today does not consist of notes in exact simple ratios. The common scale, the equal temperament (ET) scale, enables musicians to play in any key they choose, whereas with a system involving simple ratios only one key could be used. In the ET scale the octave (which still corresponds to a frequency ratio of $2:1$) is divided into 12 equal logarithmic steps, known as semitones. Each successive semitone has a frequency about 5.9% higher than its neighbour. The deviations from a simple ratio scale are small, although they are probably great enough to produce noticeable increases in the beating of harmonics of simultaneously presented complex tones at several points in the scale. For example, the musical interval of a perfect fifth corresponds to a frequency ratio of $3:2$. On the ET scale the ratio is $2.9966:2$.

While simple ratios may be preferable for simultaneously presented tones, it is not clear whether this is the case for tones presented successively. A number of experiments investigating preferred notes in performances on stringed instruments of various kinds have shown that there is no simple answer. Some workers have found preferences for simple ratios, while others have found that the preferred scale corresponds fairly closely to ET, except that notes higher than the tonic or keynote tend to be sharpened relative to that note. Boomsliter and Creel (1963) asked musicians to play familiar tunes on a monochord, a one-stringed instrument with continuously variable tuning. They found that while subjects consistently chose the same tuning for a given note within a given tune, they chose different tunings, for what is ostensibly the same note, in different melodies and in different parts of the same melody. However, Boomsliter and Creel found that the chosen patterns formed a structure of small whole number ratios to the tonic and to additional reference notes linked by small whole number ratios to the tonic. Thus within small groups of notes simple ratios are preferred, although the 'reference' point may vary as the melody proceeds.

Whether or not there is something inherently preferable about simple frequency ratios, it is clear that individual differences and cultural background can influence significantly the musical combinations that are judged to be 'pleasant' or otherwise. Thus, for example, Indian musical scales contain 'microtones' in which the conventional scale is subdivided into smaller units, producing many musical intervals which do not correspond to simple ratios. Indian music often sounds strange to Western ears, especially on first hearing, but it clearly does not sound strange to Indians; indeed, the microtones, and the various different scales which can be composed from them, are held to add considerably to the richness of the music and to the variety of moods which it can create.

While there is a psychoacoustic basis for consonance and dissonance judgements, these judgements also display individual differences and follow changes in the cultural norm. Modern classical music, for example, by Stravinsky and Stockhausen, contains many examples of chords which would have been considered dissonant 20 years ago but which are now enjoyed by many people.

B   Absolute pitch and tone deafness

Some people have the ability to recognize and name the pitch of a musical tone without reference to a comparison tone. This faculty is called absolute pitch, and is quite rare, probably occurring in less than 1% of the population. It seems to be distinct from the ability which some people develop to judge the pitch of a note in relation to, say, the lowest note which they can sing. Rakowski (1972) investigated absolute pitch by asking observers to adjust a variable signal so as to have the same pitch as a standard signal, for various time delays between the standard and variable tones. He used two groups of subjects, one group having been specially selected for their possession of absolute pitch. For long time delays the subjects without absolute pitch showed a marked deterioration in performance, presumably because the pitch sensation stored in memory was lost. The subjects with absolute pitch seemed able to recall this memory with the aid of their 'imprinted' pitch standards, so that only a small decrement in performance was observed. When the standard tone belonged to the normal musical scale (e.g. $A_2 = 110$ Hz) there was hardly any decrement in performance with increasing time delay. The subjects did not seem able to acquire new standards and never, for example, learned to remember a 1000 Hz tone 'as such'; it was always recalled as being a little lower than C_6. Attempts to improve absolute pitch identification by intensive training have met with some success (Cuddy, 1968), but the levels of performance achieved rarely equal those found in genuine cases of absolute pitch. It seems likely that absolute pitch is a faculty acquired through 'imprinting' in childhood a limited number of standards. Ward (1963a,b; 1970) has suggested that the converse is true; we may all start with a sense of absolute pitch, but the ability is trained out of us because we are reinforced for relative and not absolute pitch judgements. The limited success achieved by training in adulthood tends, at the moment, to favour the idea of some sort of imprinting.

The term 'tone deafness' is a misnomer, since nearly everyone is able to judge that two tones are different in pitch when their frequency difference exceeds a certain amount. Many people, on the other hand, have difficulty in reproducing (i.e. singing) musical notes or sequences of notes, often because the notes fall outside the normal range which they would produce in speaking. It is likely that practice effects, and musical experience in general, have a considerable influence on this ability. A second difficulty commonly experienced by naive listeners is that of assigning a direction to a pitch change; they can often hear that two tones are different, but they cannot decide which is the higher in pitch. These people show a considerable improvement with practice, and it is usually found that listeners who claim to be tone deaf are eventually able to make very fine frequency discriminations. Beckett and Haggard (1973) did, however, find large differences in initial discrimination level between self-assessed musical and nonmusical subjects, and it is of interest why such large differences arise. Very probably both genetic and environmental factors are involved.

8 GENERAL SUMMARY

In this chapter we have discussed how the pitches of stimuli are related to their physical properties, and to the anatomical and physiological properties of the auditory system. In principle, there are two ways in which the frequency of a sound may be coded; by the distribution of activity across different auditory neurones and by the temporal patterns of firing within and across neurones. It is likely that both types of information are utilized but that their relative importance is different for different frequency ranges and for different types of sounds.

The neurophysiological evidence in animals indicates that the synchrony of nerve impulses to a particular phase of the stimulating waveform disappears above 4–5 kHz. Above this frequency our ability to discriminate changes in the frequency of pure tones diminishes, and our sense of musical pitch disappears. It is likely that this reflects our use of temporal information in the frequency range below 4–5 kHz.

For complex tones two classes of theories have been popular. Temporal theories suggest that the pitch of a complex tone is derived from the time intervals between successive nerve firings evoked at a point on the basilar membrane where adjacent partials are interfering with one another. Pattern recognition theories suggest that pitch is derived by a central processor operating on neural signals corresponding to the individual partials present in the complex sound. In both theories, combination tones in the frequency region below the lowest partial may influence the pitch percept.

The pattern recognition theories are supported by the finding that low, resolvable, harmonics tend to dominate in the perception of pitch, and by the finding that a pitch corresponding to a 'missing fundamental' can be perceived when there is no possibility of an interference of partials on the basilar membrane. This has been demonstrated by presenting partials dichotically, one to each ear, or successively in time. The temporal theory is supported by the finding that (weak) pitches can be perceived when the harmonics are too close in frequency to be resolvable, and also when the stimuli have no well-defined spectral structure (e.g. interrupted noise). Thus neither of the theories can account for all of the experimental results.

We have proposed a model which incorporates features of both the temporal and the pattern recognition models. The model assumes that a complex stimulus first passes through a bank of filters (critical bands) with continuously overlapping centred frequencies. The outputs of the filters produce activity in neurones with corresponding CFs. The temporal pattern of activity in each 'channel' is analysed by a device which measures the time intervals between successive nerve impulses. Then a comparator or correlation device searches across channels looking for common time intervals. The prominent time intervals are fed to a decision device which selects among the intervals. The perceived pitch corresponds to the reciprocal of the interval selected, and will usually be the same as the pitch corresponding to the fundamental component. This model can account for the majority of experimental results presented in this chapter.

Certain aspects of the perception of music may be related to the basic mechanisms underlying pitch perception. There is some evidence, for example, that we prefer musical intervals, or pairs of tones, for which there is a similarity in the time patterns of neural discharge. On the other hand it is clear that early experience, individual differences and cultural background also play a significant role in such judgements.

FURTHER READING

The following contain quite extensive reviews of the perception of pitch, although they come to slightly different conclusions from those reached in this chapter:

de Boer, E. (1976). On the 'residue' and auditory pitch perception. In *Handbook of*

Sensory Physiology, Vol. 5 (eds W. D. Keidel and W. D. Neff). Springer-Verlag, Berlin.

Plomp, R. (1976). *Aspects of Tone Sensation*. Academic Press, London and New York.

A more recent review, concentrating on the role of frequency selectivity in pitch perception is:

Moore, B. C. J. and Glasberg, B. R. (1986). The role of frequency selectivity in the perception of loudness, pitch and time. In *Frequency Selectivity in Hearing* (ed. B. C. J. Moore), Academic Press, London.

The following collection of edited chapters reviews many aspects of the perception of music. The chapters by Rasch and Plomp and by Burns and Ward are especially relevant to this chapter:

Deutsch, D. (1982). *The Psychology of Music*. Academic Press, New York.

Demonstrations 12, 13, 15, 17, 20, 21, 22, 23, 25 and 26 of *Auditory Demonstrations on CD* are relevant to this chapter (see the list of further reading for Chapter 1).

6
Space perception

1 INTRODUCTION

The ability to localize sound sources is of considerable importance to both humans and animals; it determines the direction of objects to seek or to avoid, and indicates the appropriate direction to direct visual attention. The precision of sound localization is remarkable, particularly for brief sounds, or for those occurring in noisy or reverberant surroundings. While the most reliable cues used in the localization of sounds depend upon a comparison of the signals reaching the two ears, there are also phenomena of auditory space perception which result from monaural processing of the signals.

The term 'localization' refers to judgements of the direction and distance of a sound source. Sometimes, when headphones are worn, the sound image is located inside the head. The term 'lateralization' is used to describe the apparent location of the sound source within the head. Headphones allow precise control of interaural differences and eliminate effects related to room echoes. Thus lateralization may be regarded as a laboratory version of localization which provides an efficient means of studying direction perception.

While our binaural abilities are important for the accurate localization of sounds, this is not their only function. Using two ears, we are able to attend selectively to sounds coming from a particular direction while effectively excluding other sounds. This ability is particularly important in noisy surroundings, or when there are several sound sources competing for our attention.

As well as being able to judge the direction of a sound source, we are able, in some cases, to estimate its distance. This ability is particularly developed in blind people, who can use information from echoes and reflections to determine the positions of objects in the environment.

For some sorts of tasks, listening with two ears conveys only a small advantage over listening with one ear. Examples are: the detection of signals in quiet; intensity discrimination; and frequency discrimination.

2 THE LOCALIZATION OF PURE TONES

The cues which enable us to localize sounds may vary depending on the nature of these sounds. We consider first steady sinusoidal sounds. Later on we discuss a much more common class of sounds: those which are discontinuous or contain transients.

Consider a sinusoidal sound source located to one side of the head. The sound reaching the farther ear will be delayed in time and will be less intense relative to that reaching the nearer ear. There are thus two possible cues as to the location of the sound source. However, owing to the physical nature of the sounds, these cues are not equally effective at all frequencies. Low-frequency sounds have a wavelength which is long compared with the size of the head, and thus the sound 'bends' very well around the head. This process is known as diffraction, and the result is that little or no 'shadow' is cast by the head. On the other hand, at high frequencies, where the wavelength is short compared with the dimensions of the head, little diffraction occurs. A 'shadow', almost like that produced by a beam of light, occurs. Interaural differences in intensity are negligible at low frequencies, but may be as large as 20 dB at high frequencies. This is easily illustrated by placing a small transistor radio close to one ear. If that ear is now blocked with a finger, only sound bending around the head and entering the other ear will be heard. The sound will be much less 'tinny', since high frequencies will have been attenuated more than low; the head effectively acts like a lowpass filter. Interaural intensity differences are thus more important at high frequencies than at low.

If a tone is delayed at one ear relative to the other, there will be a phase difference between the two ears; thus, if nerve impulses occur at a particular phase of the stimulating waveform, the relative timing of the nerve impulses at the two ears will be related to the location of the sound source. However, for sounds whose wavelength is comparable with or less than the distance between the two ears, there will be ambiguity. The maximum path difference between the two ears is about 23 cm, which corresponds to a time delay of about 690 μs (see Fig. 6.1). Ambiguities occur when the half-wavelength of the sound is about 23 cm, i.e. when the frequency of the sound is about 750 Hz. A sinusoid of this frequency lying to one side of the head produces waveforms at the two ears which are in opposite phase (phase difference between the two ears of 180°). From the observer's point of view the location of the sound source is now ambiguous, since the waveform at the right ear might be either a half-cycle behind that at the left ear or a half-cycle ahead. Head movements, or movements of the sound source, may resolve this ambiguity, so that there is no abrupt upper limit in our ability to use phase

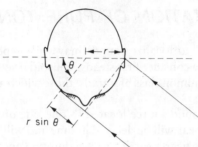

FIG. 6.1 Illustrating the difference in arrival time at the two ears for a distant sound source at an angle θ radians to the observer. If we denote the radius of the head (about 9 cm) by r, then the path difference d between the two ears is given by

$$d = r\theta + r\sin\theta$$

For a sound directly to one side of the observer, $\theta = \pi/2$ radians and $d =$ $(9 \times \pi/2) + (9 \times \sin \pi/2) = 23$ cm. Since sound takes about 30 μs to travel 1 cm, the corresponding time delay is about 690 μs.

differences between the two ears. However, when the wavelength of the sound is less than the path difference between the two ears, the ambiguities increase; the same phase difference could be produced by a number of different source locations. For periodic sounds, phase differences only provide useful cues for frequencies below about 1500 Hz.

In a classic study, Stevens and Newman (1936) investigated the localization of tone bursts with smooth onsets and offsets for observers on the roof of a building, so that reflected sounds were minimized. The listeners had to report the direction of the source, in the horizontal plane, to the nearest 15°. Although left–right confusions were rare, a low-frequency sound in front was often indistinguishable from its mirror image behind. If these front–back confusions were discounted, then the error rate was low at very low and very high frequencies, and showed a maximum for mid-range frequencies (around 3000 Hz for Stevens and Newman's data). These data were taken to indicate two different mechanisms for sound localization, one operating best at high frequencies and one at low. For middle frequencies neither mechanism operates efficiently, and errors are at a maximum.

These results have been broadly confirmed by more recent experiments (Sandel *et al.*, 1955) using anechoic chambers, except that systematic biases have been found in addition to errors; there is a tendency to underestimate the deviation of the source from the median plane (the plane connecting points which are equally distant from the two ears) when the frequency of the tone is between 1500 and 5000 Hz. When these systematic errors are eliminated, the greatest uncertainty in localization occurs at a frequency of about 1500 Hz. Sandel and co-workers also used an arrangement of two loudspeakers such that the resultant combined tone led in phase at one ear, but had a greater intensity in the other. They found that the sound was located towards the side with the phase lead for frequencies below about 1500 Hz and towards the side with greater intensity for frequencies above this. Near 1500 Hz listeners were confused.

These experiments confirm that the extent to which the cues of interaural time and intensity differences are used in the localization of pure tones is strongly related to what would be predicted from the physical nature of these cues. Intensity differences are more important at high frequencies, while phase differences only provide usable cues for frequencies below about 1500 Hz. Experiments using headphones (Mills, 1960) have shown that we are able to detect differences in intensity at the two ears even for low frequencies, and that these differences can produce a sense of location to one side. The smallest detectable difference for low frequencies is, however, larger than would occur in real life except under exceptional circumstances (e.g. holding a telephone close to one ear).

The idea that sound localization is based on interaural time differences at low frequencies and interaural intensity differences at high frequencies has been called the 'duplex theory' and it dates back to Lord Rayleigh (1907). While it appears to hold for pure tones, we shall see later that it does not apply for complex sounds.

3 BINAURAL BEATS

A phenomenon which seems to be closely related to the ability of the auditory system to process phase differences at the two ears is that of binaural beats. These may occur when a tone of one frequency is presented to one ear and a tone of slightly differing frequency is presented to the other ear. The sound appears to fluctuate or warble at a rate corresponding to the frequency difference between the two tones. Binaural beats are quite different from the physical beats which are produced when the two frequencies are mixed in an electrical or acoustical system. Such physical beats or monaural beats occur because the two frequencies are alternately in phase and out of phase, and thus alternately cancel and reinforce one another; the intensity fluctuates at a rate equal to the frequency difference between the two tones. Binaural beats, on the other hand, depend upon an interaction in the nervous system of the neural output from each ear. They provide a demonstration that the discharges of neurones in the auditory nerve preserve information about the phase of the acoustic stimulus. Neural spikes tend to occur at a particular phase of the stimulating waveform. At points in the auditory system where the signals from the two ears are combined, the trains of neural spikes from the two ears will superimpose differently depending on the relative phase of the stimuli at the two ears. There is thus a neural basis for the subjective fluctuations which occur when the relative phase at the two ears fluctuates, as it does when tones with slightly different frequencies are presented to the two ears.

Since binaural beats differ in their origin from monaural beats, it is hardly surprising that the two kinds of beats differ subjectively; binaural beats are never as distinct as monaural beats. In addition, Licklider *et al.* (1950) pointed out that there is a continuum of subjective effects associated with binaural beats depending on the frequency separation of the two tones. As the frequency separation is slowly increased from zero, the listener may hear a tone that periodically shifts in subjective location; then fluctuates in loudness; then seems 'rough'; and finally separates into two subjectively smooth tones. Monaural beats can be observed over the entire audible frequency range, whereas binaural beats are essentially a low-frequency phenomenon. Estimates of the highest frequency for which binaural beats can be observed have varied. The beats are heard most distinctly for frequencies between 300 and 600 Hz, but become progressively more difficult to hear at high frequencies. The exact upper limit depends both upon the intensity and the experimental technique used, but it is generally agreed that the beats are exceedingly difficult to hear for frequencies above 1000 Hz (Licklider *et al.*, 1950). Monaural beats are most distinctly heard when the two tones are matched for intensity, and cannot be heard when the intensities of the two tones differ greatly. Binaural beats, however, can be heard when there are large differences in intensity at the two ears (Tobias, 1963) and may even be heard when the tone to one ear is below absolute threshold (Groen, 1964). This is consistent with physiological evidence that phase locking occurs over a wide range of stimulus intensities.

One interesting feature of binaural beats is that the upper limit of the frequency at which they are perceived is higher for men than for women. Further, the upper limit for women changes with the menstrual cycle, so that just at the onset of menstrual flow the upper limit for women approaches that of men (Tobias, 1965; Haggard and Bates, 1974). These changes are presumably related to hormonal variations and variations in retained body fluid, both of which could affect nerve transmission.

4   THE LOCALIZATION OF TRANSIENTS

All sounds which occur in nature have onsets and offsets, and many also change their intensity or their spectral structure as a function of time. Interaural differences in the time of arrival of these transients provide cues for localization which are not subject to the phase ambiguities which occur for steady tones.

The detectability of interaural time differences is usually measured in a two alternative forced choice task. The stimuli delivered in the two observation intervals differ in interaural timing. For example, one stimulus might be identical at the two ears (zero interaural time delay), while the other stimulus might have an interaural time delay ΔT. The task of the subject is to say whether the first stimulus was to the left or the right of the second stimulus. In other words, the task is to identify a *shift* in location associated with a change in interaural timing.

A   The acuity of lateralizing transients

Klump and Eady (1956) measured thresholds for discriminating interaural time differences using stimuli delivered via headphones. They compared three types of stimuli: band-limited noise (containing frequencies in the range 150–1700 Hz); 1000 Hz pure tones with gradual rise and fall times; and clicks of duration 1 ms. The first stimulus varies continuously as a function of time, and thus provides transient information which is repeated many times during the presentation time of the stimulus; the pure tone provides only information relating to ongoing phase differences; while the click is effectively a single transient. The threshold interaural time differences were 9 μs, 11 μs and 28 μs. Note that an interaural time difference of 10 μs corresponds to a shift in space of about 1° in the lateral direction. Thus the greatest acuity occurred for the noise stimulus, with continuously available transient information, but the tone gave performance which was only slightly worse. The single click gave rise to the poorest performance. It is worth noting, however, that the tones in this experiment were of relatively long duration (1.4 s). For tones of shorter duration, acuity is not so great, so that cues related to onset and offset transients (which would be comparable to those provided by the clicks) become relatively more important.

For sounds with ongoing transient disparities, such as bursts of noise, the ability to detect interaural time differences improves with duration of the bursts for durations up to about 700 ms, when the threshold disparity (the smallest detectable time difference at the two ears) reaches an asymptotic level of about 6 μs (Tobias and Zerlin, 1959). It is remarkable that such small time differences between the ears are detectable, since the 'jitter' in the instant of initiation of nerve impulses has a standard deviation of about 100 μs at 1 kHz. Tobias (1972) has discussed some of the ways in which this accuracy might be achieved, including the possibility that there is a direct neural pathway from one cochlea to the other.

B   Acuity as a function of frequency

Stimuli such as noises and clicks contain energy over a wide range of frequencies. Yost *et al.* (1971) attempted to determine which frequency components were the most important, by studying the lateralization of clicks whose frequency content had been altered by filtering. The subjects were asked to discriminate a centred image (produced by identical clicks at each ear) from a displaced image (produced by delaying the click to the left ear only). They found that discrimination deteriorated for clicks which were highpass filtered, so that only energy above 1500 Hz was present, but was largely unaffected by lowpass filtering. Masking with a lowpass noise produced a marked disruption, while a highpass noise had little effect. Thus it seems that the discrimination of lateral position on the basis of time delays between the two ears depends largely on the low-frequency content of the clicks, although somewhat poorer discrimination is possible with only high frequency components.

This finding ties in rather well with the results obtained with pure tones, showing that we cannot compare phases between the two ears for frequencies above 1500 Hz. When a click is presented to the ear, it produces a waveform, at a given point on the basilar membrane, looking rather like a decaying sinusoidal oscillation (see Fig. 1.11). The frequency of the oscillation depends on which part of the basilar membrane is being observed; at the basal end the frequency is high and at the apical end it is low. For frequencies below 1500 Hz, the phases of these decaying oscillations at the two ears can be compared, thus conveying accurate information about the relative timing of the clicks at the two ears. For frequencies above 1500 Hz this 'fine-structure' information is lost; only timing information relating to the envelope of the decaying is available for binaural processing, thus reducing the accuracy with which clicks can be localized.

Henning (1974) has provided further evidence for the importance of the amplitude envelope. He investigated the lateralization of high-frequency tones which had been amplitude modulated (see Fig. 3.4 for an illustration of this waveform). He found that the detectability of interaural delays in the envelope of a 3900 Hz carrier modulated at a frequency of 300 Hz was about as good as the detectability of interaural delays in a 300 Hz pure tone. However, there were considerable differences among individual observers; the interaural delays necessary for 75% correct detections in his forced choice task had values of 20, 50 and 65 μs for three different subjects (all stimuli had 250 ms durations and 50 ms rise–fall times). Henning found that time delay of the envelope rather than time delay of the 'fine structure' within the envelope determines the lateralization. The signals could be lateralized on the basis of time delays in the envelope even when the carrier frequencies were different in the two ears. Thus it seems that for complex signals containing only high-frequency components, listeners extract the envelopes of the signals and compare the relative timing of the envelopes at the two ears. However, lateralization performance is best when the carrier frequencies are identical, and poor lateralization results when the complex waveforms at each ear have no frequency component in common. Thus factors other than the envelope can affect lateralization performance.

C   Onset disparities versus ongoing disparities

Tobias and Schubert (1959) investigated the relative importance of onset disparities and ongoing disparities in lateralization judgements by pitting one against the other. They presented bursts of noise via headphones, with a particular onset time difference, and determined the amount of ongoing disparity needed to counteract the onset information and recentre the subjective image. They found that small ongoing disparities offset much larger transient onset disparities and that for durations exceeding 300 ms the onset has no effect. Even for short bursts (10 ms) the ongoing disparity has the greater effect. For very short impulsive sounds the importance of onset disparity is much greater; for brief clicks this is the only kind of disparity. It is worth noting that for high-frequency pure tones the ongoing phase differences at the two ears are not processed by the auditory system. However, these tones can still be lateralized on the basis of onset transient disparities.

D   The phenomenon of binaural adaptation

Hafter and his colleagues (Hafter *et al.*, 1983, 1988) have recently demonstrated a form of adaptation which appears to be specific to binaural processing. They investigated the lateralization of trains of clicks which

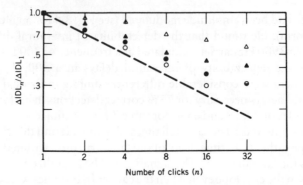

FIG. 6.2 Thresholds for detecting an interaural difference in level are plotted as a function of the number of clicks, n, in the click train. Each threshold for n clicks (ΔIDL_n) is plotted relative to the threshold for a single click (ΔIDL_1); a log scale is used. The different symbols show data for different interclick intervals: 10 ms (solid circles), 5 ms (open circles), 2 ms (solid triangles) and 1 ms (open triangles). The dashed line has a slope of -0.5 and indicates where the points would lie if each click in the train provided an equal amount of information for localization. From Hafter *et al.* (1983) by permission of the authors and *J. Acoust. Soc. Am.*

contained energy only over a limited range of high frequencies, typically around 4 kHz. They measured thresholds for detecting interaural time differences or interaural intensity differences as a function of the number of clicks in the train (n) and the interval between successive clicks (I). A sample of their results is shown in Fig. 6.2. When I was 10 ms, giving a click rate of 100/s, the thresholds decreased progressively with increasing n. The thresholds were inversely proportional to $\sqrt{n}$, which implies that all the clicks in the train provided an equal amount of information (Green and Swets, 1974). However, when I was 1 ms, giving a click rate of 1000/s, the threshold decreased only slightly with increasing n. This implies that the first click provided much more information than the subsequent clicks. The results for values of I between 1 and 10 ms showed that clicks after the first provided progressively less information as I was decreased.

In summary, for high click rates, the binaural system appears to process only the onset of the click train; it is as if there is a rapid adaptation at high click rates, so that clicks after the first convey little information for localiz-ation. The higher the click rate, the faster is the adaptation. Note that the later clicks can still be heard, even though they do not result in an improvement in localization.

Hafter *et al.* (1988) have presented evidence that a suitable 'trigger' stimulus can produce a release from adaptation. Clicks presented after the trigger are more effective for localization than clicks immediately before the trigger. Among suitable triggers are a brief low-intensity burst of noise, a brief tone burst, and a gap in the click train. Hafter and co- workers argued that the recovery from adaptation was the result of an 'active release' rather than a simple decay of the adaptation. They suggested that:

> It is as though the auditory system becomes increasingly insensitive to interaural cues past the stimulus onset while continuing to monitor for signs of new conditions. When one occurs, the slate is wiped clean and the spatial environment is sampled again.

From this point of view, the triggers described above are successful in producing a release from binaural adaptation because they signal that a change has occurred.

5 THE CONE OF CONFUSION AND THE ROLE OF HEAD MOVEMENTS

If we ignore, for the moment, the influence of the pinnae, then we may regard the head as a pair of holes separated by a spherical obstacle. If the head is kept stationary, then a given interaural time difference will not be sufficient to define uniquely the position of the sound source in space; there is a cone of confusion such that any sound source on the surface of this cone would give rise to the same interaural time difference (see Mills, 1972, and Fig. 6.3).

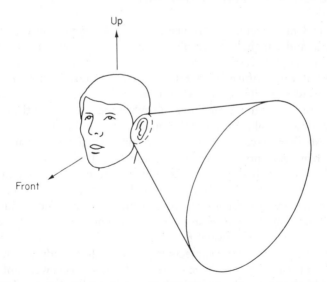

FIG. 6.3 A cone of confusion for a spherical head and a particular interaural time delay. All sound sources on the surface of the cone would produce that interaural time delay. For details of how to calculate the cone of confusion see Mills (1972).

Ambiguities related to the cone of confusion, or to the location of a sound source in the vertical direction, may be resolved by head movements. If we rotate our heads about a vertical axis by, say, 20°, and this results in a 20° shift in the apparent lateral position of the auditory image in relation to the head, then we locate the sound source in the horizontal plane. If the rotation of the head is accompanied by no change in the auditory image, then the sound is located either directly above or directly below the observer. Intermediate shifts in the location of the auditory image lead to intermediate vertical height judgements (Wallach, 1940).

Hirsh (1971) has reviewed a number of experiments showing improved localization abilities when head movements are allowed. In many cases monaural localization was as good as binaural localization (e.g. Freedman and Fisher, 1968). This suggests that head movements provide cues other than changes in interaural time and interaural intensity. For complex sounds, such as white noise, movements of either the head or the sound source produce changes in the spectral patterning at each ear (see section 6), and these changes provide cues as to the extent and direction of the movement.

6 MONAURAL LOCALIZATION AND THE ROLE OF THE PINNAE

While head movements, or movements of the sound source, are clearly important and can help to resolve ambiguities in vertical direction, our abilities at judging vertical direction are far in excess of what would be predicted if only information related to head movements or interaural differences were available. For example, we are able to judge the location of a burst of white noise in the median plane when the duration of the burst is too short to allow useful information to be gained from head movements.

Many workers have suggested that the pinnae provide information which is used in judgements of vertical location (e.g. Butler, 1969) and for the discrimination of front from back, while others (e.g. Batteau, 1967; Freedman and Fisher, 1968) have suggested that the pinnae are important for localization in every direction. To investigate the role of the pinnae, Batteau inserted microphones into casts of actual pinnae held on a bar without a model of the head in between them. The sounds picked up by the microphones were played to the subjects via high fidelity headphones. Thus the subjects had remote but realistic outer ears! The subjects were able to make reasonably accurate judgements of both azimuth (left-front-right, etc.) and elevation. When the pinnae were removed from the microphones, judgements were quite erratic.

It is noteworthy that with the artificial pinnae in place subjects reported that the sounds were actually localized out 'in space' and not, as is usually the case with headphones, lateralized inside the head. This impression persisted even when one microphone was disconnected. Clearly, then, the pinnae provide some information as to the location of sound sources.

A number of other experiments have indicated that the pinnae can play a role in sound localization. Freedman and Fisher (1968) investigated the localization of short bursts of white noise presented in an acoustically treated room. They compared three conditions: (1) with subjects listening normally, (2) with sound conducted directly to the ears via 10 cm metal tubes and (3) with casts of pinnae on the ends of the tubes. If head movements were restricted there was no significant difference between (1) and (3), while both produced significantly more accurate localization than did (2). However, if head movements were allowed, there were no differences between the three conditions, all subjects achieving nearly perfect performance. While this experiment demonstrates pinna effects, the accuracy required was not great (22.5°), and the effects were not important when head movements were allowed. It is of interest that in condition (3) the casts were not of the subject's own pinnae. Pinnae differ considerably between people, and it would be of interest to know how far we are able to use, or to learn to use, information from other people's pinnae!

Gardner and Gardner (1973) investigated localization in the median plane for wideband noise and for bands of noise with various different centre frequencies. They found that occlusion of the pinnae cavities (filling them with moulded rubber plugs) decreased localization abilities, the largest effects occurring for wideband noise and for the bands of noise with highest centre frequencies (8 and 10 kHz). However, there was still some effect at 3 kHz.

It is now generally accepted that the pinnae modify the spectra of incoming sounds in a way that depends on the angle of incidence of the sound relative to the head. This has been confirmed by measurements at the entrance to the ear canal of human observers and by measurements using realistic models of the human head (Blauert, 1983; Oldfield and Parker, 1984). The head and pinna together form a complex direction dependent filter. The frequency bands which are boosted or reduced in level depend on the direction of sound incidence. The spectral changes produced by the head and pinna can be used to judge the location of a sound source. Since it is the spectral patterning of the sound which is important, the information provided by the pinnae is most effective when the sound has spectral energy over a wide frequency range. High frequencies, above 6 kHz, are especially important, since it is only at high frequencies that the wavelength of sound is sufficiently short for it to interact strongly with the pinna.

If both ears are stimulated with identical narrowband noise signals, the direction of the sound sensation depends upon frequency only, and not upon the direction of sound incidence (Blauert, 1969/1970). Similar results have been found by Butler (1971) for the localization of tone bursts with one ear occluded. The perceived direction of the sound source depends on frequency, rather than on the actual location of the sound source. This suggests that peaks in the spectrum are a major cue for localization. However, other evidence suggests that notches in the spectrum can also play an important role (e.g. Bloom, 1977), while some studies suggest that both peaks and notches are important (Watkins, 1978).

While the spectral changes produced by the pinnae are limited to frequencies above 6 kHz, modification of the spectrum of the stimulus may occur at much lower frequencies than this, because the head, as well as the pinnae, can affect the spectrum. The effects described by Blauert and by Butler were found for frequencies between 500 Hz and 16 kHz.

If the listener is to make efficient use of spectral cues associated with the direction of a sound source, then it is necessary to distinguish spectral peaks and dips related to direction from peaks and dips inherent in the character of the stimulus itself. Thus one might expect that a knowledge of the sound source and room conditions may also be important. To some extent, the two ears provide separate sets of spectral cues, so that the difference between the two ears could be used to locate unfamiliar sound sources. However, for sound sources in the median plane (i.e. sound sources which are equidistant from the two ears) the cues at the two ears are almost identical for all locations. Plenge (1972, 1974) has presented evidence that we do, in fact, make comparisons with stored stimulus patterns in judging the location of a sound source. He showed that if subjects were not allowed to become familiar with the characteristics of the sound source and the listening room, then localization was disturbed. In many cases the sound sources were lateralized in the head rather than being localized externally. This was particularly true for sound in the median plane. However, such familiarity does not seem to require an extended learning process. We become familiar with sound source characteristics and room acoustics within a very few seconds of entering a new situation.

7   THE PRECEDENCE EFFECT

In a normal listening environment the sound from a given source, such as a loudspeaker, reaches our ears via a number of different paths. Some of the sound arrives by a direct path, but a good deal of it only reaches our ears after one or more reflections from the surfaces of the room. In spite of this, we are not normally aware of these reflections, or echoes, and they appear to have

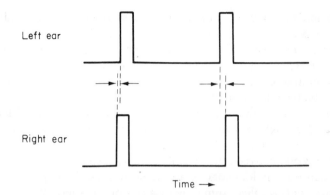

FIG. 6.4 The stimulus sequence used by Wallach *et al.* (1949) to investigate the precedence effect. The first pair of clicks arrive at the ears with a small interaural time disparity, indicated by the arrows. The second pair of clicks simulate a room echo and have a different interaural disparity. The whole stimulus sequence is heard as a single sound whose location is determined primarily by the interaural delay of the leading pair of clicks.

little influence on our judgements of the direction of the sound source. Thus we are still able accurately to locate a speaker in a reverberant room where the total energy in the reflected sound may be greater than that reaching our ears by a direct path.

Wallach *et al.* (1949) investigated the way the auditory system copes with echoes in experiments using both sound sources in free space and sounds delivered by headphones. In the experiments using headphones, pairs of clicks were delivered to each ear (two clicks in each earphone). The delay between the two clicks in a pair, and the time of arrival of the first click in a pair could be varied independently (see Fig. 6.4). Their results, and the results of more recent experiments, can be summarized as follows:

1. Two brief sounds that reach an observer's ears in close succession will be heard as a single sound if the interval between them is sufficiently short. The interval over which fusion takes place is not the same for all types of sounds. The upper limit of the interval is about 5 ms for single clicks, but may be as long as 40 ms for sounds of a complex character, such as speech or music.

2. If two brief sounds are heard as fused into a single sound, the location of the total sound is determined largely by the location of the first sound. This is known as the 'precedence effect', although it has also been called the 'Haas effect', after Haas (1951) and the 'law of the first wavefront' (Blauert, 1983). The effect is reflected in the finding that the ability to detect shifts in the location of the second sound (the echo) is reduced for a

short time following the onset of the first sound (Zurek, 1980; Perrott *et al.*, 1989).

3. The precedence effect is only shown for sounds of a discontinuous or transient character.

4. The second sound or echo can be shown to have a small but demonstrable influence. If the location of the second sound departs more and more from the location of the first sound, it 'pulls' the total sound along with it up to a maximal amount (about 7°) and then it becomes progressively less effective.

5. If the interval between the arrival of the two sounds is 1 ms or less, the precedence effect does not operate; some average or compromise location is heard. This is called 'summing localization' (Blauert, 1983).

6. If the second stimulus is made sufficiently intense (10–15 dB above the first sound), it overrides the precedence effect.

7. The precedence effect is favoured for sounds which are qualitatively similar; if the echo differs greatly from the leading sound, then fusion will not occur. In particular, the spectra of the leading sound and the echo should be similar (Divenyi and Blauert, 1987).

The precedence effect seems to be essentially a binaural phenomenon; it is the interaural differences in the leading sound which allow an accurate assessment of its location in the presence of echoes. The fusion effect itself also seems to depend on binaural interaction. A simple demonstration of this may be obtained by placing one finger in an ear while listening to a speaker in a reverberant room; immediately the characteristics of the room become more apparent. The sound becomes 'muddy' and booming, and it is difficult to locate the speaker accurately. Batteau (1968) has reported that filling the pinnae with silicone rubber produces an increase in subjective amount of reverberation, possibly indicating that the pinnae also play a role.

It is clear that the precedence effect plays an important role in our perception of everyday sounds. It enables us to locate, interpret and identify sounds in spite of wide variations in the acoustical conditions in which we hear them. Without it, listening in reverberant rooms would be an extremely confusing experience. Sometimes, on the other hand, the effect can be an inconvenience! An example of this is found in the stereophonic reproduction of music. Contrary to popular opinion, the stereo information on a record is coded almost entirely in terms of intensity differences in the two channels; time disparities are eliminated as far as possible. If the sound originates in one channel only, then the sound will be clearly located towards that channel. If the sound is equally intense in both channels, then the sound will be located in the centre, between the two channels, provided the loudspeakers are equidistant from the listener. If, however, the listener is slightly closer to one loudspeaker than to the other, the sound from that loudspeaker will lead in time, and if the time disparity exceeds 1 ms, the precedence effect will operate; the sound will appear to originate entirely from the nearer loudspeaker. In a normal room this gives the listener a latitude of about 60 cm on either side of the central position. Deviations greater than this produce significant changes in the 'stereo image'. Almost all of the sound (except that originating entirely from the farther loudspeaker) appears to come from the closer loudspeaker. Thus the notion of the 'stereo seat' is quite close to the truth.

8 TIME-INTENSITY TRADING

If identical clicks are presented to the two ears via headphones, then the sound source is usually located in the middle of the head; the image is said to be centred. If now the click in the left ear is made to lead that in the right ear by, say, 100 μs, the sound image moves to the left. However, by making the click in the right ear more intense, it is possible to make the sound image move back towards the right, so that once again the image is centred. Thus it seems possible to trade a time difference at the two ears for an intensity difference.

This finding led to the theory that time differences and intensity differences are eventually coded in the nervous system in a similar sort of way. In particular, it was suggested that the time required to evoke neural responses was shorter for more intense sounds, so that intensity differences were transformed into time differences at the neural level. Thus Deatherage and Hirsh (1957) stated:

> ... once the frame of reference becomes neural, we would hypothesize that intensity, having made its contribution to neural time, may drop out of consideration, leaving the judgement of localization almost entirely dependent upon results of comparison of neural time.

Many investigators have measured the value of the time-intensity trade, i.e. the amount of interaural time difference needed to offset a given interaural intensity difference. Its value is usually expressed in μs/dB. Reported values have varied from 1.7 μs/dB for pure tones (Shaxby and Gage, 1932), to 100 μs/dB for pulse trains (Christman and Victor, 1955). Harris (1960) measured the trading relation for clicks which had been highpass or lowpass filtered at various cutoff frequencies. He found that lowpass clicks, with cutoff frequencies below 1500 Hz, gave values of about 25 μs/dB, whereas highpass clicks gave values of about 90 μs/dB. He also noted that when an image is centred by offsetting an intensity difference with a time difference, the variability of the judgements is greater than when sounds equal in intensity are centred. Thus it seems that time differences and intensity differences may not be truly equivalent.

A number of workers have reported that, both for tones of low frequency and for clicks, observers may report two separate sound images. For tones, Whitworth and Jeffress (1961) found that one image, the 'time image', was little affected by interaural differences in level, and showed a trading ratio of about 1 μs/dB. The other, the 'intensity image', showed a trading ratio of about 20 μs/dB. For clicks, Hafter and Jeffress (1968) found ratios of 2–35 μs/dB for the 'time image', and 85–150 μs/dB for the 'intensity image'. Hafter and Carrier (1972) have confirmed that observers are able to detect differences between diotic signals (identical in each ear) and dichotic signals (different at the two ears) which have been centred by opposing a time difference with an intensity difference. Thus these experiments confirm that time and intensity differences are not truly equivalent.

Jeffress (1971) has suggested that there are at least two mechanisms underlying localization (and lateralization). One is affected by interaural differences in both level and time. It operates over the whole of the auditory frequency range and is responsible for the intensity image. The other is little affected by differences in level, but operates on interaural time differences over the frequency range below 1500 Hz. As discussed earlier, the localization of clicks on the basis of interaural time is most accurate when energy is present below 1500 Hz, since in that frequency range the timing of the 'fine structure' of the waveforms on the basilar membrane can be compared at the two ears. For frequencies above this, the fine structure information is lost, and only the envelopes of the waveforms on the basilar membrane can be compared. Physiological evidence (Kiang *et al.*, 1965) indicates that changes in the intensity of clicks produce relatively little change in the timing of phase-locked neural responses; firings still occur at a particular phase of the waveform on the basilar membrane. However, relatively more responses tend to occur on the first few deflections of the basilar membrane (recall that a click produces a waveform resembling a decaying sinusoidal oscillation), so that the mean time delay of the neural responses, a measure related more to the envelope of the signal, is shorter. This is illustrated in Fig. 6.5.

There is, then, some physiological support for Jeffress's suggestion of two mechanisms for sound localization. One, the time mechanism, operates on the interaural time differences in firing of phase locked neural fibres, which are little affected by changes in level. The second, the intensity mechanism, is affected both by interaural time differences and by differences in the mean latency of neural response to impulsive signals which result from interaural level differences. The dual sound images heard in time-intensity trading experiments probably result from a conflict between the two systems.

Taken together, the results of trading experiments make it quite clear that there is not a single simple trade between time and intensity. Rather, there

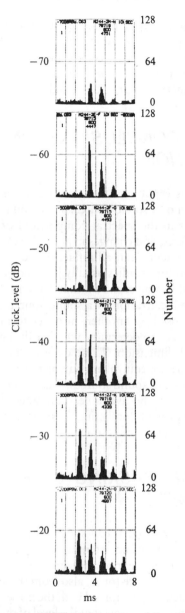

FIG. 6.5 Poststimulus time (PST) histograms of the response to click stimulation of a single auditory nerve fibre, as a function of click level. Each histogram shows the number of nerve firings occurring at a particular time after the instant of click presentation. The CF of the neurone was 630 Hz. Click level is expressed relative to a high reference level, the higher click levels being at the bottom of the figure. From Kiang *et al.* (1965), by permission of the author and MIT Press.

appear to be two different mechanisms by which time and intensity differences interact. However, it is only in the rather artificial situation of the laboratory that these two mechanisms produce sound images in widely different locations. In real life, time and intensity differences will nearly always work in conjunction to provide a single, well defined sound image.

9 GENERAL CONCLUSIONS ON SOUND LOCALIZATION

The auditory system is capable of using a great variety of physical cues to determine the location of a sound source. Time and intensity differences at the two ears, changes in the spectral composition of sounds due to head shadow and pinna effects, and changes in all of these cues produced by head or sound source movements, can all influence the perceived direction of a sound source. In laboratory studies usually just one or two of these cues are isolated. In this way it has been shown that sometimes a single cue may be sufficient for accurate localization of a sound source. In other experiments one cue has been opposed by another, in order to investigate the relative importance of the cues, or to determine whether the cues are encoded along some common neural dimension. These experiments have shown that, in some senses, the cues are not equivalent, but, on the other hand, they may also not be independent. For real sound sources, such as speech or music, all of the cues described above may be available simultaneously. However, in this situation they will not provide conflicting cues; rather the multiplicity of cues will render the location of the sound sources more definite and more accurate.

10 BINAURAL MASKING LEVEL DIFFERENCES

The masked threshold of a signal can sometimes be markedly lower when listening with two ears than when listening with one. Consider the situation shown in Fig. 6.6a. White noise from the same noise generator is fed to both ears via stereo headphones. Pure tones, also from the same signal generator, are fed separately to each ear and mixed with the noise. Thus the total signals at the two ears are identical. Assume that the level of the tone is adjusted until it is just masked by the noise, i.e. it is at its masked threshold, and let its level at this point be L_0 dB. Assume now that we invert the signal (the tone) at one ear only, i.e. we turn the waveform upside down. This is equivalent to shifting the phase of the signal by 180° or π radians (see Fig. 6.6b). The result is that

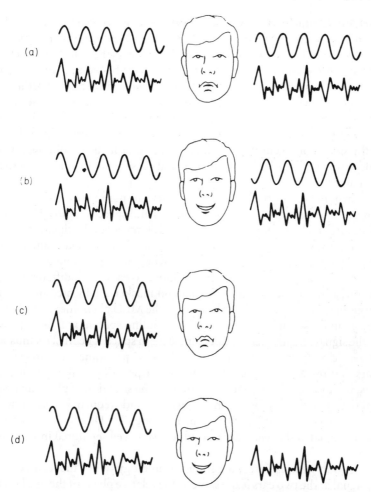

FIG. 6.6 Illustration of two situations in which binaural masking level differences (MLDs) occur. In conditions (a) and (c) detectability is poor, while in conditions (b) and (d), where the interaural relations of the signal and masker are different, detectability is good (hence the smiling faces).

the tone becomes audible again. The tone can be adjusted to a new level, L_π, so that it is once again at its masked threshold. The difference between the two levels, $L_0 - L_\pi$ (dB) is known as a masking level difference (MLD), and its value may be as large as 15 dB at low frequencies (around 500 Hz), decreasing to 2–3 dB for frequencies above 1500 Hz. Thus, simply by inverting the signal waveform at one ear we can make the signal considerably more detectable.

An example which is perhaps even more startling is given in Fig. 6.6c. The noise and signal are fed to one ear only, and the signal is adjusted to be at its masked threshold. Now the noise alone is added at the other ear; the tone becomes audible once again (Fig. 6.6d)! Thus, by adding noise at the nonsignal ear we make the tone considerably more detectable. Further, the tone disappears when it, too, is added to the second ear, making the sounds at the two ears the same. Notice that it is important that the same noise is added to the nonsignal ear; the noises at the two ears must be correlated or derived from the same noise generator. Release from masking is not obtained when an independent noise (derived from a second noise generator) is added to the nonsignal ear.

The phenomenon of the MLD is not limited to pure tones. Similar effects have been observed for complex tones, clicks and speech sounds. It seems to be the case that whenever the phase or level differences of the signal at the two ears are not the same of those of the masker, our ability to detect and identify the signals is improved relative to the case where the signal and masker have the same phase and level relationships at the two ears. Such differences only occur in real situations when the signal and masker are located in different positions in space. Thus, one implication of the MLD phenomenon is that the detection and discrimination of signals, including speech, will be improved when the signal and masker are not coincident in space. The MLD is thus seen to be very closely related to the 'cocktail party' phenomenon. However, it appears that the MLD is not merely another aspect of our ability to localize sounds, because the largest MLDs occur with the situation of phase inversion (see above) which only occurs naturally for mid-frequency pure tones at highly restricted angular locations. Further, large MLDs occur in situations where the signal and masker are not subjectively well separated in space (see later).

At this point we must introduce some terminology. When the relative phase of the signal at the two ears is the same as the relative phase of the masker, the condition is called 'homophasic'. When the phase relations are opposite (e.g. one is inverted and the other not), the term 'antiphasic' is used. In general we can describe a particular situation by using the symbols N (for noise) and S (for signal), each being followed by a suffix denoting relative phase at the two ears. A phase inversion is equivalent to a phase shift of 180° or π radians. Thus N_0S_π refers to the condition where the noise is in phase at the two ears and the signal is inverted in phase. N_u means that the noise is uncorrelated at the two ears. The suffix m indicates monaural presentation, i.e. presentation to one ear only. Table 6.1 gives the magnitude of the MLD for a variety of combinations of signal and noise. Four conditions for which there is no binaural advantage, N_0S_0, N_mS_m, N_uS_m and $N_\pi S_\pi$, all give about the same 'reference' threshold. The MLDs for the conditions shown in the table are obtained by expressing thresholds relative to this reference threshold.

Table 6.1. Values of the MLD for various interaural phase relationships of the signal and masker. These results are typical for broadband maskers and low-frequency signals.

Interaural condition	MLD in dB
N_uS_π	3
N_uS_0	4
$N_\pi S_m$	6
N_0S_m	9
$N_\pi S_0$	13
N_0S_π	15

One general finding which has emerged from studies of the MLD is that the largest effects are usually found at low frequencies. For broadband noise maskers, the MLD falls to 2–3 dB for signal frequencies above about 1500 Hz, and it is noteworthy that this is also the highest frequency for which we are able to compare phases at the two ears in localizing sounds. Thus it is likely that the MLD depends at least in part on the transmission of temporal information about the stimulus to some higher neural centre which compares the temporal information from the two ears.

A second general feature is that for a wideband masker not all of the frequency components are effective; just as was the case for monaural masking (see Chapter 3), only those components in a critical band around the signal frequency seem to be effective in masking it. Further, the release from masking in MLD conditions seems to depend only on the characterisics of the noise in a band around the signal frequency. There has been some disagreement as to whether the binaural critical bandwidth is the same as the monaural critical bandwidth. Some experiments have suggested that the binaural critical bandwidth is greater than the monaural critical bandwidth, while others have shown similar monaural and binaural critical bandwidths (Hall *et al.*, 1983; Hall and Fernandes, 1984; Zurek and Durlach, 1987; Kohlrausch, 1988). Hall *et al.* (1983) suggested that the peripheral auditory filter is the same for both monaural and binaural detection, but binaural detection may depend on the output of more than one auditory filter.

In addition to improving the detectability of tones, conditions which produce MLDs also favour other aspects of our ability to analyse signals. For example, when speech signals are presented against noisy backgrounds, speech intelligibility is better under antiphasic conditions than under homophasic conditions (e.g. Hirsh, 1950). Gebhardt and Goldstein (1972) measured frequency DLs for tones presented against noise backgrounds and found that, for a given signal-to-noise ratio, antiphasic DLs were substantially smaller than homophasic ones when the signals were close to masked threshold. Thus antiphasic conditions improve our ability to identify and discriminate signals, as well as to detect them.

The relative importance of spatial factors in the MLD was investigated by Carhart *et al.* (1969). They measured thresholds for identifying one- and two-syllable speech sounds in the presence of four simultaneous maskers. Two of the maskers were modulated white noise and two were whole sentences. They used several different listening conditions, including homophasic, antiphasic and those where the signal or the maskers were delayed at one ear relative to the other. In these latter conditions the different maskers were sometimes given opposing time delays, so that some would be located towards one ear and some towards the other. Sometimes the signal was subjectively well separated in location from the masking sounds, and under these conditions subjects reported the task of identifying the signal to be easier. However, the largest MLDs were obtained for the antiphasic condition, where there is no clear separation in the subjective locations; rather the sound images are located diffusely within the head. Thus escape from masking and lateralization/localization seem, to some extent, to be separate capacities.

It has been reported that MLDs occur for both forward and backward masking (Small *et al.*, 1972; Dolan and Trahiotis, 1972). Substantial MLDs (4–5 dB) are found for silent intervals between the signal and the masker of up to 40 ms. We shall see in the next section that this finding is inconsistent with one model of the MLD.

11 MODELS TO EXPLAIN MLDs

Several models to account for MLDs have not attempted explanations at the physiological level. Rather they have been 'black box' models, assuming that the auditory system is capable of certain types of processing without specifying exactly how it is done. We shall discuss two models of this type, and then will briefly describe models which attempt to explain MLDs in terms of neural mechanisms. None of the models is completely successful in explaining all aspects of the experimental data.

A The Webster–Jeffress model

Webster (1951) pointed out that a narrowband noise resembles a sinusoid whose amplitude and phase vary slowly from moment to moment. The band of noise which is effective in masking the tone, the critical band, may also be thought of in this way. Adding a tonal signal to this noise yields a resultant which generally differs in phase and amplitude from the original noise. If, for example, adding the signal at one ear advances the signal-plus-noise in phase, adding the signal reversed in phase at the other ear retards it. This is illustrated in Fig. 6.7a. The effects may be illustrated graphically at one instant in time by a vector diagram (Fig. 6.7b). The noise is represented by a vector whose length denotes the amplitude and whose angle denotes the phase. The signal is denoted by a second vector, whose length again denotes amplitude, but which generally differs in phase from the noise by an angle α. The figure shows the case where an antiphasic signal is added to a narrow band of noise in phase at the two ears. It may be seen that the resultant leads in phase at one ear and also has a greater amplitude at that ear. With a noise masker and a tonal signal the phase angle of addition, α, varies constantly, so that the differences in level and phase at the two ears vary from moment to moment. In some cases one ear leads in time but the other receives the more intense stimulus.

According to the Webster–Jeffress model, binaural detection is based upon the differences in phase and level at the two ears which result from the addition of the signal to the band of frequencies in the noise which contribute to the masking of the signal. Thus the cues for detection are similar to those involved in the ordinary localization and lateralization of binaural signals.

Jeffress and his colleagues (e.g. McFadden *et al.*, 1972) have described a series of experiments on MLDs where the phase angle between the signal and noise, α, was controlled, thus controlling the relative magnitude of the interaural time and level differences. They used a rather special stimulus situation, where both signal and masker were the same narrow band of noise. Consider the N_0S_π condition. When α is $0°$, the signal is added to the masker in one ear and subtracted in the other. There is no interaural phase difference, but the level difference is maximal. For this condition, substantial MLDs (up to 15 dB) occurred for frequencies of 250, 1000 and 2000 Hz. When α is $90°$, the signal vectors are at right angles to the masker vector, so that the interaural phase difference is at a maximum, but there is no interaural level difference. For this condition large MLDs were found for frequencies of 250, 500 and 1000 Hz, but not for 2000 Hz. For α between $90°$ and $180°$ the ear that is leading in time receives the weaker stimulus. Thus time and intensity are in opposition. Substantial MLDs were still found, although the subjects were sometimes not able to lateralize the signal clearly to one side. This inability to lateralize is probably not due to a cancellation of time and intensity; as we discussed earlier, the subjects tend to hear two sound images, so that responses are inconsistent. Jeffress (1971) has summarized these results as follows:

> Detection thus appears to be an aspect of lateralization. The signal is detected because it is heard as a displacement from the noise in the median plane. Even when time and level are in opposition there is movement away from the median plane, a movement which is detectable although ambiguous in direction.

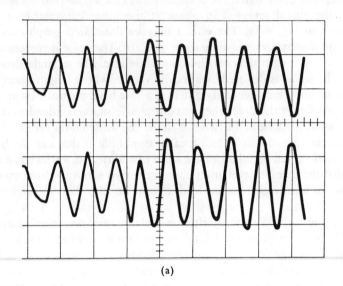

(a)

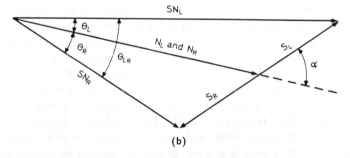

(b)

FIG. 6.7 In (a) oscilloscope traces of the signals presented to the left ear (upper) and right ear (lower) are shown. For the first part of the trace only a narrowband noise, identical in the two channels, is present. Then a tonal signal, reversed in phase in one channel relative to the other, is added. Note the resultant phase and amplitude shift between the two channels. In (b) the situation at one instant in time is represented by a vector diagram. The in-phase narrowband noise is represented by N_L and N_R. The signal in the left ear is denoted by S_L, and the signal in the right ear, which is opposite in phase, by S_R. The phase angle of addition, α, would vary randomly from moment to moment. Note that the resultant in the left ear, SN_L, differs from the resultant in the right ear, SN_R, in both amplitude and phase. From Jeffress (1971), by permission of the author.

Subjects differ in their sensitivity to the two cues, time and level differences, and at 2000 Hz only level differences can be used.

This model, when applied to the particular stimuli used by Jeffress, does explain the data rather well. However, the use of the same stimulus as both a signal and masker is a rather special case. For a tonal signal presented against a wideband random noise, the phase angle, α, varies randomly from moment to moment. Thus the subjective lateral position of the signal-plus-noise (the noise here referring to those components in a critical band around the tone) should also vary randomly from moment to moment. This does not fit in with observers' reports. Rather, if the tone can be faintly heard, it is lateralized fairly precisely in one position. Thus, for the $N_0 S_\pi$ condition, the noise is generally lateralized in the middle of the head, whereas the tone is heard towards one side. For their narrowband signals and maskers, McFadden *et al.* (1971) stated that "the phenomenology associated with detecting an S_π signal is that during a signal-plus-masker trial, there is a slight movement or shift in the auditory 'image'". If the model applied equally well to a tonal signal in wideband noise, then a part of the sound image should be heard as fluctuating in position. This does not seem to be the case.

The model also cannot explain the finding of MLDs in forward and backward masking. In order for the vector addition of signal and masker to occur, these must be present simultaneously. Thus the model deals rather well with some specific stimulus situations, but fails to account for the data in others.

B   Durlach's equalization and cancellation model

This model, presented by Durlach (1963), has four basic components, which are illustrated in Fig. 6.8. First, the stimulus in each ear is assumed to be filtered, by a mechanism analogous to the critical band. Then the total output from one filter is transformed relative to that from the other filter in such a way that the masking components become the same in both channels (the E mechanism). The output of the E mechanism in one channel is then subtracted from that in the other (the C mechanism), thus eliminating the masker. If the interaural relations of the signal are different from those of the masker, then some of the signal will remain after the C process. If the precisions of the E and C mechanisms were perfect, the signal-to-noise ratio would be improved by an infinite amount. The output from the EC mechanism is fed to a decision device which also receives inputs directly from the bandpass filters. It is assumed that the subject's detection performance is determined by the largest signal-to-noise ratio at the inputs to the decision

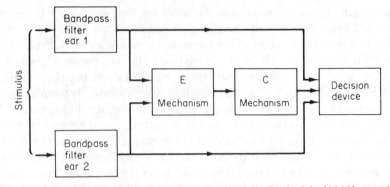

FIG. 6.8   Illustration of the major components in Durlach's (1963) equalization and cancellation model of binaural processing.

device. The ratio at the binaural input (from the EC mechanism) divided by the ratio at one of the monaural inputs gives the magnitude of the MLD.

Clearly, human observers do not show infinite MLDs. In order to account for this, it is assumed that the EC mechanisms perform imperfectly, so that there is a residue of noise at the output of the C mechanism. The imperfections are assumed to be of two types: (1) those resulting from a random jitter independent of stimulus configuration, and representable as random errors in the amplitude and time alignment of the signals at the input to the C mechanism; (2) those resulting from 'atypical' stimuli that require atypical E transformations in response. Examples of the second type might be broadband masking signals that differ by an interaural phase shift rather than an interaural time shift, or signals that differ by an interaural time shift greater than the time it takes a sound to travel around the head.

It is assumed that there are a number of possible modes of operation of the EC mechanism, but that a selector mechanism chooses that mode which gives the largest MLD. It is usually assumed that the types of operation which the E mechanism can perform are those which would be involved in the localization or lateralization of sounds, namely shifts in time and shifts in intensity. For a tone, a phase shift is equivalent to a time shift, and for a narrowband noise this is also approximately true. Thus, for the $N_\pi S_0$ condition the appropriate E process is a shift in time of the noise components around the tone. Since a narrowband noise resembles a sinusoid, a shift in time equal to half a period of the sinusoid is equivalent to inverting the phase.

A problem arises when we consider antiphasic conditions for wideband signals, such as speech sounds, in wideband maskers. If, for example, the noise is inverted in one ear with respect to the other, a shift in time only cancels the noise components in certain frequency regions, while in other frequency regions the noise actually increases. Further, such a shift in time tends to cancel the signal components in certain frequency regions. Since substantial MLDs do occur under these conditions, we must assume either that different time shifts are used in different frequency bands, or that the E mechanism is capable of a rather strange and demanding operation—that of inverting a waveform. It would seem reasonable that if such complicated transformations are required of the E mechanism, then the MLDs would be smaller than those found in the case where, for example, the masker in one ear is simply delayed in time with respect to the other. However, this does not seem to be the case. The experiments of Carhart *et al.* (1969) which we described above clearly showed that the largest MLDs are found in antiphasic conditions, rather than in conditions where the maskers are simply time delayed.

The main advantage of Durlach's model is that, with certain simple assumptions, it allows detailed quantitative predictions to be made about the outcome of experiments, some of which are as yet undone. We shall not attempt to describe these here, or to relate in detail the experimental findings to the predictions. The interested reader is referred to Durlach (1972). As with the Webster–Jeffress model, the EC model explains certain aspects of the data rather well, but fails in other cases.

C Neural models

Several workers have proposed models based on the properties of neurones in the auditory nerve and higher centres in the auditory system (Jeffress, 1948; Colburn, 1977). These models are complex, and it is beyond the scope of this book to describe them fully. Briefly, they assume that firing patterns are compared for neurones with corresponding CFs in the two ears. More specifically, it is often assumed that, at each CF, there is an array of delay lines which can delay the neural spikes from one ear relative to those from the other; each delay line has a characteristic time delay. These are followed by coincidence detectors, which count the numbers of spikes arriving synchronously from the two ears. If a sound is delayed by a time τ at the left ear relative to the right, then a delay of τ in the neural spikes from the right ear will cause the spikes from the left and right ears to be synchronous at the point of binaural interaction. Thus the interaural delay of the signal is coded in terms of which delay line gives the highest response in the coincidence detectors.

This type of model was originally proposed to account for the ability to use interaural time delays in localizing sounds (Jeffress, 1948), but it has since been extended to account for MLDs (Colburn, 1977). It is useful to think of the outputs of the coincidence detectors as providing a kind of two-dimensional display; one of the dimensions is CF and the other is the interaural delay. The response to any stimulus is a pattern of activity in this display. When a signal and a masker have the same interaural delay time, τ, then they produce activity at overlapping points in the pattern; most activity lies around a line of equal delay (τ) versus CF. When a signal and masker have different interaural delay times, the pattern is more complex. The addition of the signal to the masker may cause activity to appear at points in the pattern where there was little activity for the masker alone. This could enhance the detection of the signal, giving an MLD. For further details, the reader is referred to Colburn (1977).

12 THE SLUGGISHNESS OF THE BINAURAL SYSTEM

A number of investigators have studied the ability of subjects to follow changes in the location of stimuli over time, i.e. to perceive movements of a sound source. These studies have shown that only rather slow changes in location can be followed, a phenomenon that has been described as 'binaural sluggishness'.

Perrott and Musicant (1977) and Grantham (1986) have measured the 'minimum audible movement angle' (MAMA), defined as the angle through which a sound source has to move for it to be distinguished from a stationary source. For low rates of movement (15°/s) the MAMA is about 5°, but as the rate of movement increases, the MAMA increases progressively, to about 21° for a rate of 90°/s. Thus, the binaural system is relatively insensitive to movements at high rates.

Blauert (1972) used as a stimulus a pulse train of 80 pulses/s, presented binaurally via earphones. Either the interaural time difference (IATD) or the interaural amplitude difference (IAAD) was varied sinusoidally. For low rates of variation, the sound source was heard as moving alternately to the left and right. However, when the rate was increased, the movement could not be followed. Blauert found that the highest rate at which movement could be followed "in detail" was 2.4 Hz for the varying IATD and 3.1 Hz for the varying IAAD.

Grantham and Wightman (1978) measured the ability to follow movements in a noise lowpass filtered at 3000 Hz. The IATD was varied sinusoidally at a rate f_m. The peak IATD, determining the extent of movement, was varied to determine the threshold for distinguishing the moving stimulus from a stationary reference stimulus. The threshold IATD increased from 30 μs to 90 μs as f_m increased from 0 to 20 Hz. Again, this indicates that slow movements can be followed well, but rapid movements are more difficult to follow.

The sensitivity to changes in interaural cues has also been determined by measuring MLDs. Grantham and Wightman (1979) measured thresholds for detecting a brief tone which was phase inverted at one ear relative to the other (S_π). The masker was a noise whose correlation between the two ears could be varied continuously between +1 (N_0) and −1 (N_π). The correlation was made to vary sinusoidally at rate f_m. The signal was presented at various points on the masker's modulation cycle. For $f_m = 0$ Hz (fixed interaural correlation), the signal threshold decreased monotonically as the masker's interaural correlation changed from −1 to +1. The decrease, corresponding to an MLD ($N_\pi S_\pi - N_0 S_\pi$), was 20, 16 and 8 dB for signals at 250, 500 and 1000 Hz, respectively. For $f_m > 0$, the function relating signal threshold to the masker's interaural correlation at the moment of signal presentation became progressively flatter with increasing f_m for all signal frequencies. For $f_m = 4$ Hz, the function was flat; there was no measurable effect of masker interaural correlation on the signal threshold. Again, these results indicate that the binaural system is slow in its response to changes in interaural stimulation.

In summary, results from a variety of experiments indicate that the binaural system responds sluggishly to changes in interaural time, intensity, or correlation. Thus, the auditory system is relatively insensitive to the motion of sound sources.

13 THE INFLUENCE OF VISION ON AUDITORY LOCALIZATION

Many everyday experiences indicate that auditory localization can be influenced by conflicting visual cues. At a cinema the loudspeakers are usually placed behind the screen, in its centre (except where stereo or multichannel sound is used), yet the sound still appears to come from the actor's mouth as he moves about the screen. Similarly, the loudspeaker in a television set is usually located to one side of the screen, but the sound does not appear to be 'detached' from the visual image.

A number of experiments have shown that exposure to conflicting auditory and visual cues for a period of time may lead to an after-effect in which the localization of sounds is systematically displaced. This may indicate that connections between the 'frames of reference' for auditory space and for spaces in other modalities (vision, balance and touch) are modifiable to some extent.

Young (1928) and later Willey *et al.* (1937) attempted to distort auditory space using a 'pseudophone'; this has a tube from each ear leading to a trumpet on the opposite side of the head. With this arrangement, sounds from the left are heard as coming from the right, and vice versa. Although the listeners were able to learn to respond appropriately, for example to point to the left when a sound was on the left, no genuine auditory reorientation appeared to take place, even after a week of exposure. Held (1955) used an electronic pseudophone which displaced the interaural axis by 22° about the vertical axis of the head. After wearing this for a day, listeners were tested with the pseudophone set to give no displacement. They reported that a single sound source produced two images, one near the normal position and one displaced from it in the opposite direction to the original direction of rotation of the pseudophone. Kalil and Freedman (1967) found that after wearing a pseudophone which displaced a sound 15° to the right of a visible source, subjects heard a sound presented straight in front of them (from a concealed source) as displaced a few degrees to the left. Freedman *et al.* (1967) have reported similar effects for subjects exposed to discrepant auditory and kinaesthetic cues. Overall, these and other results (Weerts and Thurlow, 1971) suggest that auditory space can be 'recalibrated' to some extent on the basis of visual information.

Some experiments of Wallach (1940) indicate another way in which vision is important for auditory localization. His subjects had their heads fixed in the vertical axis of a cylindrical screen which rotated about them. The screen was covered in vertical stripes and, after watching the movement of these for a few moments, the observers would perceive themselves as in constant rotation and the screen as at rest. A stationary sound source was then activated straight ahead of the observers. Since the observers in this situation perceive themselves as moving, they have to interpret the sound source as lying directly above or below them. If the sound source is at a constant azimuth (e.g. 20° to the left of the observer), the sound source cannot be interpreted as lying above the observer, since interaural differences of time and intensity now exist. Instead the source is perceived as rotating with the observer at an elevation which is approximately the complement of the constant azimuth (in this case at an elevation of about 70°). Thus our interpretation of auditory spatial cues is strongly influenced by our perceived visual orientation. Or, more correctly, the highest level of spatial representation involves an integration of information from the different senses.

14 THE PERCEPTION OF DISTANCE

Just as was the case for judgements of lateral position, there are a number of cues which we can use in judging the distance of a sound source. For familiar sounds, sound level may give a crude indication of distance from the listener. This cue appears to be most effective when multiple sound sources are present, so that comparison of the levels of different sources is possible (Mershon and King, 1975). Over moderate distances the spectrum of a complex sound source may also be changed, owing to the absorbing properties of the air; high frequencies are attenuated more than low. However, judgements again depend on familiarity with the sounds (Coleman, 1962, 1963).

The cues described above could be used to judge the distance of a sound source in free space. Normally we listen in rooms with reflecting walls. In this case the ratio of direct to reflected sound, and the time delay between direct and reflected sound, provide cues to distance. Von Békésy (1960) showed that altering these ratios produced the impression of sounds moving towards or away from the listener. The work of Wallach *et al.* (1949) and others on the precedence effect (section 7) showed that we exhibit little direct awareness of room echoes; rather these are fused with the leading sound. However, we are still able to use information related to echoes to judge distance, in spite of this perceptual fusion. Mershon and Bowers (1979) have shown that the ratio of direct to reflected sound can be used to judge absolute as well as relative distance, and that this cue can be used even for the first presentation of an unfamiliar sound in an unfamiliar environment.

We may conclude that, just as was the case for judgements of the direction of sound sources, judgements of distance may depend on a multiplicity of cues. Absolute sound level, spectral changes and reflected sounds may all influence judgements of distance. The effective use of the first two of these cues depends strongly on familiarity with the sound source and the listening environment, and they are most effective for judgements of the relative distance of sound sources. However, the ratio of direct to reflected sound can be used to judge the distance of unfamiliar sounds. In general, localization of sounds in depth is relatively inaccurate, and errors of the order of 20% are not uncommon for unfamiliar sound sources.

15 OBSTACLE DETECTION AND THE BLIND

Many blind people, and some blindfolded sighted people, are able to detect the presence of obstacles in the environment and to judge their distance. However, such people are not often able to explain how they do this, and the descriptions which are used, such as 'feeling the objects on my face', are not particularly helpful. Supa *et al.* (1944) carried out a series of experiments to determine the cues involved in what they called 'facial vision'. In an initial experiment they found that blindfolded normal subjects could learn to avoid objects after a short learning period, but that blind subjects could normally detect objects at greater distances. Both normal and blind subjects could distinguish between the first perception of an object at a distance and the 'near approach' to it.

There have been two types of cues suggested as the basis for facial vision. These are cutaneous sensation due to air currents and auditory sensation based on the reflection of sound from obstacles. Supa and his co-workers attempted to eliminate each of these cues in turn: cutaneous cues were removed by covering the skin with veils and sleeves while auditory cues were removed by plugging the ears or by using a background masking noise. They concluded that stimulation of the face and other areas of the skin is neither a necessary nor a sufficient condition for obstacle detection, whereas auditory stimulation is both necessary and sufficient. Subjects make use either of sounds which they emit themselves or of sounds occurring in the environment in order to locate objects.

Wilson (1967) has pointed out that, in the neighbourhood of an obstacle, sound reaches the observer both directly and by reflection from the obstacle. Interference between these signals introduces a series of maxima and minima in the spectrum, the frequencies of which depend on the path difference. For a sound containing a wide range of frequencies a pitch is heard (sometimes called the 'reflection tone') which becomes higher as the obstacle is approached. Thus the value of this pitch, and its rate of change as the obstacle is approached, provide cues as to the distance of the object. In addition, the spectrum of the reflected sound is modified according to the size of the obstacle; a large object reflects both high and low frequencies, whereas a small object only reflects high frequencies. Thus, spectral changes in the reflected sound provide at least a crude estimate of the size of the object.

Further changes in spectrum may result if the obstacle absorbs certain portions of the spectrum, or if it introduces frequency-dependent phase shifts. Thus a crude form of obstacle recognition may even be possible. Tests using blind subjects have shown that objects subtending an angle as small as 3.5° can be detected, and that changes in distance of the order of 20% and in area of the order of 30% can be discriminated (Kellog, 1962). Kellog also investigated the discrimination of discs covered with different types of material. He found that some materials could be discriminated with high accuracy (plain wood and velvet could be discriminated 99.5% of the time) while others, such as painted wood and glass, could not be discriminated at all. In general, discrimination was good between 'soft' and 'hard' materials, but, surprisingly, denim cloth and velvet could be distinguished with 86.5% accuracy. Rice (1967) found that some subjects could distinguish between a circle, a square and a triangle of the same surface area with an accuracy of about 80%. In order to achieve these discriminations most subjects emitted both normal vocal sounds and clicking and hissing sounds.

16 GENERAL CONCLUSIONS

In this chapter we have discussed the cues and the mechanisms involved in the localization of sounds. Our acuity in locating sounds is greatest in the horizontal plane, fairly good in the vertical direction and poorest for distance. For each of these, we are able to use a number of distinct cues, although the cues may differ depending on the type of sound.

For localization in the horizontal plane, the cues of interaural time and intensity difference are most important. Interaural time is most useful at low frequencies, while interaural intensity is most useful at high frequencies. However, transient sounds, or periodic sounds with low repetition rates, can be localized on the basis of interaural time delay even when they contain only high frequencies. For periodic sounds, the binaural system shows a form of adaptation, so that judgements of position in space depend mostly on the leading part of the sound, and less on later parts. This adaptation is more rapid for stimuli with high repetition rates. A recovery from adaptation may be produced by a weak 'trigger' whose spectral characteristics differ from that of the test sound.

The direction dependent filtering produced by the pinnae is important for judgements of location in the vertical direction, and for front-back discrimination. It is also important for creating the percept of a sound being outside the head, rather than inside.

The multiplicity of cues to sound location provides a certain redundancy in the system, so that even under very difficult conditions (reverberant rooms or brief sounds) we are still capable of quite accurate localization.

Binaural processing, using information relating to the differences of the signals at the two ears, can improve our ability to detect and analyse signals in noisy backgrounds. This is illustrated by laboratory studies of the binaural masking level difference (MLD). Binaural processing also helps us to suppress room echoes, and to locate sound sources in reverberant rooms.

The binaural system is rather sluggish in responding to changes in interaural time or intensity. Thus we are relatively insensitive to the motion of sound sources.

Our judgements of auditory location may be influenced by visual or kinaesthetic stimulation. Such stimulation may also lead to after-effects in which the apparent position of a sound source is slightly displaced from its 'true' position. These effects may indicate that there is some 'plasticity' in the relations between auditory, visual and kinaesthetic space, so that a 'recalibration' of auditory space can occur on the basis of information from other modalities.

Blind people, and blindfolded normal subjects after some practice, are able to detect obstacles in the environment, and to make crude estimations of their distance and of their size and nature. This ability depends upon the reflections of sound from the obstacles, although subjects are not always aware of this. Again, a number of possible cues may be used in this situation, but the most important one is probably the 'reflection tone' which results from the interference of direct and reflected sound, and whose pitch depends on path difference.

FURTHER READING

The following chapter by Mills gives a clear, but slightly dated review of sound localization:

Mills, A. W. (1972). Auditory Localization. In *Foundations of Modern Auditory Theory*, Vol. 2 (ed. J. V. Tobias), Academic Press, New York.

Extensive reviews of data and models related to binaural hearing can be found in:

Blauert, J. (1983). *Spatial Hearing*, MIT Press, Cambridge, Mass.
Yost, W. A. and Gourevitch, G. (1987). *Directional Hearing*, Springer, New York.

Demonstrations 35, 36, 37 and 38 of *Auditory Demonstrations* on CD are relevant to this chapter (see the list of further reading for Chapter 1).

7

Auditory pattern and object perception

1 INTRODUCTION

So far we have described several attributes of auditory sensation such as pitch, subjective location and loudness, which can be related in a reasonably straightforward way to the physical properties of stimuli. In many cases we have discussed the neural code which may underly the perception of these attributes. In everyday life, however, we do not perceive these attributes in isolation. Rather, the auditory world is analysed into discrete sound sources or auditory objects, each of which may have its own pitch, timbre, location and loudness. Sometimes the source may be recognized as familiar in some way, such as a particular person talking; often the 'object' perceived may be identified, for example as a particular spoken word. In this chapter we will discuss four related aspects of auditory object and pattern perception. Firstly, we will discuss the factors involved in the identification of a single object among a large set of possible objects. Secondly, we will discuss some of the cues we use to analyse a complex mixture of sounds into discrete sources. Thirdly, we will discuss the perception of sequences of sounds. Finally, we will describe a number of general 'rules' which govern the perceptual organization of the auditory world.

2 TIMBRE PERCEPTION AND OBJECT IDENTIFICATION

Many of the attributes of sensation we have described so far, such as pitch and loudness, may be considered as unidimensional: if we are presented with a large variety of sounds with different pitches it is possible to order all of the sounds on a single scale of pitch going from low to high (this is not quite true for complex tones; see Shepard, 1964). Similarly, sounds differing in loudness can be ordered on a single scale going from quiet to loud. Our ability to identify one object from among a large set of objects depends upon there being several dimensions along which the objects vary. When a set of stimuli vary along a single dimension we can only name the individual stimuli in the set when their number is less than about 5–6. For example, Pollack (1952) investigated the ability of subjects to name musical tones with different pitches, as a function of the number of possible tones. He found that they could only do this reliably when the number of possible tones was less than 5–6. This was true whether the tones were spread over a wide frequency range of several octaves, or were concentrated in a relatively narrow range, say one octave (subjects with absolute pitch do better in this task).

In order for us to be able to identify more stimuli than this, extra dimensions are required. In hearing, the extra dimensions arise in two main ways. Firstly, for complex stimuli the patterning of energy as a function of frequency is important. Secondly, auditory stimuli typically vary with time, and the temporal patterning can be of crucial importance to perception. Auditory space, or location, can sometimes provide extra dimensions, for example, by indicating the size of an object, but usually it defines where, rather than what, an object is. Thus auditory pattern or object perception depends primarily on structures in frequency and time.

A   Time-invariant patterns and timbre

If a single frequency component is presented, then the sound pattern can be described by just two numbers, specifying frequency and intensity. However, almost all of the sounds that we encounter in everyday life are considerably more complex than this, and contain a multitude of frequencies with particular levels and relative phases. The distribution of energy over frequency is one of the major determinants of the quality of a sound or its timbre. Timbre has been defined by the American Standards Association (1960) as "that attribute of auditory sensation in terms of which a listener can judge that two sounds similarly presented and having the same loudness and pitch are dissimilar". Differences in timbre enable us to distinguish between the same note played on, say, the piano, the violin or the flute.

Timbre as defined by the ASA depends upon more than just the frequency spectrum of the sound; fluctuations over time can play an important role, and we will discuss the effects of these in section 2B. For the purpose of this section we can adopt a more restricted definition suggested by Plomp (1970): "Timbre is that attribute of sensation in terms of which a listener can judge that two steady complex tones having the same loudness, pitch and duration are dissimilar". Timbre defined in this way depends mainly on the relative magnitudes of the harmonics of the tones.

Unlike pitch or loudness, which may be considered as unidimensional, timbre is multidimensional; there is no single scale along which we can compare or order the timbres of different sounds. Thus, we need some way of describing the spectrum of a sound which takes into account this multidimensional aspect, and which can be related to the subjective timbre. A crude first approach is to look at the overall distribution of spectral energy. For example, complex tones with strong lower harmonics (below the 6th) sound mellow, whereas tones with strong harmonics beyond the 6th or 7th sound sharp and penetrating. However, a much more quantitative approach has been described by Plomp and his colleagues (Plomp *et al.*, 1967; Plomp, 1970). They used a statistical technique which is similar to 'factor analysis' (Slater, 1960), and which allows the determination of the principal dimensions of variation in a set of stimuli. Firstly, a spectrum is characterized with a set of numbers representing the levels in 18 third-octave frequency bands. This relatively broadband analysis achieves a basic economy consistent with the frequency analysing power of the peripheral auditory system; critical bands are roughly one third-octave in width over a fairly wide frequency range. A representative sample of spectra is then obtained (e.g. the vowels of a language spoken by a set of speakers with subjectively different voices). The level in each third-octave band varies as a function of vowel or speaker, but the levels in different bands are not entirely independent, particularly for bands of adjacent centre frequency. Thus, the information about the vowel or speaker conveyed by the levels in the 18 third-octave bands is redundant, or partially duplicated. This redundancy can be eliminated by statistical procedures that yield the chief higher order dimensions underlying the differences between sounds in the sample chosen. Each higher order dimension is a weighted function of each of the original 18 dimensions. Different sets of higher order dimensions are obtained according to whether we emphasize the differences between vowels or the differences between speakers.

This procedure results in a reduction in the number of dimensions needed to account for the differences between the spectra in the set. In general, the more the number of dimensions is reduced, the less satisfactorily are those differences accounted for. For the vowels described above, three dimensions are sufficient to account for about 82% of the total variation. Thus, with a reasonably small error, each vowel can be represented as a point in a three-dimensional space. If we take into account variations between different speakers, or between the same speaker on different occasions, the representation of each vowel becomes a 'blob' of a certain volume in this three-dimensional space.

Consider now the subjective significance of these higher order dimensions. To investigate this, Pols *et al.* (1969) carried out perceptual analyses of the vowel stimuli, using a technique based on triadic comparison. In this method the subject has to decide, for each possible group of three stimuli, which pair is most similar and which pair is least similar. On the basis of these judgements a multidimensional perceptual space can be constructed for the different vowel sounds. (The exact method by which this is done is rather complex. The interested reader is referred to Shepard, 1962, and Kruskal, 1964.) Each vowel is represented as a point in the multidimensional space, and the greater the distance between these points the more dissimilar are the vowels judged to be. As was the case for the physical analysis, the number of dimensions can be reduced at the expense of a loss of 'goodness of fit'. When Pols *et al.* (1969) compared the three-dimensional physical configuration with the three-dimensional perceptual configuration, they found a close correspondence; the correlation coefficients for the three dimensions were 0.992, 0.971 and 0.742. When six dimensions were used, the correlation coefficients were even higher. Pols and co-workers summed up these results as follows:

> From this remarkable correspondence, it can be concluded that the subjects used for their perceptual judgements information comparable with that present in the physical representation of these signals. The perceptual differences between the stimuli, to be considered as timbre differences, appear to be qualified by their differences in frequency spectra.

It should not be assumed that the dimensions derived by Pols and co-workers would be applicable to other sorts of sounds, or that the number of dimensions involved in timbre judgements is necessarily small. It is likely that the number of dimensions required is limited by the number of critical bands required to cover the audible frequency range. This would give a maximum of about 30 dimensions. For a restricted class of sounds, however, a much smaller number of dimensions may be involved. It appears to be generally true, both for speech and nonspeech sounds, that the timbres of steady tones are determined primarily by their magnitude spectra, although their phase spectra may also play a small role (Plomp and Steeneken, 1969; Darwin and Gardner, 1986; Patterson, 1987a).

B   Time-varying patterns

Although differences in static timbre may enable us to distinguish between two sounds which are presented successively, they are not always sufficient to allow the absolute identification of an 'auditory object', such as a musical instrument. One reason for this is that the magnitude and phase spectrum of the sound may be markedly altered by the transmission path and room reflections. In practice, the recognition of a particular timbre, and hence of an 'auditory object', may depend upon several other factors. Schouten (1968) has suggested that these include: (1) whether the sound is periodic, having a tonal quality for repetition rates between about 20 and 20 000 per second, or irregular, and having a noise-like character; (2) whether the waveform envelope is constant, or fluctuates as a function of time, and in the latter case what the fluctuations are like; (3) whether any aspect of the sound (spectrum, periodicity or envelope) is changing as a function of time; (4) what the preceding and following sounds are like.

The recognition of musical instruments, for example, depends quite strongly on onset transients and on the temporal structure of the sound envelope. The characteristic tone of a piano depends upon the fact that the notes have a rapid onset and a gradual decay. If a recording of a piano is reversed in time, the timbre is completely different. It now resembles that of a harmonium or accordion, in spite of the fact that the long-term magnitude spectrum is unchanged by time reversal. In addition, many instruments have noise-like qualities which strongly influence their subjective quality. A flute, for example, has a relatively simple harmonic structure, but synthetic tones with the same harmonic structure do not sound flute-like unless each note is preceded by a small 'puff' of noise. In general, tones of standard musical instruments are poorly simulated by the summation of steady component frequencies, since such a synthesis cannot produce the dynamic variation with time characteristic of these instruments. Thus traditional electronic organs (pre-1965), which produced only tones with a fixed envelope shape, could produce a good simulation of the bagpipes, but could not be made to sound like a piano. Modern synthesizers shape the envelopes of the sounds they produce, and hence are capable of more accurate and convincing imitations of musical instruments. For a simulation to be completely convincing, it is sometimes necessary to give different time envelopes to different harmonics within a complex sound (Risset and Wessel, 1982).

3 INFORMATION USED TO SEPARATE AUDITORY OBJECTS

It is hardly ever the case that the sound reaching our ears comes from a single source. Usually the sound arises from several different sources, but we have little difficulty in assigning the different frequency components in the sound to their appropriate sources. Our ability to do this is greater than we might expect from simple studies of masking, and the critical band. In this section we will consider some of the physical cues which are used to achieve this perceptual separation. In section 5 we will consider the perceptual rules which can be derived from this, and the rules which govern the perception of auditory sequences. The physical cues which we will describe are not completely independent of one another, and not one of them always works perfectly. The ways in which the cues are used provide pointers to the rules governing perceptual organization.

A Fundamental frequency

When we listen to two steady complex tones together (e.g. two musical instruments or two vowel sounds), we do not generally confuse which harmonics belong to which tone. Rather we hear each tone as a separate source, even though the harmonics may be interleaved, and sometimes overlapping. We can do this only if the two tones have different fundamental frequencies (F_o). Broadbent and Ladefoged (1957), in an experiment using synthetic vowels, showed that the normal percept of a single fused voice occurs only if all the harmonics have the same F_o. If the harmonics are split into two groups, with different F_o's, then two separate sounds are heard. Scheffers (1983) has shown that if two vowels are presented simultaneously, they can be identified better when they have F_o's differing by more than 6% than when they have the same F_o.

F_o appears to be important in two complementary ways. Firstly, a common F_o causes a series of sinusoidal components to fuse together, being heard as a single sound. Secondly, if a sinusoidal component does not share this common F_o, it tends to be heard as a separate sound. This is illustrated by some experiments of Moore et al. (1986). They investigated the effect of mistuning a single low harmonic in a harmonic complex tone. When the harmonic was mistuned sufficiently it was heard as a separate pure tone standing out from the complex as a whole. The degree of mistuning required varied somewhat with the duration of the sounds; for 400 ms tones a mistuning of 3% was sufficient to make the harmonic stand out as a separate tone. Darwin and Gardner (1986) have demonstrated a similar effect for vowel sounds. They also showed that mistuning a harmonic could reduce the contribution of that harmonic to the timbre of the vowel; the effect of the mistuning was similar to the effect of reducing the harmonic in level.

The results described above can be explained in a qualitative way by extending the model of pitch perception presented in Chapter 5. Assume that the pitch of a complex tone results from a correlation or comparison of time intervals between successive nerve firings in neurones with different CFs. Only those 'channels' which show a high correlation would be classified as 'belonging' to the same sound. Such a mechanism would automatically group together components with a common F_o.

This simple extension is not entirely satisfactory since, when two complex tones are presented, there will be many channels in which the responses are influenced by harmonics from both tones. In these channels the temporal pattern of firing may be dominated by one harmonic, or may reflect the presence of more than one harmonic. The auditory system may be capable of partitioning the temporal information within a channel, assigning part to one tone and part to the other. We do not know how this is achieved. However, it is even more difficult to see how such an analysis could be achieved by a mechanism operating only on the spatial pattern of neural activity (Assmann and Summerfield, 1989).

B   Onset disparities

Rasch (1978) investigated the ability to hear one complex tone in the presence of another. One of the tones was treated as a masker and the level of the other (the higher in F_o) was adjusted to find the point where it was just detectable. When the two tones started at the same time, and had exactly the same temporal envelope, the threshold of the variable tone was between 0 and -20 dB relative to the level of the masking tone (see Fig. 7.1a). Thus, when a difference in F_o was the only cue, the tone with the higher F_o could not be heard when its level was more than 20 dB below that of the other tone.

Rasch also investigated the effect of starting the high tone just before the low tone (Fig. 7.1b). He found that threshold depended strongly on onset asynchrony, reaching a value of -60 dB for an asynchrony of 30 ms. Thus, when the high tone started 30 ms before the low tone, it could be heard much more easily, and with much greater differences in levels between the two tones.

Although the percept of his subjects was that the high tone continued throughout the low tone, Rasch showed that this percept was not based upon sensory information received during the presentation time of the low tone. He found that identical thresholds were obtained if the high tone terminated immediately after the onset of the low tone (Fig. 7.1c). It appears that the perceptual system 'assumes' that the high tone continues, since there is no evidence to the contrary. This effect is related to the continuity phenomenon which was described in Chapter 3, section 8, and we will discuss it further in this chapter (section 5).

Rasch (1978) showed that if the two tones have simultaneous onsets but different rise times, this also can give very low thresholds for the high tone, provided the higher tone has the shorter rise time. Under these conditions, and those of onset asynchronies up to 30 ms, the notes sound as though they start synchronously. Thus, we do not need to be consciously aware of the

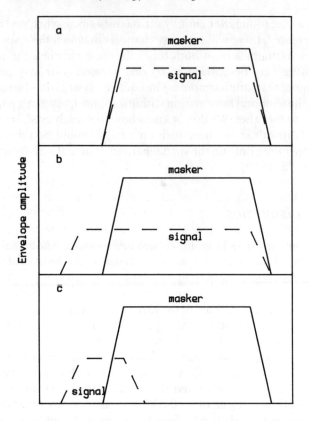

FIG. 7.1   Schematic illustration of the stimuli used by Rasch (1978). Both the signal and the masker were periodic complex tones, with the signal having the higher fundamental frequency. When the signal and masker were gated on and off synchronously (panel a), the threshold for the signal was relatively high. When the signal started slightly before the masker (panel b) the threshold was markedly reduced. When the signal was turned off as soon as the masker was turned on (panel c), the signal was perceived as continuing through the masker, and the threshold was the same as when the signal did continue through the masker.

onset differences for the auditory system to be able to exploit them in the perceptual separation of complex tones. Rasch also pointed out that, in ensemble music, different musicians do not play exactly in synchrony even if the score indicates that they should. The onset differences used in his experiments correspond roughly with the onset asynchronies of nominally 'simultaneous' notes found in performed music. This supports the view that the asynchronies are an important factor in the perception of the separate parts or voices in polyphonic music.

One modern-day example of the role of onset differences in aiding perceptual separation comes from electronic organs which have a synthesizer section. If the same note is played on the synthesizer section (set to, say, piano) and on the more conventional section (set to, say, violins), then the two notes remain perceptually separate even though they have exactly the same F_0. The main reason for this is that the shape and rise time of the envelope at onset is different for the two notes.

Onset asynchronies can also play a role in determining the timbre of complex sounds. Darwin (1984) showed that a tone that stops or starts at a different time from a vowel is less likely to be heard as part of that vowel than if it is simultaneous with it. For example, incrementing the level of a single harmonic can produce a significant change in the quality (timbre) of a vowel. However, if the incremented harmonic starts before the vowel, the change in vowel quality is markedly reduced.

C Contrast with previous sounds

The auditory system seems particularly well suited to the analysis of changes in the sensory input. The perceptual effect of a change in a stimulus can be roughly described by saying that the preceding stimulus is subtracted from the present one, so what remains is the change. The changed aspect stands out perceptually from the rest. Alternatively we might say that steady stimulation results in some kind of adaptation. When some aspect of a stimulus is changed, that aspect is freed from the effects of adaptation, and thus will be enhanced perceptually. While the underlying mechanism is a matter of debate, the perceptual effect certainly is not.

A powerful demonstration of this effect may be obtained by listening to a stimulus with a particular spectral structure and then switching rapidly to a stimulus with a flat spectrum, such as white noise. A white noise heard in isolation may be described as 'colourless'; it has no pitch and has a neutral sort of timbre. However, when a white noise follows immediately after a stimulus with spectral structure, the noise sounds 'coloured'. The coloration corresponds to the inverse of the spectrum of the preceding sound. For example, if the preceding sound is a noise with a bandstop or notch (Fig. 7.2a), the white noise (Fig. 7.2b) has a pitch-like quality, with a pitch value corresponding to the centre frequency of the notch (Zwicker, 1964). It sounds like a noise with a small spectral peak (Fig. 7.2c). A harmonic complex tone with a flat spectrum may be given a speech-like quality if it is

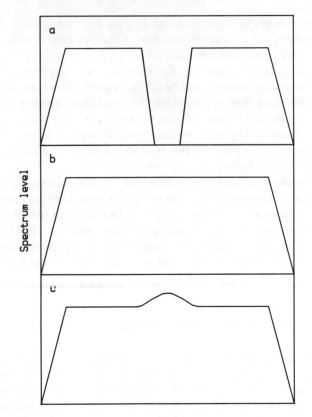

FIG. 7.2 Schematic illustration of the spectra of stimuli used to demonstrate the effect of contrast with previous sounds. A noise with a spectral notch is presented first (panel a). The stimulus is then changed to a noise with a flat spectrum (panel b). Normally this noise is perceived as 'colourless'. However, following the noise with the spectral notch it sounds like a noise with a spectral peak, such as that shown in panel c.

preceded by a harmonic complex having a spectrum which is the inverse of that of a speech sound, such as a vowel (Summerfield *et al.*, 1987).

A second demonstration of the effects of a change in a stimulus can be obtained by listening to a steady complex tone with many harmonics. Usually such a tone is heard with a single pitch corresponding to F_o, and the individual harmonics are not separately perceived. However, if one of the harmonics is changed in some way, either by altering its relative phase or its level, then that harmonic stands out perceptually from the complex as a whole. For a short time after the change is made, a pure-tone quality is perceived. The perception of the harmonic then gradually fades, until it merges with the complex once more. Notice that a decrease in level of a harmonic can produce this effect; the direction of the change is not crucial. Our ability to hear out harmonics when they change in some way is in excess of what would be expected on the basis of the critical bandwidth, or on the basis of direct studies of this ability for steady, unchanging, complex tones (see Chapter 3, section 2F). This illustrates the powerful nature of the change detection mechanisms.

Change detection is obviously of importance in assigning sound components to their appropriate sources. Normally we listen against a background of sounds which may be relatively unchanging, such as the humming of machinery, traffic noises, and so on. A sudden change in the sound is usually indicative that a new source has been activated, and the change detection mechanisms enable us to isolate the effects of the change and interpret them appropriately.

D   Correlated changes in amplitude or frequency

In section 3B we described the work of Rasch (1978) showing that the perceptual separation of two complex tones could be enhanced by introducing an onset asynchrony. The threshold of detection of the tone with the higher F_0 could be markedly reduced if that tone started 30 ms before the other tone. Rasch also showed that, even when the two tones started synchronously, it was possible to enhance their perceptual separation by frequency modulating the upper tone. This modulation was similar to the vibrato which often occurs for musical tones, and it was applied so that all the components in the higher tone moved up and down in synchrony. Rasch found that the modulation could reduce the threshold for the higher tone by 17 dB. Thus, when two complex tones are presented simultaneously, their perceptual separation can be enhanced if the components of one or the other are frequency modulated in a coherent way. A similar enhancement of perceptual separation can be produced by amplitude modulation of one of the tones.

Modulations in frequency or in amplitude can be effective not only in separating different groups of components, but also in producing a perceptual fusion of components (McAdams, 1982, 1989). This may occur even when those components are not harmonics of a common F_0. For example, if we present a steady complex sound containing many components with randomly distributed frequencies, a single noise-like sound will be heard, with a certain timbre. A subgroup of components in the complex can now be made to stand out perceptually from the rest by making them vary in a coherent way in either frequency, amplitude or both. This group will be perceived as a prominent 'figure' against a steady background, and both the figure and the background will have a timbre different from that of the original, unvarying sound.

The fusion of components which vary in a coherent way can also affect the perception of a single harmonic complex tone. Say, for example, we present the 3rd, 4th and 5th harmonics of a 200 Hz fundamental, namely 600, 800 and 1000 Hz. This complex may be perceived in two ways. We may listen in an analytic mode, hearing the pitches of one or more individual components (Chapter 3, section 2F) or we may listen in a synthetic mode, hearing a single pitch corresponding to the missing fundamental (Chapter 5, section 4). The analytic mode is more likely if the complex is presented continuously, or if we build up the complex by adding one component at a time. However, the synthetic mode is more likely if all the components in the complex are turned on and off together; the coherent behaviour of the components causes them to be fused into a single percept.

E   Sound location

It is a matter of everyday experience that components coming from the same direction tend to be assigned to a single source, whereas those coming from different directions are assigned to different sources. Thus the cues used in sound localization also help in the analysis of complex auditory inputs. We described in Chapter 6 a phenomenon that was related to this, namely the binaural masking level difference (MLD). The phenomenon can be summarized as follows: whenever the phase or level differences of a signal at the two ears are not the same as those of a masker, our ability to detect the signal is improved relative to the case where the signal and masker have the same phase and level relationships at the two ears. The practical implication is that a signal is easier to detect when it is located in a different position in space from the masker. Although most studies of the MLD have been concerned with threshold measurements, it seems clear that similar advantages of binaural listening can be gained in the identification and discrimination of signals presented against a background of other sound.

An example of the use of binaural cues in separating an auditory 'object' from its background comes from an experiment by Kubovy *et al.* (1974). They presented eight continuous sinusoids to each ear. The sinusoids had frequencies corresponding to the notes in a musical scale and each component had the same phase in the two ears. By shifting the phase of one of the sinusoids, relative to its counterpart in the opposite ear, that component could be displaced in subjective space from the rest, and was heard to stand out perceptually. A sequence of phase shifts in different components was clearly heard as a melody. This melody was completely undetectable when listening to the input to one ear alone. Thus, differences in relative phase at the two ears can allow an auditory 'object' to be isolated in the absence of any other cues.

4 THE PERCEPTION OF TEMPORAL PATTERNS

A The perception of rhythm

Just as sounds can be patterned according to the amount of energy in different frequency regions, so also can they be patterned according to how they vary as a function of time. Many of the auditory sequences occurring naturally are rhythmic, so that one might reasonably expect that the perceptual mechanisms are designed to make use of these rhythms (Sturgess and Martin, 1974). If an auditory pattern is rhythmic, then certain elements in the pattern are temporally redundant, so that once early elements of the pattern are heard, later elements, and possibly the end of the pattern, can be anticipated.

A number of workers have investigated the 'perceptual organization' or subjective grouping of repeating sequences of two elements (e.g. a high pitched buzz and a low pitched buzz). Royer and Garner (1966, 1970) required subjects to give verbal reports of the way such sequences were perceived. They found that subjects usually organized the pattern beginning at specific elements. These elements, termed preferred start points, either began a run of identical elements or were chosen to produce a pattern ending in a run of identical elements (HHHLHLHL or LHLHLHHH). If the temporal patterns were made more complex by the addition of features such as temporal pauses or intensity accents, organization could be either by these features or by the pattern structure of the elements. If the pattern structure was made to conflict with the pause organization by inserting a temporal pause before a nonpreferred start point (HHLHLHLH HHLHLHLH ...) the pause organization was dominant.

These experiments indicate a powerful subjective tendency for such patterns to be perceived as organized wholes. The physical characteristics which determine the organization are arranged in a hierarchical manner, timing being the most important characteristic. Handel (1973) has confirmed that if repeating patterns are segmented by temporal pauses, the pattern perception is based on the structure of the temporal grouping rather than on the structure of the pattern elements. In other words, the exact timing of the elements is more important in determining the subjective rhythm than is the patterning of the elements themselves (produced by pitch variations in this case). A review of the perception of rhythm is given in Fraisse (1982).

B   Auditory streaming

In the experiments on temporal patterning that we have described so far, the rate of presentation of elements was relatively slow (3–4 elements per second), and all the elements in the pattern were perceived as being part of a single pattern. When we listen to fast tone sequences (say 10 per second), this does not always happen. The tones are not grouped simply according to their physical temporal order, but according to their attributes, e.g. their pitches. When the tone sequence is perceived as a coherent whole, this is called fusion. When the sequence appears to split into a number of separate patterns, this is called rhythmic fission. Van Noorden (1971) investigated this phenomenon using a tone sequence where every second B was omitted from the regular sequence ABABAB ..., producing a sequence ABA ABA ... He found that this could be perceived in two ways, depending on the frequency separation of A and B. For small separations a single rhythm, resembling a gallop, is heard (fusion). For larger separations two separate tone sequences can be heard, one of which (A A A) is running twice as fast as the other (B B B) (fission). Van Noorden found that for some conditions either fusion or fission could be heard, according to the instructions given and the 'attentional set' of the subject.

Bregman and Campbell (1971) called the fission of the sound into perceptually separate tone sequences 'primary auditory stream segregation'. Bregman (1978) has suggested that each stream corresponds to an auditory 'object', and that stream segregation reflects the attribution of different components in the sound to different sources (see section 5). Components are more likely to be assigned to separate streams if they differ widely in frequency, or if there are rapid jumps in frequency between them.

Dowling (1968, 1973) has shown that stream segregation may also occur when successive tones differ in intensity or in spatial location. He presented a melody composed of equal-intensity notes, and inserted between each note of the melody a tone of the same intensity, with a frequency randomly selected from the same range. He found that the resulting tone sequence produced a meaningless jumble. Making the interposed notes different from those of the melody, either in intensity, frequency range, or spatial location, caused them to be heard as a separate stream, enabling subjects to pick out the melody.

A number of composers have exploited the fact that stream segregation occurs for tones widely separated in frequency. By playing a sequence of tones in which alternate notes are chosen from separate frequency ranges, an instrument such as the flute, which is only capable of playing one note at a time, can appear to be playing two themes at once. Many fine examples of this are available in the works of Bach. There are also cases where composers intend interleaved notes played by different instruments (e.g. the first and second violins) to be heard as a single melody. This only works when the different instruments have similar timbres and locations, and play in similar pitch ranges.

C Judgement of temporal order

A phenomenon which is probably related to that of stream segregation occurs in judgements of the temporal order of sounds. Ladefoged and Broadbent (1960) reported that extraneous sounds in sentences were grossly mislocated, so that a click might be reported as occurring a word or two away from its actual position. Surprisingly poor performance was also reported by Warren *et al.* (1969) for judgements of the temporal order of three or four unrelated items, such as a hiss, a tone and a buzz. Most subjects could not identify the order when each successive item lasted as long as 200 ms. Naive subjects required that each item lasted at least 700 ms to identify the order of four sounds presented in an uninterrupted series of repeated sequences. These durations are well above those which are normally considered necessary for temporal resolution in speech and music. For example, Winckel (1967) reported that the temporal order of musical notes is resolvable down to about 50 ms per note. Further, it is known that for smaller numbers of items the threshold duration for discrimination is much smaller; Hirsh (1959) found that for pairs of unrelated items durations as small as 20 ms still allowed correct order discrimination.

The poor order discrimination described by Warren *et al.* is probably a result of stream segregation. The sounds they used do not represent a coherent class. They have different temporal and spectral characteristics, and, as for tones widely differing in frequency, they do not form a single perceptual stream. Items in different streams appear to float about with respect to each other in subjective time, in much the same way as a click superimposed on speech. Thus, temporal order judgements are difficult. It should be emphasized that the relatively poor performance reported by Warren *et al.* (1969) is found only in tasks requiring absolute identification of the order of sounds, and not in tasks which simply require the discrimination of different sequences. Further, with extended training and feedback subjects can learn to distinguish between and identify orders within sequences of nonrelated sounds lasting only 10 ms or less (Warren, 1974). For sequences of tones, the component durations necessary for correct order identification may be as low as 2–7 ms (Divenyi and Hirsh, 1974).

To explain these effects Divenyi and Hirsh suggested that two kinds of perceptual judgements are involved. At longer component durations the listener is able to hear a clear sequence of steady-state sounds, whereas at shorter durations a change in the order of components introduces qualitative changes that are capable of being discriminated by trained listeners. Similar explanations have been put forward by Green (1973) and Warren (1974) (see also Chapter 4).

Bregman and Campbell (1971) investigated the factors that make temporal order judgements for tone sequences difficult. They used naive subjects, so that performance presumably depended on the subjects actually perceiving the sounds as a sequence, rather than on their learning the overall sound pattern. They found that in a repeating cycle of mixed high and low tones subjects could discriminate the order of the high tones relative to one another, or of the low tones among themselves, but they could not order the high tones relative to the low ones. The authors suggested that this was because the two groups of sounds split into separate perceptual streams, and that judgements across streams are difficult.

In a further investigation of this effect, Bregman and Dannenbring (1973) used tone sequences in which successive tones were connected by frequency glides. They found that these glides reduced the tendency for the sequences to split into high and low streams, while at the same time order perception was easier. Conditions using partial glides also showed decreased stream segregation, although the partial glides were not quite as effective as complete glides. Thus, complete continuity between tones is not required to reduce stream segregation; a frequency change 'pointing' towards the next tone allows the listener to follow the pattern more easily.

The effects of frequency glides and other types of transitions in preventing stream segregation or fission are probably of considerable importance in the perception of speech. Speech sounds may follow one another in very rapid sequences, and the glides and partial glides observed in the acoustic components of speech may be a strong factor in maintaining the speech as a unified stream (see Chapter 8).

5   GENERAL PRINCIPLES OF PERCEPTUAL ORGANIZATION

Bregman (1978), and Bregman and Pinker (1978) have suggested that it is useful to make a distinction between two concepts in hearing: source and stream. A source is some physical entity which gives rise to acoustic pressure waves, for example a violin being played. A stream, on the other hand, is the percept of a group of successive and/or simultaneous sound elements as a coherent whole, appearing to emanate from a single source. For example, it is the percept of hearing a violin being played. A great many different sorts of physical cues may be used to derive separate perceptual streams corresponding to the individual sources which give rise to a complex acoustic input. Bregman and Pinker (1978) describe this acoustic factoring as parsing; the acoustic information is parsed to form separate streams in the same way that visual information falling on the retina is parsed to form objects and backgrounds. The parsing has two aspects: "the grouping together of all the simultaneous frequency components that emanate from a single source at a given moment, and the connecting over time of the changing frequencies that a single source produces from one moment to the next".

The Gestalt psychologists (e.g. Koffka, 1935) described many of the factors which govern perceptual organization and, as we shall see, their descriptions and principles apply well to the way physical cues are used to achieve the parsing of the acoustic input. It seems likely that the 'rules' of perceptual organization have arisen because, on the whole, they tend to give the right answers. That is, use of the rules generally results in a grouping of those parts of the acoustic input that arose from the same source, and a segregation of those that did not. No single rule will always work, but it appears that the rules can generally be used together, in a coordinated and probably quite complex way, in order to arrive at a correct interpretation of the input. In the following sections we will outline the major principles or rules of perceptual organization. We should note that these generally apply both to vision and hearing, and that they were mostly described first in relation to vision.

A Similarity

This principle is that elements will be grouped if they are similar. In hearing, similarity usually implies closeness of timbre, pitch, loudness, or subjective location. We have already seen examples of this principle in studies of the perception of tone sequences. If we listen to a rapid sequence of pure tones, say 10 tones per second, then tones which are closely spaced in frequency, and are therefore similar, form a single perceptual stream, whereas tones which are widely spaced form separate streams.

In the case of complex tones the basis of 'similarity' is not so clear. Van Noorden (1975) investigated the perception of sequences of complex tones each of which was composed of a group of harmonics of a missing fundamental. When the (missing) fundamentals were different, but the harmonics fell in the same frequency region, fusion occurred; the tones formed a single perceptual stream. When the (missing) fundamentals were the same, but the harmonics fell in different frequency regions, fission took place; the harmonics in different frequency regions formed separate perceptual streams. Thus for sequences of complex tones it appears that pitch does not provide the basis for similarity; tones with the same (missing) fundamental, and therefore the same pitch, do not necessarily form a single stream, whereas tones with similar timbres do, even if the pitches are different. This demonstration of van Noorden is not entirely clear cut, however, since some of the complex tones he used contained only a few high harmonics, and hence had a rather weak, ambiguous pitch (see Chapter 5).

A final example of grouping on the basis of similarity comes from a study by van Noorden (1975) of the perception of a sequence of tones with the same frequency but with an intensity which alternated between two values. When there was a large difference between the two intensity values, the sequence of loud tones formed a separate perceptual stream from the soft tones, and attention could be directed either to the loud tones or the soft tones. When the tones were similar in intensity, a single stream was perceived with a tempo twice that of either the loud or the soft tones. Thus similarity in loudness can form the basis of perceptual grouping.

B   Good continuation

This principle exploits a physical property of sound sources, that changes in frequency, intensity, location or spectrum tend to be smooth and continuous, rather than abrupt. Hence a smooth change in any of these aspects indicates a change within a single source, whereas a sudden change indicates that a new source has been activated. Again, we have already seen examples of this in the perception of tone sequences. Bregman and Dannenbring (1973) showed that the tendency of a sequence of high and low tones to split into two streams was reduced when successive tones were connected by frequency glides. Such glides are commonly found in speech sounds (see Chapter 8), and probably help to hold the speech together as a single perceptual stream.

A second example comes from studies using synthetic speech (see Chapter 8). In such speech, large fluctuations of an unexpected kind in F_o (and correspondingly in the pitch) give the impression that a new speaker has stepped in to take over a few syllables from the primary speaker. However, it appears that, in this case, the smoothness of the F_o contour is not the sole factor which determines whether an intrusion is perceived. A single speaker's F_o's cover a range of about one octave, but the intrusion effect is observed for much smaller jumps than this, provided they are inconsistent with the changes in F_o required by the linguistic and phonetic context. Thus it appears that the assignment of incoming spectral patterns to particular speakers is done partly on the basis of F_o, but in a manner which requires a knowledge of the 'rules' of intonation; only deviations which do not conform to the 'rules' are interpreted as a new speaker.

Darwin and Bethell-Fox (1977) have reported an experimental study of this effect. They synthesized spectral patterns which changed smoothly and repeatedly between two vowel sounds. When the F_o of the sound patterns was constant they were heard as coming from a single source, and the speech sounds heard included glides (l as in let) and semivowels (w as in we). When a discontinuous, step-like F_o contour was imposed on the patterns, they divided into two perceptually distinct speech sources, and the speech was perceived as containing predominantly stop consonants (e.g. b as in be, and d as in day) (see Chapter 8 for a description of the characteristics of these speech sounds). Apparently a given group of components is usually only perceived as part of one stream (section 5D). Thus, the perceptual segregation produces illusory silences in each stream during the portions of the signal attributed to the other stream, and these silences are interpreted, together with the gliding spectral patterns in the vowels, as indicating the presence of stop consonants (see Chapter 8). It is clear that the perception of speech sounds can be strongly influenced by stream organization.

C   Common fate

The different frequency components arising from a single sound source usually vary in a highly coherent way. They tend to start and finish together, to change in intensity together, and to change in frequency together. This fact is exploited by the perceptual system, and gives rise to the principle of common fate: if two or more components in a complex sound undergo the same kinds of changes at the same time, then they are grouped and perceived as part of the same source. This is a powerful principle, and it gives rise to perceptual abilities in excess of what would be expected from studies using steady stimuli.

There are two examples of common fate which we have described, and which are of importance in the perceptual analysis of sounds such as speech and music. The first concerns the role of the onsets of sounds. Components will be grouped together if they start synchronously; otherwise they will form separate streams. The onset asynchronies necessary to allow the separation of two complex tones are not large, about 30 ms being sufficient. The asynchronies which are observed in performed music are typically as large as, or larger than this, so that when we listen to polyphonic music we are easily able to hear separately the melodic line of each instrument.

Our second example concerns modulations; components which are amplitude or frequency modulated in a synchronous way will be grouped together. Again, this has its counterpart in performed music. The notes produced by musical instruments are often amplitude or frequency modulated (tremolo, vibrato), and this helps us to assign the appropriate harmonics to each instrument. Although our examples have both been drawn from the perception of music, very similar considerations apply to the case where several people are talking at once. The components from any single voice usually start and finish together, and, at least over short periods of time, vary together in amplitude and frequency. This contributes to our ability to hear out one voice from a mixture of voices.

D Disjoint allocation

Broadly speaking, this principle, also known as 'belongingness', is that a single component in a sound can only be assigned to one source at a time. In other words, once a component has been 'used' in the formation of one stream, it cannot be used in the formation of a second stream. For certain types of stimuli, the perceptual organization may be ambiguous, there being more than one way to interpret the sensory input. When a given component might belong to one of a number of streams, the percept may alter depending on the stream within which that component is included.

An example is provided by the work of Bregman and Rudnicky (1975). They presented a sequence of four brief tones in rapid succession. Two of the tones, labelled X, had the same frequency, but the middle two, A and B, were different. The four-tone sequence was either XABX or XBAX. The listeners had to judge the order of A and B. This was harder than when the tones AB occurred in isolation (Fig. 7.3a) because A and B were perceived as part of a longer four-tone pattern, including the two 'distractor' tones, labelled X (Fig. 7.3b). They then embedded the four-tone sequence into a longer sequence of tones, called 'captor' tones (Fig. 7.3c). When the captor tones had frequencies close to those of the distractor tones, they 'captured' the distractors into a separate perceptual stream, leaving the tones AB in a stream of their own. This made the order of A and B easy to judge. It seems that the tones X could not be perceived as part of both streams. When only one stream is the subject of judgement and hence of attention, the other one may serve to remove distractors from the domain of attention.

It should be noted that the principle of disjoint allocation does not always work, particularly in situations where there are two or more plausible perceptual organizations (Bregman, 1987). In such situations, a sound element may sometimes be heard as part of more than one stream. Some examples will be given in Chapter 8.

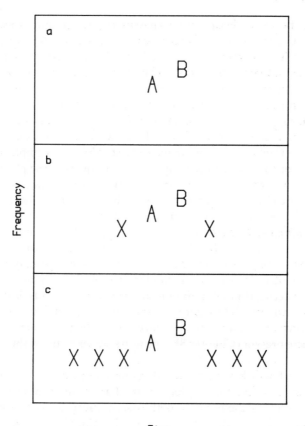

Time

FIG. 7.3 Schematic illustration of the stimuli used by Bregman and Rudnicky (1975). When the tones A and B are presented alone (panel a) it is easy to tell their order. When the tones A and B are presented as part of a four tone complex XABX (panel b) it is more difficult to tell their order. If the four tone complex is embedded in a longer sequence of X tones (panel c), the X's form a separate perceptual stream, and it is easy to tell the order of A and B.

E   Closure

In everyday life the sound from a given source may frequently be temporarily obscured by other sounds. While the obscuring sound is present there may be no sensory evidence which can be used to determine whether the obscured sound has continued or not. Under these conditions the obscured sound still tends to be perceived as continuous. The Gestalt psychologists called this process 'closure'. One example of this occurs when reception of FM radio is disturbed by ignition noise from passing traffic. The interference is perceived as a series of clicks or a buzz superimposed on the continuous speech or music signal. In fact, what happens is that the interference temporarily captures the response of the radio, so that while each interfering click is present nothing at all of the desired signal gets through. The perceptual system fills in the missing parts of the signal.

A laboratory example of this phenomenon is the continuity effect described in Chapter 3, section 9. When a sound A is alternated with a sound B, and B is more intense than A, then A may be heard as continuous, even though it is interrupted. The sounds do not have to be steady. For example, if B is noise, and A is a tone which is gliding upwards in frequency, the glide is heard as continuous even though certain parts of the glide are missing. Notice that, for this to be the case, the gaps in the tone must be filled with noise. In the absence of noise, discrete jumps in frequency are clearly heard.

The continuity effect also works for speech stimuli alternated with noise. In the absence of noise to fill in the gaps, interrupted speech sounds hoarse and raucous. When noise is presented in the gaps, the speech sounds more natural and continuous (Miller and Licklider, 1950). For connected speech at moderate interruption rates the intervening noise actually leads to an improvement in intelligibility (Dirks and Bower, 1970). This may be because the abrupt switching of the speech produces misleading cues as to which speech sounds were present (Chapter 8). The noise serves to mask these misleading cues.

It is clear from these examples that the perceptual filling in of missing sounds does not take place solely on the basis of evidence in the acoustic waveform. Our past experience with speech, music and other stimuli must play a role, and the context of surrounding sounds is obviously important. We should note, however, that the filling in only occurs when one source is perceived as masking or occluding another. This percept must be based on acoustic evidence that the occluded sound has been masked. Thus, if a gap is not filled by a noise or other sound, the perceptual closure does not occur; a gap is heard.

F   The figure-ground phenomenon and attention

Several times in this chapter we have referred to the role of attention. It seems that we are not generally capable of consciously attending to every aspect of the auditory input (or indeed of other sensory inputs); rather, certain parts are selected for conscious analysis. In principle, we might think it possible to attend to and compare any arbitrary small group of elements in a complex acoustic signal. However, this does not appear to be the case. Rather, it appears that the complex sound is analysed into streams, and we attend primarily to one stream at a time. This attended stream then stands out perceptually, while the rest of the sound is less prominent. The Gestalt psychologists called the separation into attended and unattended streams the 'figure-ground phenomenon'.

At a crowded cocktail party, we attend to one conversation at a time, and the other conversations form a kind of background. Similarly, when we listen to a piece of polyphonic music, we attend primarily to one melodic line at a time. We can, of course, switch attention from one conversation to another, or from one melodic line to another, and we may have some awareness of the other voices, but it appears that one stream at a time is selected for a complete conscious analysis. Neisser (1967) has suggested that attention may be brought to bear after the preliminary analysis into streams has occurred. The 'pre-attentive' processes involved thus place constraints upon attention: it is difficult to attend simultaneously to, or to make relative judgements about, elements which form parts of two separate perceptual streams.

Although the formation of auditory streams places constraints upon attention, we should not view this as an entirely one-way process; attention may also influence the formation of streams. For example, when we listen to a sequence of alternating tones, with an interval of about seven semitones between the tones, we may hear either fission or fusion depending on our attentional 'set' (van Noorden, 1975). We can listen selectively, trying to hear either the upper tones or the lower tones, or we can listen comprehensively, trying to hear all the tones together. The associated percepts seem to be mutually exclusive. When we listen without any particular set, we may hear first one percept and then the other. The change occurs at irregular intervals, and appears spontaneous. This is an example of a perceptual reversal, resulting from an ambiguity in the interpretation of the sensory input.

We may interpret the importance of changes in stimuli (section 3C) in the context of the figure-ground phenomenon. Whenever some aspect of a sound changes, while the rest remains relatively unchanging, then that aspect is drawn to the listener's attention: it becomes the figure, while the steady part forms the background. This is of practical value since events of significance in the world are usually associated with a change of some kind. Our sensitivity to change provides a way of directing our attention to new and potentially important events in the environment.

Finally, we should note that our ability to direct attention to one stream among a number, and indeed to form the stream in the first place, does not depend only upon information available in the acoustic waveform. The Gestalt rules themselves constitute a form of knowledge, but other sources of information or knowledge may also be involved. An example of this comes from the 'cocktail party' phenomenon, our ability to attend selectively to one conversation among many. It turns out that we can follow a conversation more successfully if the subject matter of that conversation is different from that of the other conversations. Clearly, this involves relatively high level processes. We shall discuss this point further in Chapter 8.

6   GENERAL CONCLUSIONS

In everyday life the sound reaching our ears generally arises from a number of different sound sources. The auditory system is usually able to parse the acoustic input, so that the components deriving from each source are grouped together and form part of a single perceptual stream. Thus, each source may be ascribed its own pitch, timbre, loudness and location, and sometimes a source may be identified as familiar.

The identification of a particular sound source depends on the recognition of its timbre. For steady sounds, the timbre depends primarily on the distribution of energy over frequency. The perceptual differences in the timbres of sounds can be represented as distances in a multidimensional space. This space correlates highly with that derived from a physical analysis of the sound using filters whose bandwidths approximate the critical bandwidths of the ear. The time structure of sounds can also have an influence on their timbres; onset transients are particularly important.

Many different physical cues can be used to achieve the perceptual separation of the components arising from different sources. These include differences in fundamental frequency, onset disparities, contrast with previous sounds, changes in frequency and intensity, and sound location. No single cue is effective all of the time, but used together they generally provide an excellent basis for the parsing of the acoustic input.

When we listen to rapid sequences of sounds, the sounds may be perceived as a single perceptual stream, or they may split into a number of perceptual streams, a process known as primary auditory stream segregation or fission. Fission is more likely to occur if the elements making up the sequence differ markedly in frequency, amplitude, location or spectrum. Such elements would normally emanate from more than one sound source. When two elements of a sound are grouped into two different streams, it is more difficult to judge their temporal order than when they form part of the same stream.

The general principles which govern the perceptual organization of the auditory world correspond well to those described by the Gestalt psychologists. The principle of similarity is that sounds will be grouped into a single perceptual stream if they are similar in pitch, timbre, loudness or subjective location. The principle of good continuation is that smooth changes in frequency, intensity, location or spectrum will be perceived as changes in a single source, whereas abrupt changes indicate a change in source. The principle of common fate is that if two components in a sound undergo the same kinds of changes at the same time, then they will be grouped and perceived as part of a single source. The principle of disjoint allocation is that a given element in a sound can only form part of one stream at a time. The principle of closure is that when parts of a sound are masked or occluded, that sound will be perceived as continuous, provided there is no direct sensory evidence to indicate that it has been interrupted.

Usually we attend primarily to one perceptual stream at a time. That stream stands out from the background formed by other streams. Stream formation places constraints upon attention, but attention may also influence the formation of streams. Stream formation may also depend upon information not directly available in the acoustic waveform.

FURTHER READING

This is an area in which there is no authoritative text. However, the forthcoming book by Bregman promises to provide such a text:

Bregman, A. S. (1990). *Auditory Scene Analysis: The Perceptual Organization of Sound*, MIT Press, Cambridge, Mass. (in preparation).

The following provide some useful additional material:

Bregman, A.S. (1978). The formation of auditory streams. In *Attention and Performance* Vol.7 (ed. J. Requin), Lawrence Erlbaum, New Jersey.
Bregman, A. S. and Pinker, S. (1978). Auditory streaming and the building of timbre. *Can. J. Psychol.* 32, 19–31.
Kubovy, M. and Pomerantz, J.R. (1981). *Perceptual Organization*, Erlbaum, New Jersey.
Hartmann, W. M. (1988). Pitch perception and the segregation of auditory entities. In *Auditory Function* (eds G. M. Edelman, W. E. Gall and W. M. Cowan), Wiley, New York.
Yost, W. A. and Watson, C. S. (1987). *Auditory Processing of Complex Sounds*, Erlbaum, New Jersey.

Demonstrations 19, 28, 29 and 30 of *Auditory Demonstrations* on CD are relevant to the contents of this chapter (see list of further reading for Chapter 1).

8
Speech perception

1 INTRODUCTION

In this chapter we shall be concerned with the problem of how the complex acoustical patterns of speech are interpreted by the brain and perceived as linguistic units. The details of this process are still not fully understood, despite a large amount of research carried out over the past 40 years. What has become clear is that speech perception does not depend on the extraction of simple invariant acoustic patterns directly available in the speech wave-form. This has been illustrated both by perceptual studies and by attempts to build machines which recognize speech (see Holmes, 1988). A given speech sound is not represented by a fixed acoustic pattern in the speech wave; instead the speech sound's acoustic pattern varies in a complex manner according to the preceding and following sounds.

For continuous speech, perception does not depend solely on cues present in the acoustic waveform. Part of a word which is highly probable in the context of a sentence may be 'heard' even when the acoustic cues for that part are minimal or completely absent. For example, Warren (1970b) has shown that when an extraneous sound (such as a cough) completely replaces a speech sound in a recorded sentence, listeners report that they hear the missing sound. Clearly, the linguistic context is of considerable importance. This phenomenon is probably related to the continuity effect described in Chapters 3 and 7; when a weak sound is alternated with a louder sound of similar frequency, the weak sound may appear continuous even though it is, in fact, pulsating. The effect reported by Warren has been shown to depend on similar factors; the listeners only 'hear' the missing sound if the cough is relatively intense and contains frequency components close to those of the missing sound. This kind of filling-in process is obviously of importance when listening in noisy environments, and it illustrates the importance of non-acoustic cues in speech perception. On the other hand, we are able to recognize words spoken in isolation, provided they are clearly articulated, so linguistic context is not a *necessary* requirement for the perception of speech.

It is far beyond the scope of this book to give more than a brief description of certain selected aspects of speech perception. We shall not emphasize the aspects of speech recognition related to semantic cues (the meaning of preceding and following words and the subject matter), syntactic cues (grammatical rules) and circumstantial cues (speaker identity, listening environment, etc.), even though these may be of considerable importance, especially in noisy environments. We shall concentrate rather on the perceptual processing of patterns in the acoustic waveform.

The study of the perception of acoustic patterns in speech has been greatly aided by the use of speech synthesizers. These devices allow the production of acoustic waveforms resembling real speech to varying degrees; the closeness of the resemblance depends upon the complexity of the device and the trouble to which the experimenter is prepared to go. In contrast to real speech, these waveforms have controlled and precisely reproducible characteristics. Using a speech synthesizer, the experimenter can manipulate certain aspects of the speech waveform, leaving all the other characteristics unchanged, making it possible to investigate what aspects of the waveform determine how it is perceived. The results of such experiments have been instrumental in the formulation of theories of speech perception.

2 THE NATURE OF SPEECH SOUNDS

The most familiar units of speech are words. These can often be broken down into somewhat smaller units, that is, into syllables. However, linguists generally consider that syllables can in turn be analysed in terms of sequences of smaller units – the speech sounds or phonemes. To clarify the nature of phonemes, consider the following example. The word 'bit' is composed of three phonemes: an initial, a middle and a final phoneme. By altering just one of these phonemes at a time we can create three new words: 'pit', 'bet' and 'bid'. Each of these three words differs from 'bit' by just one phoneme. Thus, for the linguist, the phonemes are the smallest units of sound that in any given language differentiate one word from another. Phonemes on their own do not have a meaning or symbolize an object (some are not even pronounceable in isolation), but in relation to other phonemes they distinguish one word from another, and in combination they form syllables and words. Note that phonemes are defined in terms of what is perceived, rather than in terms of acoustic patterns. Thus, they are abstract, subjective entities, rather like pitch. However, they are also sometimes specified in terms of the way they are produced.

Not all linguists or psychologists would accept that it is appropriate to consider phonemes as 'the basic units' of speech perception (Mehler, 1981), and indeed some would deny that the phoneme has any perceptual reality as a unit (e.g. Warren, 1976). However, the analysis of speech in terms of phonemes has been widespread and influential, and we shall continue to use the concept for the purposes of discussion. English has around 40 different phonemes which are represented by a set of symbols. Some symbols are the letters of the Roman alphabet, and others are special characters. When a character is used to represent a phoneme this is indicated by a slash (/) before and after the character. For example, /s/ is the first and /i/ is the final phoneme of the word 'see'.

Some workers have suggested that speech perception may proceed via the extraction of certain phonetic features which are descriptive of the way that the speech sounds are produced (Jakobson *et al.*, 1963). These phonetic features might in turn be derived from certain acoustic patterns or properties of the speech. We will return to this point later.

A simple view of speech perception would hold that speech is composed of a series of acoustic patterns or properties, and that each pattern or set of patterns corresponds to a particular phoneme. Thus, the acoustic patterns would have a one-to-one correspondence with the phonemes, and a sequence of patterns would be perceived as a sequence of phonemes, which would then be combined into words and phrases. Unfortunately, this view is not tenable. To understand why, we must consider in more detail the characteristics of speech sounds. The following paragraphs outline the relationship between the way in which speech sounds are produced and the acoustic characteristics of the speech.

Speech sounds are produced by the vocal organs, namely the lungs, the windpipe, the larynx (containing the vocal folds), the throat or pharynx, the nose and nasal cavities, and the mouth. The part of this system lying above the larynx is called the vocal tract, and its shape can be varied extensively by movements of various parts such as the tongue, the lips and the jaw.

The space between the vocal folds is called the glottis. The vocal folds can open and close, varying the size of the glottis. This affects the flow of air from the lungs. The term 'glottal source' refers to the sound energy produced by the flow of air from the lungs past the vocal folds as they open and close quite rapidly in a periodic or quasi-periodic manner. Sounds produced while the vocal folds are vibrating are said to be 'voiced'. The glottal source is a periodic complex tone with a relatively low fundamental frequency, whose spectrum contains harmonics covering a wide range of frequencies, but with more energy at low frequencies than at high (see Fig. 8.1a). This spectrum is subsequently modified by the vocal tract. The vocal tract behaves like a rather complex filter, introducing resonances (called formants) at certain frequencies. The formants are numbered, the one with the lowest frequency being called the first formant (F1), the next the second (F2) and so on. The centre frequencies of the formants differ according to the shape of the vocal tract.

The speech sounds which are characterized most easily are the vowels. These are usually voiced (but they can be whispered) and they have formants that are relatively stable over time. Figure 8.1(b) shows cross sections of the vocal tract for three different vowels, and Fig. 8.1(c) shows the filter functions or transfer functions for those vocal tract shapes. Figure 8.1(d) shows the spectra of the vowels resulting from passing the glottal source through the vocal tract. Notice that the vowels contain peaks in their spectra at the frequencies corresponding to the formants.

Many speech sounds are produced by a narrowing or constriction of the vocal tract at some point along its length. Such sounds are classified into a number of different types according to the degree and nature of the constriction. The major types are fricatives, stops, affricates and nasals.

Fricatives are produced by forcing air past a narrow constriction, which gives a turbulent air flow. They have a noise-like quality, and may consist of that noise alone (as in /s/), or may consist of that noise together with a glottal source, as in /z/, the voiced counterpart of /s/.

Stops are produced by making a complete closure somewhere in the vocal tract. The closure may remain for some time, but the closing and opening are rapid. The closure stops the flow of air for a certain time, with a consequent reduction or cessation of acoustic energy, after which the airflow and energy abruptly resume. As with fricatives, stops may be voiced (as in /b/, /d/ or /g/) or voiceless (as in their counterparts /p/, /t/ or /k/). For a voiced stop, the vocal folds are vibrating at or close to the moment when the release of the closure occurs; they may also vibrate during the closure. For voiceless stops, the vocal folds stop vibrating during closure and usually for some time after the release.

Affricates are like a combination of stop and fricative; they are characterized by a closure, giving silence, followed by a narrow constriction giving turbulence. An example is /tʃ/ as in the first and last sounds of 'church'.

Many voiceless sounds do not show a distinct pattern of formants, particularly when they are produced by a constriction close to the outer end of the vocal tract (e.g. /s/). However, they do generally have a distinct spectral shape, which is determined by the shape of the vocal tract during their articulation, and this determines how they sound.

Nasals, such as /m/ and /n/, are produced by allowing air to flow through the nasal passages, keeping the oral cavity completely closed. This can produce one or more extra resonances and also an antiresonance. The latter reduces the energy of the glottal source over a certain frequency range. The net effect is a broad low-amplitude, low-frequency spectral prominence.

The different classes of consonants described above differ from each other

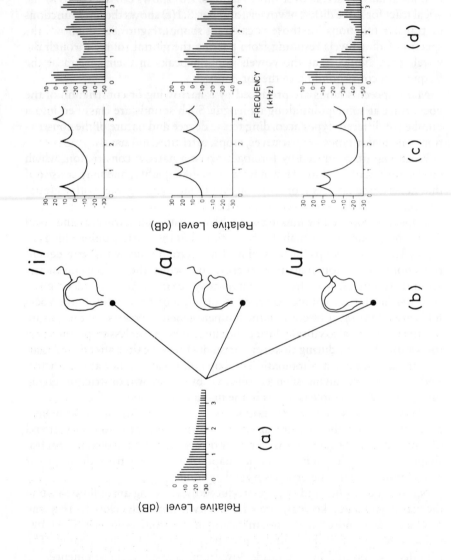

in the *manner* in which they are produced. The manner of articulation refers to the degree and type of constriction of the vocal tract. In addition, there are, within each class, differences in the *place* of articulation (the place at which maximum constriction occurs, e.g. teeth, lips, roof of the mouth). All of these differences are reflected in the acoustic characteristics of the speech wave, as revealed by the spectrum. However, for nearly all speech sounds, the spectra are not static, but change as a function of time. For further details of the relationship between articulation and the acoustic characteristics of speech, the reader is referred to Pickett (1980, an introductory text) and Fant (1960, a technical treatment of the subject).

Speech, then, is composed of acoustic patterns which vary in frequency, intensity and time. In order to show these variations simultaneously a display known as the spectrogram is used. In this display the amount of energy in a given frequency band is plotted as a function of time. Essentially, the short-term spectrum is determined for a series of successive samples of the speech. Time is represented on the abscissa, frequency on the ordinate, and intensity by the darkness used. In a display like this, it is impossible to have high resolution both in frequency and in time; one is traded against the other. In a 'wideband' spectrogram the bandwidth of the analysis used is typically 300 Hz. This gives good time resolution, often showing individual glottal pulses of voiced speech but not the individual harmonics of the voice fundamental frequency (when the fundamental is below 300 Hz; exceptions may occur for children and the upper ranges of women's voices). In a 'narrowband' spectrogram the bandwidth of analysis is typically 45 Hz. This is usually sufficient to resolve individual harmonics, but it gives poorer resolution in time, and does not usually show individual glottal pulses. Note that neither wideband nor narrowband spectrograms are representative of the way that the ear analyses sounds; the bandwidths of the auditory filters vary with centre frequency (see Chapter 3), whereas the spectrogram usually uses a fixed bandwidth and a linear frequency scale.

An example of a wideband spectrogram is given in Fig. 8.2. Very dark areas indicate high concentrations of energy at particular frequencies, while very light areas indicate an absence of energy. Dark bands running roughly

---

FIG. 8.1 Illustration of how three different vowel sounds are produced. Part a shows the spectrum of the sound produced by vibration of the vocal folds. It consists of a series of harmonics whose levels decline with increasing frequency. Part b shows schematic cross-sections of the vocal tract in the positions appropriate for the three vowels. Part c shows the filter functions or transfer functions associated with those positions of the vocal tract. Part d shows the spectra of the vowels resulting from passing the glottal source in panel a through the filter functions in panel c. From Bailey (1983) by permission of the author.

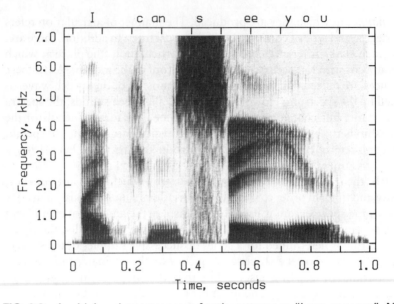

FIG. 8.2 A wideband spectrogram for the utterance "I can see you". Notice the concentration of energy at particular frequencies (corresponding to formants), except for the /s/ sound, and the lack of silent intervals between successive words. The vertical striations correspond to individual periods of vocal fold vibration, and their spacing depends on the rate of this vibration.

horizontally can be clearly seen; these correspond to the formants. Several formants are visible in this example, but experiments using synthetic speech suggest that the first three are the most important for the purpose of identifying speech sounds. Indeed, many researchers consider that the frequencies of the formants, and not some other characteristic such as their bandwidths or amplitudes, are the most important determinant of vowel quality (e.g. Klatt, 1982). There are, of course, other ways of analysing vowel sounds, as we saw in Chapter 7 (e.g. the dimensional analysis approach by Plomp and his colleagues), but analysis in terms of formants has been by far the most common and most influential technique.

A marked characteristic of speech sounds is that there are often rapid changes in the frequency of a given formant or set of formants. These changes, known as formant transitions, reflect the changes in the shape of the vocal tract as the articulators move from one position to another. For some speech sounds, such as stop consonants, the formant transitions are an inherent property of the sounds; stops are produced by rapid movements of the articulators. The formant transitions in such sounds have been found to be important acoustic cues for determining their identity. For other sounds, the formant transitions occur as a consequence of the smooth movement of the articulators from the position appropriate for one sound (the /i/ as in see) to the position appropriate for another (the /u/ as in you). This effect is known as coarticulation. A consequence of coarticulation is that the acoustic properties of a given speech sound are influenced by the preceding and following sounds.

The spectrogram of a complete sentence may show a number of time intervals where there is little or no spectral energy. However, these silent intervals do not generally correspond to 'spaces' between words, as we do not pause between each word when speaking. Rather, they usually indicate the presence of particular types of speech sounds, particularly the stop consonants and affricates. Thus, in explaining speech perception we have to specify not only how (or whether) the acoustic patterns in the speech sound are 'decoded' into individual phonemes, but also how the sequence of sounds is segmented into individual words and syllables. This has turned out to be a major difficulty for models of speech perception, and also for attempts to build machines to recognize speech. For example, most such machines would have great difficulty in distinguishing the utterances 'recognize speech' and 'wreck a nice beach' if these were spoken in a normal conversational manner.

3 SPEECH PERCEPTION – WHAT IS SPECIAL ABOUT SPEECH?

Some researchers have argued that special mechanisms have evolved for the perception of speech sounds, and that the perception of speech differs in significant ways from the perception of nonspeech sounds. In particular, it has been argued that there is a special 'speech mode' of perception which is engaged automatically when we listen to speech sounds. In this section we will compare some aspects of the perception of speech and nonspeech sounds, and evaluate the extent to which speech perception appears to require special decoding mechanisms.

A The rate at which speech sounds occur

Liberman *et al.* (1967) pointed out that in rapid speech as many as 30 phonemes per second may occur. It was argued that this would be too fast for resolution in the auditory system; the sounds would merge into an unanalysable buzz and so a special decoding mechanism would be required. However, recent evidence does not support this point of view. We saw in Chapters 4 and

7 that listeners can, in fact, learn to identify sequences of sounds when the individual items are as short as 10 ms (corresponding to a rate of 100 items per second), but that at these short durations the listeners do not perceive each successive item separately but rather learn the overall sound pattern. It is likely that for continuous speech something similar occurs. The successive acoustic patterns in speech are probably not perceived as discrete acoustic events. Rather the listener recognizes the sound pattern corresponding to a group of acoustic patterns. The size of this larger sound pattern remains unclear, but it might, for example, correspond to a whole syllable.

B The variable nature of acoustic cues

A central problem in understanding speech perception is the variable nature of the acoustic patterns which can be perceived as any particular phoneme. Consider as an example the phoneme /d/ as in 'dawn'. A major cue for the perception of /d/ is the form of second formant transition which occurs at the release of the sound. Consider the highly simplified synthetic spectrographic patterns shown in Fig. 8.3. When these are converted into sound, the first formant transition (the change in frequency of the lowest formant at the beginning of the sound) indicates that the sound is one of the voiced stops /b, d, g/. Some other aspect of the sounds determines which of these three is

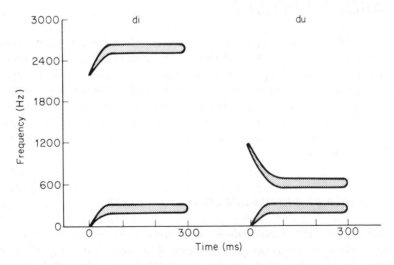

FIG. 8.3 Highly simplified spectrographic patterns which are perceived as /di/ and /du/ when they are converted into sound. From Liberman *et al.* (1967), by permission of the authors and the American Psychological Association.

actually heard. The sounds illustrated are actually identified as /di/ and /du/ when presented to listeners. On the basis of a number of perceptual experiments using such synthetic speech sounds, Liberman *et al.* (1967) concluded that the second formant transitions in the patterns are the cues for the perception of /d/ as opposed to /b/ or /g/. Notice that, although listeners identify both /di/ and /du/ as beginning with the phoneme /d/, the acoustic patterns at the beginning of the sounds are vastly different for the two sounds. In the case of /di/ the second formant rises from about 2200 to 2600 Hz; in /du/ it falls from 1200 to 700 Hz. These differences occur because the formants always glide towards the values appropriate for the vowels following the /d/. Different vowels inevitably give rise to different formant transitions. Thus the same phoneme can be cued, in different contexts, by acoustic patterns that are vastly different.

It should be noted that highly simplified patterns such as those in Fig. 8.3 do not produce very convincing speech sounds; the /di/ and /du/ are not clearly heard. In natural speech, there may be many cues other than the second formant transition to signal the distinction between the two sounds. We will return to this point later.

Liberman and his colleagues (e.g. Liberman and Mattingly, 1985) have argued that the context-dependent restructuring of the acoustic patterns seen here for the /d/ phoneme occurs quite generally for consonant sounds. It is rarely possible to find invariant acoustic cues corresponding to a given consonant. For steady-state vowels the frequencies of the formants do provide more or less invariant cues, but vowels are rarely steady state in normal speech. Usually vowels are articulated between consonants at rather rapid rates, so that "vowels also show substantial restructuring – that is, the acoustic signal at no point corresponds to the vowel alone, but rather shows, at any instant, the merged influences of the preceding or following consonant" (Liberman *et al.*, 1967). The general conclusion is that a single stretch of acoustic signal may carry information about several neighbouring phonemes. Thus, there is a complex relation between acoustic pattern and phoneme. Liberman and his colleagues have argued that this implies that phoneme perception requires a special decoder. Liberman *et al.* (1967) refer to those phonemes whose acoustic patterns show considerable context-dependent restructuring as 'encoded', while those phonemes for which there is less restructuring are called 'unencoded'. They suggested that the perception of encoded phonemes (such as stops) should differ from the perception of unencoded phonemes (such as vowels) and from the perception of nonspeech sounds. However, it is generally held that there is no clear dichotomy between encoded and unencoded phonemes. Encodedness can be regarded as a dimension going from more contextually dependent to less contextually dependent.

C   Categorical perception

For highly encoded phonemes it is found that certain small changes to the acoustic signal may make little or no difference to the way the sound is perceived, while other equally small changes produce a distinct change, altering the phoneme identity. Liberman *et al.* (1967) demonstrated this using simplified synthetic speech signals in which the second formant transition was varied in relatively small, acoustically equal steps through a range sufficient to produce the percept of the three syllables /bi/, /di/ and /gi/. Subjects did not hear a series of small changes in the acoustic signal, but "essentially quantal jumps from one perceptual category to another" (Liberman *et al.*, 1967). It was found that subjects did not hear changes within one phoneme category, but only changes from one phoneme to another. This was called categorical perception. Notice that categorical perception does not normally occur for nonspeech sounds. For an acoustic signal varying along a single dimension, such as frequency, we are normally able to discriminate many more stimuli than we can identify absolutely (see Chapter 7, section 2).

In order to demonstrate categorical perception in the laboratory, both identification and discrimination tasks must be performed. The identification task establishes the boundaries between phonetic categories. In the discrimination task, three or four successive stimuli are presented, one of which is different from the others. The listener is required to pick the odd one out. For the ideal case of categorical perception, discrimination would be high for stimuli that straddle category boundaries, but would drop to chance level for pairs of stimuli falling within one category. In practice the situation is rarely as straightforward as we have described here but, whenever discrimination of acoustic changes is good across phoneme boundaries and poor within phoneme categories, this is taken as evidence of categorical perception.

The perception of steady-state vowels is very different. Small physical changes in the acoustic stimulus are easily perceived, so that one vowel may be heard to shade into another, and many intraphonemic variations are heard. Liberman *et al.* (1967) suggested that this is because vowels are much less encoded than consonants, so that they may be perceived in the same way as nonspeech sounds. However, as noted above, vowel sounds in rapidly articulated speech do show restructuring, and there is evidence (Stevens, 1968) that perception of certain vowels in their proper dynamic context is more nearly categorical than is found for steady state vowels.

Although categorical perception has been considered to reflect the operation of a special speech decoder, there is evidence that categorical perception can occur for nonspeech signals. Locke and Kellar (1973) obtained identification and discrimination functions for chords consisting of three simultaneous pure tones, using both musicians and nonmusicians as subjects. Of the three tones in the chord, only the middle tone was varied, in small steps over a range sufficient to produce a chord of A minor (440, 523 and 659 Hz) at one end of the range, and a chord of A major (440, 554 and 659 Hz) at the other end. Categorization was considerably more prominent among the musicians; they tended to recognize the chords as either A minor or A major. Further, the discrimination curves for musicians paralleled predictions from categorization more closely than did the curves for nonmusicians. In other words, the discrimination performance of musicians was better for frequency changes which altered the identity of the chord than for changes that did not alter the identity.

A second example of categorical perception for nonspeech stimuli is provided by the work of Miller *et al.* (1976). They presented a low level noise stimulus whose onset could occur at various times in relation to the onset of a more intense buzz stimulus (a filtered squarewave). In one part of the experiment subjects labelled single stimuli with either of two responses: 'no noise' or 'noise'. They found that labelling shifted abruptly around a noise lead time of about 16 ms, so that when the noise onset occurred more than 16 ms before that of the buzz the label 'noise' was applied. Otherwise the label 'no noise' was applied. Subjects were also required to discriminate among stimuli differing in relative noise onset time. They found that discrimination was best for pairs of stimuli which lay on either side of the 16 ms boundary. These findings resemble the categorical perception found for synthetic speech stimuli.

These demonstrations of categorical perception for nonspeech stimuli indicate that the phenomenon is not unique to speech, and that its explanation does not depend on the existence of a special speech decoder. However, it appears to occur commonly for speech sounds, whereas it is rare for nonspeech sounds. How, then, can it be explained? We will consider three explanations, which are not mutually exclusive.

The first suggests that the differences in perception which are observed for 'encoded' consonants and relatively 'unencoded' vowels may be explained in terms of differences in the extent to which the acoustic patterns can be retained in acoustic memory (see Darwin and Baddeley, 1974 and Pisoni, 1973). The acoustic patterns corresponding to the consonant parts of speech sounds often have a lower intensity than those for vowel sounds. In addition, the acoustic patterns associated with consonants fluctuate more rapidly and often last for a shorter time than those for vowels. Consequently, auditory memory for the acoustic patterns of consonants may decay rapidly. It may be that by the time these acoustic patterns have been processed in the identification of the phoneme they are lost from auditory memory. Thus, finer discrimination of stimuli within phoneme categories is not possible. However, for longer and more intense speech sounds such as vowels, the acoustic patterns may be retained in acoustic memory for longer periods, so that additional discriminations, based upon these stored patterns, can be made.

A second possible explanation for categorical perception is that categories and boundaries in speech have evolved in order to exploit the natural sensitivities of the auditory system (Stevens, 1981). Thus, the boundaries which separate one speech sound from another tend to lie at a point along the acoustic continuum where discrimination is optimal. Demonstrations of categorical perception using synthetic speech stimuli typically use a series of stimuli which vary in 'acoustically equal steps'. However, the definition of 'acoustically equal' is somewhat arbitrary. For example, if the dimension being varied is frequency, it is not clear whether the steps should have an equal size on a linear scale, a logarithmic scale or some other scale. Similarly, it is not clear whether the steps should be defined in absolute terms or relative to some baseline frequency. The latter would be more in accord with Weber's law, but it has seldom been done in speech research. Similar difficulties apply to the choice of equal steps in time. Thus, steps which are physically equal on some arbitrary scale may not be equal in psychoacoustic terms. At category boundaries, 'physically equal' steps may be larger than average in perceptual terms.

A third explanation for categorical perception is that it arises from extensive experience with our own language. When we learn to understand the speech of a particular language, we learn to attend to acoustic differences which affect the meanings of words and to ignore acoustic differences which do not affect word meanings. Once we have learned to do this, it may be difficult to *hear* acoustic differences which do not affect word meanings. Categorical perception will arise as a natural consequence of this. This explanation can account for the fact that it is sometimes difficult to hear differences between phonemes of an unfamiliar language, differences which are perfectly obvious to a native speaker. For example, native Japanese speakers may have difficulty distinguishing /r/ and /l/, since the acoustic patterns that distinguish these for an English listener are not used for phonetic distinctions in Japanese.

D   Evidence for brain specialization

One line of evidence indicating that the perception of speech is special is provided by studies establishing that different regions in the brain play a role in the perception of speech and nonspeech sounds. These studies are based on the assumption that the crossed neural pathways from the ear to the brain (i.e. from the right ear to the left cerebral cortex, and vice versa) are generally more effective than the uncrossed pathways. If competing stimuli are presented simultaneously to the two ears (e.g. two different spoken messages), then (for most people) speech stimuli presented to the right ear are better identified than those presented to the left, while the reverse is true for melodies (Broadbent and Gregory, 1964; Kimura, 1964). This suggests that encoded speech signals are more readily decoded in the left cerebral hemisphere than in the right. Studies of deficiencies in speech perception and production for people with brain lesions have also indicated that the left hemisphere plays a primary role in speech perception (Kimura, 1961).

It is hardly surprising that there are areas of the brain specialized for dealing with speech. We have to learn the phonemes, words and grammar of our own language, and this knowledge has to be used in understanding speech. However, it could still be the case that the initial auditory processing of speech sounds is similar to that of nonspeech sounds.

E Evidence for a speech mode from sinewave speech and other phenomena

When we listen to sounds with the acoustical characteristics of speech, we seem to engage a special way of listening, called the 'speech mode'. Evidence for this comes from studies of the perception and identification of sounds which vary in the extent to which their acoustic characteristics approach those of speech. House *et al.* (1962) required subjects to learn to associate members of various ensembles of acoustic stimuli with buttons on a response box. They found that stimuli with spectral and temporal properties similar to those of speech are learned more readily than simpler stimuli but only if the speech-like stimuli are actually identified by the listener as speech. Thus, as Stevens and House (1972) have put it,

> ... although one can imagine an acoustic continuum in which the sounds bear a closer and closer relation to speech, there is no such continuum as far as the perception of the sounds is concerned – the perception is dichotomous. Sounds are perceived either as linguistic or as nonlinguistic entities.

In some cases, the speech mode can be engaged by highly unnatural signals, provided those signals have the temporal patterning appropriate for speech. An example is provided by the work of Remez and his colleagues on 'sinewave speech' (Remez *et al.*, 1981). They analysed natural spoken utterances to determine how the frequencies and amplitudes of the first three formants varied over time. They then generated synthetic signals consisting of just three sinusoids. The frequencies and amplitudes of the sinusoids were set equal to those of the first three formants of the original speech, and changed over time in the same way. Such signals are quite different from natural speech, lacking the harmonic structure of speech, and not having the pulsing structure associated with voicing.

Remez *et al.* (1981) found that these artificial signals could be perceived in two ways. Listeners who were told nothing about the stimuli heard science-fiction like sounds, electronic music, computer beeps and so on. Listeners who instead were instructed to transcribe a "strangely synthesized English sentence" were able to do so. They heard the sounds as speech, even though the speech sounded unnatural. Apparently, instructions to the listener can help to engage the speech mode. However, once that mode is engaged, it is difficult to reverse the process. Listeners who have heard the stimuli as speech tend to continue to do so. It should be emphasized that the temporal patterning of the sinewaves is critical. Speech is not heard if isolated vowels are presented.

In summary, when we are presented with speech-like sounds, there is a perceptual dichotomy: either the sounds are perceived as speech or they are not. Stevens and House (1972) suggested that "the listener need not be set for speech prior to his hearing the signal; his prepared state is triggered by the presence of a signal that has appropriate acoustic properties". Very probably there is a strong involuntary component to this 'triggering' of the speech mode; no matter how hard we try, when we listen to natural (as opposed to synthetic) speech, it is impossible to hear it in terms of its acoustical characteristics, i.e. as a series of hisses, whistles, buzzes, etc. Rather we perceive a unified stream of speech sounds.

Like most of the other phenomena indicating that speech perception is 'special', listening in a specific perceptual mode is not unique to speech perception. For example, Chapter 5 and Chapter 7 (section 3D) described how a harmonic complex tone can be perceived in two modes. We may listen in an analytic mode, hearing the pitches of one or more individual partials, or we may listen in a synthetic mode, hearing a single pitch corresponding to the fundamental component. The latter is the more usual mode of perception. However, the speech mode is unusual in that it operates for an entire class of highly complex and varied acoustic signals, whose main common feature is that they were produced by a human vocal tract.

F   Duplex perception

This phenomenon was first described by Rand (1974) and it has been explored subsequently by Liberman and his colleagues (Liberman, 1982; Mann and Liberman, 1983). Consider the simplified synthetic stimuli whose spectrograms are shown in Fig. 8.4. The upper part shows the case where the

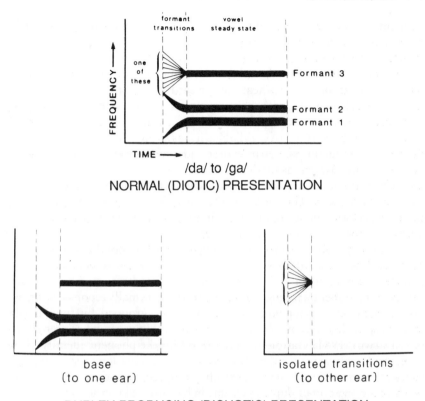

FIG. 8.4 Schematic spectrograms of the stimuli used to demonstrate 'duplex perception'. The upper section shows the spectrogram of a complete sound, which is presented diotically (the same sound to each ear). By varying the transition in the third formant, the percept can be changed from /ba/ to /ga/. In the lower section the stimulus is separated into two parts. The 'base', consisting of the first and second formants with their transitions and the steady state part of the third formant, is presented to one ear. The transition in the third formant is presented to the other ear. Adapted from Mann and Liberman (1983) by permission of the authors and Elsevier Sequoia.

same stimuli are presented to the two ears. All stimuli are identical in their first and second formants, including the formant transitions. The transition in the third formant can be varied to produce the percept of either /da/ or /ga/. Consider now the case shown in the lower part of the figure. The stimulus is split into two parts. One part, the 'base' consists of the first and second formants with their transitions, plus the steady-state part of the third formant. The base is presented to one ear only. The other part consists of the isolated third formant transition. This is presented to the other ear.

These stimuli are perceived in two ways at the same time. A complete syllable is perceived, either /da/ or /ga/ depending on the form of the isolated formant transition, and it is heard at the ear to which the base is presented. Simultaneously a nonspeech chirp is heard at the other ear. Thus, the transition is heard separately, but at the same time it is combined with the base to give the percept of a syllable; it has a duplex role in forming the percept. Note that the base on its own sounds like a stop-vowel syllable which is ambiguous between /da/ and /ga/.

Other examples of duplex perception can be found in the work of Darwin and his co-workers. Gardner and Darwin (1986) showed that frequency modulation of a single harmonic near to a formant frequency made that harmonic appear to stand out as a separate tone. However, this did not prevent that harmonic from contributing to the identity of the vowel. Thus, a harmonic can be heard separately but still contribute to vowel quality.

If the formants of a speech sound are separated into two groups with different fundamental frequencies, then listeners normally report hearing two sounds with different pitches. The sounds are grouped by fundamental frequency, as described in Chapter 7, section 3A. However, it has been shown (e.g. Darwin, 1981; Gardner *et al.*, 1989) that the phonetic identity of the sound is not always altered by this perceptual segregation. Listeners sometimes report two sound images but only one speech sound.

The phenomenon of duplex perception has aroused considerable interest, partly because it violates the principle of disjoint allocation described in Chapter 7, section 5. This principle states that a given acoustic element cannot be assigned to more than one source at a time. The violation was thought to indicate that there are specialized and separate 'modules' for dealing with speech and nonspeech sounds (Liberman and Mattingly, 1985). The principle of disjoint allocation would then apply within a module, but it would be possible for different modules to share the same acoustic element. In fact, Bregman (1987) has pointed out that the principle of disjoint allocation does not always apply even for nonspeech stimuli (or visual stimuli). For example, if a single low harmonic in a complex tone is mistuned in frequency by more than about 3%, it tends to be heard as a pure tone standing out from the complex tone as a whole (Moore *et al.*, 1986). However, that harmonic may still make a contribution to the residue pitch of the whole sound (Moore *et al.*, 1985c). As discussed in Chapter 7, the 'rules' of perceptual organization do not always work. However, violations seem more common for speech sounds than for nonspeech sounds. It appears that the speech perception mechanism sometimes groups acoustic elements together even when the acoustic properties of the elements suggest that they come from different sources.

One interesting aspect of duplex perception has been revealed by studies of the ability to discriminate changes in the isolated third formant transition (Mann and Liberman, 1983). When listeners are asked to attend to the speech percept, discrimination is best for stimuli that straddle the phoneme boundary. In other words, categorical perception occurs. When listeners are asked to attend to the nonspeech chirp, there is no peak in the discrimination function. Thus, the same stimuli are discriminated differently depending on whether listeners are attending to the speech or the nonspeech percept.

G Cue trading

Some of the synthetic signals described in this chapter contain only a single cue to signal the phonetic contrast between two sounds, such as the third formant transition distinguishing /da/ and /ga/ in the experiment of Mann and Liberman (1983). However, in natural speech almost every phonetic contrast is cued by several distinct acoustic properties of the speech signal (e.g. Bailey and Summerfield, 1980). Within limits, a change in the setting or value of one cue, which would normally lead to a change in the phonetic percept, can be offset by an opposed setting of a change in another cue so as to maintain the original phonetic percept. This is known as 'cue trading' or 'phonetic trading'. It has been argued (e.g. Repp, 1982) that the properties of cue trading can only be explained by assuming that listeners make use of their tacit knowledge of speech patterns.

Studies of particular interest are those where different patterns of results are obtained depending on whether the same stimuli are perceived as speech or nonspeech. For example, Best *et al.* (1981) constructed sinewave analogues of a 'say'-'stay' continuum by following a noise resembling an /s/ with varying periods of silence and then three sinusoids imitating the first three formants of the periodic portion of the speech signal (/ei/). They investigated the trading relation between two cues to the distinction between 'say' and 'stay'. The first cue is the length of the silent interval. The second cue is the initial frequency of the tone simulating the first formant (F1); a high onset indicates 'say' and a low onset indicates 'stay'. A sequence of three stimuli – AXB – was presented on each trial. A and B were analogues of a clear 'say' (no silence, high F1 onset) and a clear 'stay' (long silence, low F1 onset). The stimulus X contained various combinations of the duration of silence and the F1 onset frequency, and subjects were required to say whether X sounded more like A or more like B. Several subjects were tested, and it was found that after the experiment they could be divided into two groups: those who reported that the stimuli were heard as 'say' and 'stay', and those who reported various nonspeech impressions or inappropriate speech percepts. Only the subjects in the first group showed a trading relation between the silent interval and the F1 onset frequency. The other subjects based their judgements either on the duration of silence or on the F1 onset frequency. It seems that a trading relation only occurred with these stimuli when the subjects were listening in the speech mode.

It should not be assumed that trading relations never occur for nonspeech stimuli. For example, Parker *et al.* (1986) have shown that trading relations can be found for stimuli which have some speech-like properties but are not actually perceived as speech. Similarly, in Chapter 6 we described how interaural time differences may be traded for interaural level differences in sound localization. However, the fact that trading relations differ according to whether stimuli are perceived as speech or nonspeech provides support for the concept of a special speech mode of perception.

H Audiovisual integration

The movements of a speaker's face and lips can have a strong influence on our perception of speech signals; what we hear is influenced by what we see. A dramatic example of this is provided by the work of McGurk and MacDonald (1976). They prepared videotape recordings of a person saying bisyllables such as 'baba' and 'mama'. The video and audio tracks were then rearranged such that the audio recording of one bisyllable was synchronized with the video recording of a different bisyllable. Most observers perceived syllables which were not present in either the audio or the video recordings. For example, the combination of acoustical 'mama' and optical 'tata' was typically perceived as 'nana'. Notice that most observers were not aware of the conflict between auditory and visual cues. They 'heard' the sound 'nana' and were surprised when they closed their eyes and the percept changed to 'mama'.

The interpretation of these results is not clear. The acoustical and optical information are combined in complex manner which is not always easy to account for (for a review see Summerfield, 1987). Some authors have argued that audiovisual integration provides evidence for a speech-specific mode of perception that makes use of articulatory information (Repp, 1982; Liberman and Mattingly, 1985). However, we should bear in mind that audiovisual integration can occur for nonspeech sounds. For example, we described in Chapter 6 (section 13) how sound localization can be influenced by vision.

I Interim summary of work on the special nature of speech perception

We have described above several phenomena which have been used to support the argument that speech perception is special. Some of these phenomena were thought to be unique to the perception of speech stimuli when they were first discovered. However, subsequent work, or further consideration of existing work, has indicated that comparable phenomena often exist for the perception of nonspeech sounds. Nevertheless, the evidence for the existence of a special speech mode of perception is compelling. It is also clear that certain areas of the brain are specialized for dealing with speech sounds, and that speech itself is special by virtue of the special way in which it is produced.

4 MODELS OF SPEECH PERCEPTION

There are many models of speech perception, but no model is generally accepted and no model is specified in enough detail to allow rigorous experimental testing. It is beyond the scope of this book to describe any of these models in detail, but we will briefly describe two influential models which may be considered as representing the extreme ends of the 'spectrum' of models.

One model is the 'motor theory' of speech perception proposed by Liberman and his colleagues (Liberman *et al.*, 1967; Liberman and Mattingly, 1985). In its most recent form, the model claims that "the objects of speech perception are the intended phonetic gestures of the speaker, represented in the brain as invariant motor commands that call for movements of the articulators through certain linguistically significant configurations" (Liberman and Mattingly, 1985). In other words, we perceive the articulatory gestures the speaker is intending to make when producing an utterance. The intended gestures "are not directly manifested in the acoustic signal or in the observable articulatory units". A second claim of the motor theory is that speech perception and speech production are intimately linked and that this link is innately specified. Perception of the intended gestures occurs in a specialized speech mode whose main function is to make the conversion from acoustic signal to articulatory gesture automatically.

The proponents of this model have argued that it can account for a large body of phenomena characteristic of speech perception, including the variable relationship between acoustic patterns and perceived speech sounds, duplex perception, cue trading, evidence for a speech mode, and audiovisual integration (Liberman and Mattingly, 1985). However, the model is incomplete in that it does not specify how the translation from the acoustic signal to the perceived gestures is accomplished. In this sense, it is more a philosophy than a theory of speech perception (Klatt, 1989).

A very different type of model proposes that there is a sequence of stages of processing, one of which includes an array of phonetic feature detectors (Stevens, 1986; see Klatt, 1989, for a review). The speech signal first undergoes analysis in the peripheral auditory system. There is some evidence that this analysis, including filtering, lateral suppression, adaptation, and phase locking, can enhance some of the less variable acoustic characteristics of phonetic features, while suppressing irrelevant variability (Delgutte and Kiang, 1984; Goldhor, 1985). The next stage is an array of acoustic property detectors, including onset detectors, spectral change detectors, formant frequency detectors and periodicity detectors. These property detectors are assumed to compute relational attributes of the signal, for example changes in spectrum or periodicity across different parts of the signal, which tend to be more invariant than absolute attributes. The next stage is an array of phonetic feature detectors. These examine the set of auditory property values over a chunk of time, and make decisions as to whether a particular phonetic feature, such as voicing or nasality, is present. These decisions are language specific, i.e. the detectors are tuned to the phonetic contrasts of the language in question. However, the decisions may be similar in many languages owing to constraints imposed on all speakers and listeners by the speech production mechanism (Stevens, 1989) and by the auditory system (Stevens, 1981). A phonetic feature detector may make a decision based on the input from a single acoustic property detector, or it may combine information from several property detectors. Finally, there are stages of segmental analysis and lexical search. It is beyond the scope of this book to describe these stages; the reader is referred to Klatt (1989) for details.

The philosophy underlying this model is that it should be possible to find a relatively invariant mapping between acoustic patterns and perceived speech sounds, provided the acoustic patterns are analysed in an appropriate way. This point is elaborated in the following section.

5   THE SEARCH FOR INVARIANT ACOUSTIC CUES AND THE MULTIPLICITY OF CUES

Some workers have suggested that the role of encoded or overlapping cues in speech perception has been somewhat overstated (e.g. Fischer-Jørgensen, 1972). Cole and Scott (1974) have noted that speech perception involves the simultaneous identification of at least three qualitatively different types of cues: invariant cues, context-dependent cues (e.g. formant transitions) and cues provided by the waveform envelope (see below). In a review of the literature on consonant phonemes, traditionally considered as highly encoded speech sounds, Cole and Scott (1974) conclude that *all* consonant phonemes are accompanied by invariant acoustic patterns, i.e. by acoustic patterns which accompany a particular phoneme in any vowel environment. In some cases the invariant patterns are sufficient to define the consonant uniquely, while in other cases the invariant patterns limit possible candidates to two or three phonemes. They show, further, that context-dependent cues are also present in all consonant-vowel syllables. In other words, any given syllable contains both invariant and context-dependent cues. The context-dependent cues may sometimes be necessary to discriminate between two phoneme candidates which have been indicated by the invariant cues.

Stevens (1980) and Blumstein and Stevens (1979) have pointed out several of the acoustic properties which may be used to distinguish between different phonemes in natural, as opposed to synthetic, speech. Some of these properties are illustrated in Fig. 8.5, which shows several representations of the acoustic attributes of the utterance 'the big rabbits'. The oral and nasal stops, fricatives and affricates, such as /p m s z tʃ/, are characterized by a rapid change in spectrum over a time period of 10–30 ms following the release. This is shown in the top left of the figure for the consonant /b/. Vowels, glides (/j/ as in the first sound of 'yet') and semi-vowels (/w/ as in 'we'), on the other hand, are characterized by much slower changes in the spectrum. Thus, rapidity of spectrum change is the crucial property for distinguishing these classes of sounds.

A second property is the abruptness of amplitude change accompanying a consonant. A rapid amplitude change together with a rapid spectrum change is indicative of the stop consonants /p t k b d g/. These rapid amplitude changes may be seen in the lower part of Fig. 8.5 for the /b/ and /t/ sounds. Note that stops are also associated with an interval of silence or near silence during the closure.

Periodicity also serves to distinguish between certain pairs of speech sounds. For example, the voiced consonant /b/ may be distinguished from the unvoiced consonant /p/ by the presence of low frequency periodicity during the closure interval. Also, for the unvoiced consonant /p/, noise alone is present for a period of time following the release of closure and then voicing begins. The delay between the release of the consonant and the start of voicing is known as the voice onset time (VOT). Thus voiced and unvoiced consonants may be distinguished by the presence or absence of low frequency periodicity during the closure interval, and by the duration of the VOT. Many other cues to consonant voicing have been described.

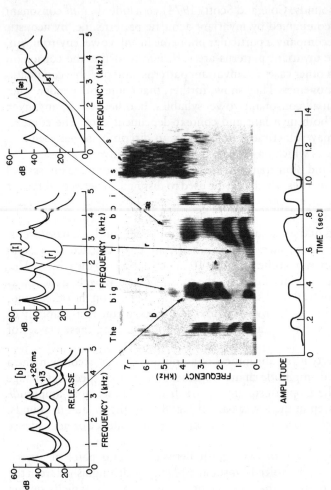

FIG. 8.5 Several representations of the utterance 'The big rabbits'. The middle section shows a spectrogram like that in Fig. 8.2. At the top are short term spectra sampled at various points during the utterance. At the bottom is the variation in overall amplitude with time. The spectra have been 'pre-emphasized', by boosting the high frequencies relative to the low frequencies. From Stevens (1980), by permission of the author and *J. Acoust. Soc. Am.*

For stop consonants, another distinguishing property is the gross shape of the spectrum at the release of the consonant, which can serve to define the place of articulation of the consonant. For example, the spectra for /p/ and /b/ show spectral prominences that are spread out or diffuse in frequency, and are flat or falling, as seen in the top left corner of Fig. 8.5. The spectra for /d/ and /t/ show prominences that are spread out, but whose amplitudes increase with increasing frequency, while the spectra for /g/ and /k/ show a distinctive peak in the midfrequency range, with other spectral peaks being smaller and well separated from the central peak. Blumstein and Stevens (1980) showed that sounds with onset spectra having these general shapes will be categorized appropriately by human listeners. However, later work (e.g. Kewley-Port *et al.*, 1983) showed that dynamic changes in the spectra were more important. It seems that the important property is not simply the gross spectral shape at any one time, but rather the relationship between the spectral shape around the release and the spectral shape of the following sound.

The features described above, when taken together, serve to define uniquely any stop consonant. Thus the phonemes described by Liberman *et al.* (1967) as being highly 'encoded' do seem to be identifiable from relatively invariant acoustic cues.

The bottom part of Fig. 8.5 shows the variation of overall amplitude with time during the utterance. However, there is considerably more detail present in the time waveform than is indicated by this smoothed outline. Imagine that we plot the speech waveform in terms of pressure variations as a function of time. Such a plot could be obtained as a display on an oscilloscope if the pressure variations were converted into voltage variations using a microphone. The envelope is the curve produced by drawing a smooth line passing through the peaks in the waveform; it is a kind of 'outline' of the waveform. An example of a speech waveform is given in Fig. 8.6, for the utterance 'I'm a waveform'. Notice that for much of the time the envelope shows peaks which are fairly regularly spaced. This indicates that the speech sounds are periodic and involve the vibration of the vocal folds (i.e. they are voiced). The time intervals between these peaks in the envelope are the same as the corresponding periods of vibration of the vocal folds. The part of the envelope corresponding to the /f/ in 'form' does not show these periodic peaks, because of the noise-like nature of this sound, and it also has a lower amplitude. Variations in amplitude, and therefore in loudness, also occur during the voiced parts of the speech.

Clearly, then, the waveform envelope gives us information about fluctuations in amplitude as a function of time. Both amplitude and duration have been demonstrated to be of considerable importance in determining the prosodic features of speech (those concerned with intonation and stress). A

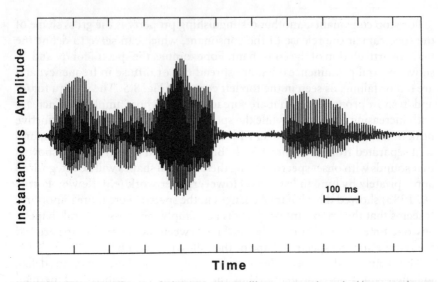

FIG. 8.6 The waveform of the utterance 'I'm a waveform'. The envelope would be a smooth curve joining the peaks of the wave.

period of silence can provide cues for stress, enabling us to distinguish between such phrases as 'lighthouse keeper' and 'light housekeeper'. However, such cues are only useful if they are evaluated in relation to duration and amplitude cues from adjacent syllables; speech rates and average intensities vary considerably, so that a measurement of amplitude or duration taken in isolation would have little significance. Thus our use of amplitude and duration cues in determining prosodic features indicates that information relating to the waveform envelope can be retained in memory for relatively long time periods.

There is good evidence that the waveform envelope also provides information about the phonemic composition of speech. Many experiments have shown that the durations of speech sounds, short periods of silence and relative amplitude can influence the perception of particular phonemes. All of these can be extracted from the waveform envelope. An indication of the amount of information which may be carried in the waveform envelope is provided by an experiment of Katz and Berry (1971). They imposed the waveform envelopes of various speech stimuli on a white noise 'carrier'. The intelligibility scores for this 'speech-modulated' white noise were quite good, although words in sentences were discriminated better than words in isolation.

Van Tasell *et al.* (1987) studied the importance of envelope cues by extracting the envelopes of nonsense syllables and using these envelopes to modulate noise. The envelopes were extracted by rectifying and then lowpass filtering the speech (compare the model of temporal resolution described in Chapter 4, section 5A). Three different cutoff frequencies were used for the lowpass filter: 20, 200 and 2000 Hz. The lowest cutoff preserved only the slow variations in envelope amplitude, like those shown in the lower part of Fig. 8.5. The higher cutoff frequencies preserved more rapid fluctuations including those associated with the fundamental frequency of the male talker's voice. They found that identification of the nonsense syllables improved significantly as the cutoff frequency increased from 20 to 200 Hz, but did not increase significantly thereafter. The pattern of the results indicated that subjects were able to make use of three main types of envelope cues: those distinguishing voiced from voiceless sounds; those indicating the amplitude of the consonant relative to the vowel; and those to do with the shape of the envelope and which distinguish the voiceless stops /p t k/ from other consonants.

These results show that, to some extent, the auditory system is able to decode speech stimuli on the basis of time-amplitude variations alone. The ability to extract information from the waveform envelope is not, of course, unique to speech; we saw in Chapter 5 that periodically interrupted white noise has a pitch corresponding to the envelope repetition rate, and in Chapter 6 that the envelope of high frequency, amplitude modulated tones can be used in the lateralization of such sounds.

It is clear that in the perception of speech the human listener makes use of a great variety of types of information which are available in the speech wave. Many different cues may be available to signal a given phoneme, but the cues may not be constant and may differ in relative importance from utterance to utterance. Many kinds of context-dependent variations in the acoustic cues occur, and accurate speech recognition may depend upon the listener's ability to allow for the effects of context. The multidimensional nature of the acoustic cues allows for a high level of redundancy in the speech wave; there may be several different acoustic cues for a given phoneme, of which just one or two might be sufficient for recognition. This redundancy can be used to overcome the ambiguities inherent in the speech; to lessen the effects of interfering stimuli; to compensate for distortions in the signal (for example, when the speech is transmitted over a telephone line); and to allow for poor articulation on the part of the speaker. At a higher level of processing, errors made in identifying a speech sound from its acoustic pattern can be corrected using: knowledge of the kinds of speech signals which can be produced by the human vocal tract; linguistic rules; the 'sense' of the message; and a knowledge of the characteristics of the speaker, e.g. their accent or sex.

6   THE RESISTANCE OF SPEECH TO CORRUPTING INFLUENCES

One way to assess the degree of redundancy in the speech wave is to eliminate or distort certain features and to determine the effect on the intelligibility of the speech. The results of such experiments have indicated that speech is remarkably resistant to many kinds of quite severe distortions. Most of the experimental data have been obtained using articulation-testing methods: subjects listen to a spoken list of syllables, words or sentences and the percentage of items correctly recognized is called the articulation score.

One factor which can affect speech intelligibility is the amount of background noise. For satisfactory communication the average speech level should exceed that of the noise by 6 dB (i.e. the S/N ratio should be +6 dB). When speech and noise levels are equal (0 dB S/N ratio), the word articulation score reaches about 50%. However, speech may be intelligible at negative S/N ratios (where the speech level is below that of the noise) for connected speech, particularly if the listener is familiar with the subject matter, or if the speech and the noise come from different directions in space (this is an example of the MLD phenomenon which was discussed in Chapter 6). In many real-life situations the noise is intermittent rather than continuous. This decreases the effectiveness of the noise in masking the speech by an amount depending on the on–off ratio of the noise and the interruption rate. At high interruption rates (above about 200/s) the noise has effects similar to those of continuous noise. At rates between 1 and 200/s it is possible to patch together the bits of speech heard between the noise, so that the noise is not a very effective masker. At very slow interruption rates whole words or groups of words may be masked, while others are heard perfectly. Thus, articulation scores drop once more.

A second factor which may affect speech intelligibility is a change in frequency spectrum. Many transmission systems (e.g. a telephone line) pass only a limited range of frequencies. Some of the first investigations of speech intelligibility were conducted by engineers of the Bell Telephone Laboratories, in an attempt to assess the importance of frequency range. Experiments using filters with variable cutoff frequencies have shown that no particular frequency components are essential for speech recognition. For example, if a lowpass filter is used to remove all frequency components above 1800 Hz, then the syllable articulation score is about 67%, while normal conversation is fully intelligible. However, speech is equally intelligible if instead a highpass filter is used to remove all frequency components below 1800 Hz. Experiments using bandpass filters have shown that, over a fairly wide range of centre frequencies, a surprisingly narrow band of frequencies is sufficient for satisfactory recognition. For example, a band of frequencies from 1000 Hz to 2000 Hz is sufficient to give a sentence articulation score of about 90%. Clearly, the information carried by the speech wave is not confined to any particular frequency range. This fits in very well with the notion that there are normally multiple acoustic cues to signal phonetic distinctions in speech.

A third kind of disrupting influence which commonly occurs is peak clipping. If an amplifier or other part of a transmission system is overloaded, then the peaks of the waveform may be flattened off, or clipped. In severe cases the clipping level can be only 1 or 2% of the original speech wave's peak values, with the result that the original speech wave, with its complex waveform shape, is transformed into a series of rectangular pulses. This severe distortion does degrade the quality and naturalness of speech, but it has surprisingly little effect on intelligibility; word articulation scores of 80 or 90% are still obtained.

We see, then, that speech is intelligible under a wide variety of conditions where we might have expected rather poor performance. It remains intelligible in the presence of large amounts of background noise, when all but a small part of the speech spectrum is removed, and when time-amplitude variations in the waveform are destroyed by peak-clipping. Once again we are led to the conclusion that no single aspect of the speech wave is essential for speech perception. Thus the speech wave is highly redundant. Each of the distortions described will destroy some of the cues carried in the speech waveform, but the remaining cues are sufficient to convey the message. This is of great practical advantage. If speech perception depended on a near-perfect transmission of sound from speaker to listener, then speech communication in most real situations would become extremely difficult, and devices like the telephone would have to be much more elaborate and costly than they are. Nature has designed the speech communication process so that it can operate under a great variety of adverse conditions.

7   GENERAL CONCLUSIONS

Speech is a multidimensional stimulus varying in a complex way in both frequency and time. Although the speech wave can be described in terms of amplitude and time, this does not seem to be the most appropriate description from the point of view of the auditory system. Nor is a description in terms of static spectra satisfactory. To achieve a description consistent with the known functioning of the auditory system, the dimensions of intensity, frequency and time should be shown simultaneously. A display of this type which has been widely used is the spectrogram, which shows how the short-term spectrum of the speech, usually plotted on a linear frequency scale, varies with time. However, displays which take into account the frequency-resolving power of the auditory system may be more appropriate.

A basic problem in the study of speech perception is to relate the properties of the speech wave to specific linguistic units. It is still not clear whether the basic unit of perception is the syllable, the phoneme, or some other unit such as the phonetic feature. For rapid connected speech, the psychoacoustic evidence indicates that the acoustic patterns signalling individual phonetic features or phonemes would occur too rapidly to be separately perceived in correct temporal order. Thus the recognition of the overall sound pattern corresponding to a longer segment, such as a syllable, is more likely. It is possible that the units of perception are phonemes or phonetic features, but information about several phonemes or features is extracted in parallel over relatively long stretches of sound.

A second problem is that of finding cues in the acoustic waveform which indicate a particular linguistic unit unambiguously. It is possible to find a number of relatively invariant cues for phonemes or phonetic features in single words or syllables articulated clearly in isolation, but these cues are not so apparent in rapid connected speech. In many cases a phoneme will only be correctly identified if information obtained from a whole syllable or even a group of several words is utilized. The complex relationship between the speech wave and the linguistic units of speech has been one of the central problems in the study of speech perception, and has had a powerful influence on the development of theories of speech perception.

There is good evidence that speech is a special kind of auditory stimulus, and that speech stimuli are perceived and processed in a different way from nonspeech stimuli; there is a special 'speech mode' of perception. The evidence includes: categorical perception, the phenomenon that speech sounds can be better discriminated when they are identified as being linguistically different; studies of cerebral asymmetry, which indicate that certain parts of the brain are specialized for dealing with speech; duplex perception which demonstrates that a single acoustic pattern such as a formant transition can be heard both as part of a speech sound and as a separate nonspeech sound; the fact that cue trading has different properties depending on whether signals are perceived as speech or as nonspeech; studies of audiovisual integration showing that the perceived identity of speech sounds is influenced both by what is heard and by what is seen on the face of the talker; and the finding that speech-like sounds are either perceived as speech or as something completely nonlinguistic. Examples of this latter effect are provided by 'sinewave speech' in which the first three formants are replaced by sinusoids at the formant frequencies. These are either heard as artificial nonspeech sounds, or as speech. Many of these phenomena are not unique to speech, but taken together they provide good evidence for a special mode of speech perception.

The complex and variable relationship between the acoustic waveform and the phoneme, and the various phenomena indicating that speech perception is 'special', have led to the development of the 'motor theory'. This holds that speech perception depends on the listener inferring the intended articulatory gestures of the talker. However, there are many alternative models. One assumes analysis through a sequence of stages including: analysis in the peripheral auditory system; an array of acoustic property detectors; and an array of phonetic feature detectors. This type of model emphasizes the fact that some invariant acoustic cues do exist if the signal is analysed appropriately and if the analysis takes into account the relational properties of the signal, as it changes over time.

It is clear that speech perception involves processing at many different levels and that separate information at each level may be used to resolve ambiguities or to correct errors which occur at other levels. The initial analysis of speech sounds into features, phonemes or syllables can be checked and readjusted using knowledge of the ways in which speech sounds can follow one another. Our knowledge of syntactics (grammatical rules) and semantics (word meanings) allows further adjustments and corrections, while situational cues such as speaker identity and previous message content provide yet further information. It is likely that the processing of speech does not occur in a hierarchical way from one level to the next, but that there are extensive links between each level. Thus, the information at any level may be reanalysed on the basis of information from other levels. Even some details of the speech wave itself may be retained for a short time in 'echoic memory' so that the signal can be reanalysed.

The multidimensional nature of speech sounds, and the large amount of independent information which is available at different levels of processing, produce a high level of redundancy in speech. This is reflected in the finding that speech intelligibility is relatively unaffected by severe distortions of the signal. Speech can be accurately understood in the presence of large amounts of background noise, or when it is severely altered by filtering, interruption or peak clipping. Thus speech is a highly efficient method of communication which remains reliable under difficult conditions.

FURTHER READING

The following papers provide comprehensive reviews of phenomena and issues in speech perception, each from a slightly different viewpoint:

Pisoni, D. B. and Luce, P. A. (1987). Acoustic-phonetic representations in word recognition. *Cognition* 25, 21–52.

Repp, B. H. (1982). Phonetic trading relations and context effects: New experimental evidence for a speech mode of perception. *Psych. Bull.* 92, 81–110.

The following chapter provides a detailed review of many aspects of speech perception:

Jusczyk, P. (1987). Speech perception. In *Handbook of Perception and Human Performance. Vol. II. Cognitive Processes and Performance*, Wiley, New York.

The following chapter provides a detailed review and evaluation of models of speech perception:

Klatt, D. H. (1989). Review of selected models of speech perception. In *Lexical Representation and Process* (ed. W. D. Marslen-Wilsen), MIT Press, Cambridge, Mass. (in press).

The following chapter reviews the role of frequency selectivity in speech perception, for both normal and impaired hearing:

Rosen, S. and Fourcin, A. J. (1986). Frequency selectivity and the perception of speech. In *Frequency Selectivity in Hearing* (ed. B. C. J. Moore), Academic Press, London.

9

Practical applications

1 INTRODUCTION

It is the purpose of this chapter to describe a few of the practical applications of auditory research. The topics chosen are by no means exhaustive, but are meant to be illustrative of the range of possible applications.

2 APPLICATIONS OF PSYCHOACOUSTIC RESEARCH IN THE ALLEVIATION OF DEAFNESS

A Psychoacoustics and audiology

Audiology is the science of the evaluation of hearing, particularly in relation to the hearing impaired. On the basis of an audiological examination, particular types of hearing disorders may be diagnosed and particular types of hearing aids recommended. Psychoacoustics is the scientific basis of audiology, and most tests in clinical audiology are based on the findings of psychoacoustic research and on changes in psychoacoustic phenomena which may occur in different disorders of the auditory pathways. Some of these have been discussed already in Chapter 2.

The basic difference between audiology and psychoacoustics lies in the methodology employed. A psychoacoustician may have an interest in quite small and subtle effects, and may be willing to test individual subjects for many hours and/or to average results across a large number of subjects, in order to investigate these effects. The audiologist, on the other hand, requires tests which can be applied quickly and simply to a particular patient, in order to determine the nature of the disorder and determine where in the auditory pathway the disorder lies. This difference in approach, although it is quite obvious, has nevertheless considerably impeded the interchange of results and ideas between the two disciplines.

There are several areas in which psychoacoustics may be able to make useful contributions in the diagnosis and treatment of the hearing impaired. One is in the development of new tests which can be used in clinical situations to investigate particular aspects of hearing disorders. The need for such tests is particularly evident in cases of sensorineural hearing loss, where at the present time there may be problems both in diagnosing the site of the disorder and in predicting the extent of the difficulties which the patient may encounter in everyday life.

Measures of frequency selectivity have already proved to be useful. We discussed in Chapter 3 the finding that impairments in frequency selectivity are commonly associated with hearing losses of cochlear origin. The degree of impairment in frequency selectivity provides a sensitive indicator of the amount of damage to the cochlea, and in addition may be useful in predicting the difficulties experienced by the patient in everyday life. One measure which has been applied in the clinic is the psychophysical tuning curve (Chapter 3, section 3A and Fig. 3.5). However, the exact method of measurement has not yet been standardized. Further, the maskers used have most often been sinusoids, whereas narrowband noises might be preferable, since they prevent the listener using beats as a cue.

An alternative to the psychophysical tuning curve is to measure the auditory filter shape using notched noise maskers (see Chapter 3, section 3B and Figs. 3.6 and 3.7). In a clinical test it is not necessary to measure the entire filter shape. Indeed, just two threshold measurements, one for a notch width of zero, and the other for a notch width of 80% of the centre frequency, give a good indication of the degree of frequency selectivity. For a normal listener, these two thresholds typically differ by 35–40 dB for a centre frequency of 1 kHz. For an impaired listener, the difference may be much less, so that the normal and abnormal ears are easily and clearly distinguished.

B   Hearing aid design

Psychoacoustic research can help in the design of new types of hearing aids to compensate for some of the abnormalities of perception which occur in the impaired ear. These abnormalities include loudness recruitment (Chapter 2, section 8A) and reduced frequency selectivity (Chapter 3, section 10). Psychoacoustics has two roles to play in this. The first is in the characterization of the perceptual abnormalities. This is essential for deciding what type of compensation should be used. The second is in the design and evaluation of particular compensation schemes.

An example of this approach is found in attempts to compensate for loudness recruitment. In a recruiting ear, the absolute threshold is elevated, but the level at which sounds become uncomfortably loud may be almost normal. That is, the growth of loudness with increasing intensity is more rapid than normal. A hearing aid which amplifies all sounds equally is not satisfactory in such cases. If the gain of the aid is set so as to make faint sounds audible, then more intense sounds will be over-amplified, and will be uncomfortably loud.

One method of compensating for loudness recruitment is to use a hearing aid which compresses the dynamic range of the input, so that low-level sounds are amplified more than high-level sounds. This can be done in a crude way simply•by peak-clipping the output above a certain level, but this introduces a considerable amount of distortion. An alternative method is to use an amplifier whose gain is adjusted automatically according to the overall level of the input. This is often called automatic gain control (AGC). Although this idea sounds simple, it has turned out to be rather difficult to design effective AGC systems for hearing aids. To understand why, we have to consider the reasons why a wide dynamic range is necessary.

One reason is that the average level of speech varies from one situation to another over a range of at least 30 dB. The person with recruitment may only be able to hear comfortably over a much smaller range of sound levels. This problem can be dealt with by using AGC in which the gain changes slowly from one situation to another. Unfortunately, it is also necessary for the gain to be rapidly reduced in response to a sudden intense sound, such as a door slamming, or a cup being dropped. With slow-acting AGC, this means that the aid goes 'dead' for a certain time after the intense sound, which is very annoying for the user. Recently, Moore and Glasberg (1988c) have described a new type of AGC which changes gain slowly from one situation to another, but which can selectively reduce the gain for sudden intense sounds. As soon as the intense sound is over, the gain returns quickly to what is was before the sound occurred. This type of AGC is very effective in dealing with variations in overall sound level from one situation to another.

A second reason why a wide dynamic range is important is that, even for speech at a constant average level, individual acoustic elements may vary over a range of 30 dB or more. Typically, the acoustic elements associated with vowels are more intense than those associated with consonants. Thus, a person with recruitment may be able to hear the vowel sounds, but weaker consonants may be inaudible. To deal with this, it is necessary to use AGC whose gain changes rapidly, so that the levels of weak consonants can be increased relative to those of vowels. This is often called 'syllabic compression'.

One problem in implementing syllabic compression is that the amount of recruitment is usually not constant as a function of frequency. For example, the rate of growth of loudness with intensity may be almost normal at low frequencies, but markedly abnormal at high frequencies, where the threshold elevation is usually greatest. Thus, the compression appropriate at one frequency will be inappropriate at other frequencies. One way of getting round this problem is to split the input into a number of frequency bands, using a bank of bandpass filters, and to apply the appropriate amount of compression to the output of each filter. The compressed signals are then recombined.

Evaluations of multiband compression systems have given mixed results. Some studies have shown distinct advantages for multiband compression (e.g. Villchur, 1973), while others have shown no advantage (e.g. Barford, 1978). However, many studies have used speech stimuli in which the range of levels has been very restricted. When the level of the speech is allowed to vary somewhat from one word to the next, as would occur in everyday life, multiband compression does have advantages (Lippmann *et al.*, 1981).

Adequate compensation for recruitment can probably be achieved with a small number of bands, say, two or three. Indeed, there may be a disadvantage in using a large number of bands, since the compression tends to reduce spectral contrasts in complex stimuli. In a multiband compression system, the differences in level between peaks and dips in the spectrum of the input are reduced. If the impaired ear has reduced frequency selectivity, as is often the case (Chapter 3, section 10), then the reduction in spectral contrast compounds the difficulties experienced in picking out the spectral features of complex sounds. For example, the formants in speech sounds (Chapter 8) may not be resolved, so that speech recognition is impaired. To avoid this problem, the bands in a compression aid should have bandwidths which are broad in comparison to the 'auditory filters' of the impaired listener. In practice, this means that only a few bands should be used, probably no more than three.

Laurence *et al.* (1983) have described a hearing aid which incorporates two forms of AGC. Initially, a slow-acting AGC operates on the whole signal, to compensate for variations in overall sound level from one situation to another. Then the signal is split into two frequency bands, with fast-acting AGC (syllabic compression) in each band. The aid was shown to have significant advantages for the understanding of speech both in quiet and in background noise in comparison to a similar aid without AGC.

In summary, although there has been some controversy over the benefits of compression in hearing aids (Plomp, 1988), there is evidence that it can give benefits in well designed systems (Moore, 1989).

A second way in which the pre-processing of sounds could be useful, is in reducing the deleterious effects of background noise or reverberation. We described in Chapter 3 the common experience of hearing impaired people, that they can understand speech well in a quiet situation with one speaker, but that understanding is difficult when there is background noise or reverberation. Several groups of researchers are working on methods of signal processing for reducing the effects of background noise and/or reverberation. Although these methods have mostly failed to improve speech intelligibility (Lim, 1983), a scheme for enhancing spectral features of speech in noise has shown promise (Simpson *et al.*, 1989).

C Cochlear implants

Over the past two decades considerable progress has been made in research aiming to bring help to those people who are totally deaf through disorders of the cochlea. The number of people in this category is not certain, but may be considerable. In the USA there are 200 000–300 000 people (0.1% of the whole population) who are so deaf that they cannot hear anything using a conventional hearing aid. In a large proportion of these, the disorder is in the cochlea rather than in the central nervous system, and the auditory nerve is partially intact (but degenerated to some extent) in the majority of individuals. In such people it is possible to create a sensation of sound by direct electrical stimulation of the auditory nerve. This occurs because of the way in which the auditory nerve is connected to the central nervous system; nerve impulses in the auditory nerve lead to activity in those parts of the brain that are normally concerned with the analysis and perception of sounds, and are interpreted as having arisen from acoustic stimulation.

There are now several commercially available systems which attempt to restore some useful hearing to totally deaf people by electrical stimulation of the auditory nerve. These systems are usually known as cochlear implants. Their design has been strongly influenced by psychoelectrical studies, i.e. by studies of the ability to detect and discriminate electrical stimuli. For stimuli applied to a single stimulating electrode, the most important findings are as follows. 'Sounds' can be heard for a wide range of electrical frequencies of stimulation (25–16 000 Hz), but changes in sensation with changes in rate of stimulation only occur for rates below about 600 Hz. The apparent pitch of electrical stimuli increases regularly with frequency for frequencies up to 300–500 Hz, but then flattens off. The smallest detectable change in frequency varies considerably from patient to patient. Some patients can detect changes of 5% or less for frequencies up to a few hundred Hz, others require changes of around 30%, and a few appear to have hardly any ability to detect frequency changes (Merzenich *et al.*, 1973b; Fourcin *et al.*, 1979). The range of currents between the threshold for detection and the point at which the stimulus becomes uncomfortable is very small, especially for high stimulating frequencies. Thus, an extreme form of loudness recruitment is present.

Some researchers have implanted several electrodes, either within the cochlea or directly into the auditory nerve. If current is passed between a closely spaced pair of electrodes, then it is possible selectively to stimulate groups of neurones within the auditory nerve. These studies have shown that different electrode pairs are associated with different sensations. For electrodes which stimulate neurones in the base of the cochlea the sensation is described as 'sharp', whereas stimulation of neurones close to the apex gives a 'dull' sensation (Clark *et al.*, 1987). Thus, different places of stimulation are associated with different timbres. Unfortunately, it is difficult to isolate the current produced by stimulation of a given electrode pair to the neurones closest to the pair; there is always a spread of current to adjacent neurones. This limits the effective number of separate 'channels' for electrical stimulation.

The results summarized above show that the discrimination of electrical stimuli by a deaf person is much less acute than the discrimination of acoustical stimuli by a normally hearing person. This means that careful thought has to be given to the way in which speech should be 'coded' into electrical form, so as to convey as much information as possible. Speech-coding strategies can be classified into three main categories. In the first, the aim is to produce in the auditory nerve patterns of activity which resemble as closely as possible those which would occur in a normally hearing person in response to the same sounds (e.g. Merzenich *et al.*, 1974; Merzenich, 1983). The speech is passed through a bank of bandpass filters intended roughly to approximate the filtering which takes place in a normal cochlea. The output from each filter is used to derive a signal which is fed to the appropriate electrode in a multi-electrode array.

In the second strategy, which has been used particularly with single-electrode implants, the analogue waveform is fed more or less directly to the stimulating electrode, sometimes after compression (AGC) and after frequency response shaping. The idea is to squeeze as much information as possible into the single electrode, hoping that the patient will somehow make sense of the information, even if at first the sensation is highly unnatural (House, 1976; Hochmair and Hochmair-Desoyer, 1983).

In the third strategy, the input to the patient is simplified by extracting simple patterns from the speech and presenting only those patterns to the implanted electrode(s) (e.g. Moore *et al.*, 1985a; Clark *et al.*, 1987). An advantage of this approach is that the patterns can be transformed so as to make them more discriminable for the patient. Clark *et al.* (1987) have developed a system using a multi-electrode array implanted within the cochlea. The fundamental frequency of speech is extracted and coded as the rate of stimulation with brief pulses of current. The two most prominent peaks in the low- and mid-frequency portions of the spectrum are also extracted. Often these correspond to the first and second formants of the speech. The frequencies of the spectral peaks are coded in terms of which electrodes are activated. Two electrodes are activated in rapid succession, one for each of the spectral peaks. Finally, the intensity of the sound is coded by the magnitude of each pulse of current.

Clinical evaluations of implant systems have shown that there can be large individual differences, even for patients using the same implant system. Most patients find the implants useful for recognizing environmental sounds and as an aid to lip reading. Some patients are able to understand speech without lipreading, provided the speech is clearly enunciated in a quiet situation. A few can understand speech reasonably well even in moderate levels of background noise. The results have not provided a clear answer to the question of which type of speech coding strategy is best, although there is increasing evidence that multi-electrode systems give better results than single-electrode systems (Gantz *et al.*, 1987; Tyler *et al.*, 1989; Spillman and Dillier, 1989). It seems likely that cochlear implants will become more and more widely used in the treatment of total deafness.

3 PSYCHOACOUSTIC CONSIDERATIONS IN CHOOSING YOUR HI-FI

The last few years have seen a considerable expansion in the sale of sound-reproducing equipment while at the same time manufacturers have been competing with one another in their efforts to produce 'better' amplifiers, loudspeakers, compact disc (CD) players and so on. Unfortunately, the criterion for 'better' has not usually been clearly defined, and in most cases there has been little effort to investigate the extent to which improvements in technical specification actually produce audible improvements. We will define the objective of high fidelity as the reproduction of sounds corresponding as closely as possible to the intention of the record producer/performer. Thus the emphasis is on accuracy or fidelity of reproduction.

Any high fidelity (hi-fi) reproduction system contains several different components, each of which may alter or distort signals in various ways. Common system components include: record players (pickup, arm and turntable); CD players; cassette players; amplifiers; and loudspeakers (usually two). Each of these can distort the signal in one or more ways, and for any particular type of distortion the performance of the chain as a whole is determined by the performance of its weakest link. In the following sections we start by considering the ways in which the performance of hi-fi components is specified, and give some guidelines as to the perceptual relevance of these specifications. We then consider in turn each of the major components in a sound-reproducing system, emphasizing those aspects of performance which are likely to be most important in determining how the system sounds.

A   The interpretation of specifications

One specification which is commonly quoted is frequency response. This is measured by using as input to the component a sine wave of constant amplitude but variable frequency. Ideally, the output of the component should not vary as a function of frequency, so that all frequencies are reproduced to an equal extent. In practice there is a limit to the range of frequencies which the component reproduces, and there may also be some irregularities in the response. The degree to which the response differs from the ideal response can be specified by using the output in response to a given frequency (often 1 kHz) as a reference level. The output at other frequencies can then be specified in relation to this level, and the overall response can be specified in terms of the range of frequencies over which the variations in output level fall within certain limits. Thus, the frequency response for a reasonably good loudspeaker might be stated as 50–15 000 Hz ± 5 dB. This would mean that the sound level did not vary over more than a 10 dB range for any frequency from 50 Hz to 15 000 Hz.

Two aspects of the response are of perceptual relevance. The first is the overall frequency range. There is little point in having a response which extends below about 30 Hz, since there is little energy in music below that frequency, and in any case it is impractical to reproduce frequencies below 30 Hz in domestic environments. At the high-frequency end, while some people can hear up to 20 kHz or so, most people cannot detect the effect of lowpass filtering speech or music at 16 kHz (Ohgushi, 1984). Even when they can, the lowpass filtering does not result in any degradation of sound quality. Thus, a frequency response extending from 30 to 16 000 Hz is perfectly adequate for hi-fi reproduction.

The other important aspect of the response is its regularity. If the frequency response has large peaks and dips, then these affect the timbre of the reproduced sound, introducing 'coloration'. Psychoacoustic studies suggest that, under ideal conditions, subjects can detect changes in spectral shape when the level in a given frequency region is increased or decreased by 1–2 dB relative to other frequency regions (Bucklein, 1962; Green, 1988; Moore *et al.*, 1989). Thus, a response flat within ±1 dB will not be detectably different from a perfectly flat response.

To summarize the important features to look for in a frequency response: ideally the response should be flat within ±1 dB over the range 30 to 16 000 Hz. A response flat within ±2 dB over the range 40 to 14 000 Hz would still be very good.

Most components distort signals to some extent. Usually the distortion is specified in terms of the extent to which frequency components are present at the output which were not present at the input. Unfortunately, distortion is not usually specified in a way which allows an easy estimate of its audibility. The most common method is to specify harmonic distortion. A pure tone of a particular frequency is used as input to the component. If the component distorts the signal, the output will not be exactly sinusoidal, but will be a periodic waveform of the same repetition rate as the input. This periodic waveform can be expressed as a fundamental component (of frequency equal to that of the input sinusoid) and a series of harmonics. The total amplitude of the second and higher harmonics, expressed as a percentage of the amplitude of the fundamental, is called the 'harmonic distortion'.

The audibility of harmonic distortion is not predictable from this simple percentage, because audibility depends upon the distribution of energy among the different harmonics. If the energy of the distortion products is mainly in the second and third harmonics, then these harmonics will be masked to some extent by the fundamental, and if the signal is a piece of music, they will in any case be masked by the harmonics which are normally present in the input signal. In this case distortion of 2–3% would not normally be noticed. If, on the other hand, the distortion produces high harmonics, then these will be much more easily audible, and subjectively more objectionable. Distortion in this case should be kept below about 0.1%.

A different way of measuring distortion is to apply two tones of differing frequency to the input of the component and to measure the amplitudes of other, spuriously generated, frequencies at the output. Again, the amplitudes of the distortion products are usually expressed as a percentage of the amplitudes of the primary tones. Each tone produces its own harmonic distortion products but, in addition, there are frequency components produced by the nonlinear interaction of the two tones. If the frequencies of the two input tones are f_1 and f_2, then 'combination' products will be produced with frequencies such as $f_1 - f_2$, $f_1 + f_2$, $2f_1 - f_2$, $2f_1 + f_2$. This type of distortion is called 'intermodulation distortion' (note that the auditory system produces similar distortion products, particularly $2f_1 - f_2$; see Chapters 1, 3 and 5). Once again, it is difficult to predict the audibility of a given percentage of intermodulation distortion in a normal listening situation, since the figures quoted by a manufacturer depend upon the exact frequencies and relative levels of the tones chosen for the test. In general, intermodulation distortion is more easily audible than harmonic distortion, but values of less than 0.5% are unlikely to be detected.

Many components add a certain amount of undesired noise to the signal. This noise usually takes the form of a low-frequency hum (related to the frequency of the alternating current supply) and a high-frequency hiss. The performance of a component in this respect is usually specified as the ratio of the output power with a relatively high-level input signal to the output power due to hum and noise alone. The ratio is normally expressed in decibels. Sometimes the hum and noise are 'weighted' to reflect the sensitivity of the ear to different frequencies. This is rather like the weighting used in the sound level meters described in Chapter 2, and it usually results in a higher signal-to-noise ratio. A ratio of 70 dB unweighted, or 80 dB weighted is adequate for most purposes, although for source material with a very wide dynamic range (as is sometimes found on CDs), slightly higher ratios may be desirable.

B   Amplifiers

The basic performance of even a moderately priced hi-fi amplifier is likely to be so good that improvements in technical specification would make little audible difference. For example, a moderately good amplifier will have a frequency response from 20 to 20 000 Hz ±1 dB, distortion less than 0.1% and a signal-to-noise ratio greater than 80 dB. These values are better than the limits required by the ear. Nevertheless, some aspects of performance are worth considering.

The necessary power output of an amplifier can only be determined in relation to the loudspeakers with which it will be used. Loudspeakers vary considerably in the efficiency with which they convert electrical energy into sound energy; 'horn' loudspeakers may have efficiencies of 30% or more, while 'transmission line' loudspeakers may convert less than 1% of the electrical energy into sound (see below). Thus it is nonsense to say, as one manufacturer has done, that an amplifier produces "forty-four watts of pure sound". In fact, even one acoustic watt, in a normal-sized room, would correspond to an extremely loud sound. There are many loudspeakers available which produce high sound levels (in excess of 90 dB SPL) with quite moderate electrical inputs, say 1 W. In other words, given loudspeakers of reasonable efficiency, it is quite unnecessary to spend a lot of money on a high-power amplifier. Additionally, it is worth remembering that a doubling of power (which might mean a doubling in price) produces only a 3 dB change in sound level, which is only just noticeable (see Chapter 2).

C Loudspeakers

Efficiency is an important aspect of loudspeaker performance. As mentioned in the previous section, loudspeakers vary considerably in the efficiency with which they convert electrical energy into sound energy. Unfortunately, manufacturers have not yet standardized their methods of specifying efficiency, but a common way is in terms of the electrical input (in watts) required to produce a sound level of 90 dB SPL at a distance of 1 m from the loudspeaker. An alternative is to specify the sound level produced at a distance of 1 m by an input of one watt. This level can vary from as little as 77 dB SPL to over 100 dB SPL. A 200 W amplifier would be needed to produce the same sound level in the first case as a 1 W amplifier in the second case.

Most loudspeakers have frequency responses which are considerably less regular than those of amplifiers. Many loudspeakers are so bad that the manufacturers do not specify decibel limits in quoting a 'frequency range' for their loudspeakers. *A frequency response without decibel limits is meaningless.*

The frequency response of a loudspeaker is normally measured in an anechoic chamber, so that there is no reflected sound from walls, ceiling or floor which could affect the results. In domestic situations, reflected sound is always present and influences the perceived sound quality to some extent. High frequencies are usually absorbed more than low frequencies, so that the relative level of the low frequencies is boosted. Additionally, at certain low frequencies room resonances may occur giving the music an unpleasant 'coloured' sound. Finally, at high frequencies, complex interference patterns are set up, so that the sound entering the ears depends strongly on the exact position of the head.

Given that room acoustics are bound to have an influence on the 'effective' frequency response of a loudspeaker, one might think that the response of a loudspeaker measured in an anechoic chamber is not particularly relevant to how the loudspeaker will sound. This is not in fact the case, because peaks and dips in the 'anechoic' frequency response combine with peaks and dips produced by room acoustics to produce an overall response which is more irregular than either alone. To minimize this irregularity the 'anechoic' frequency response should be as smooth as possible. In addition, listeners appear to compensate for the characteristics of a room in judging the nature of a sound source. This is shown by the everyday experience that the quality of the voice of a familiar person does not change markedly with changes in the room in which the person is heard. The effect is an example of perceptual constancy; the properties of an object (in this case a voice) as perceived by an observer vary little with quite large changes in the conditions of observation.

It may be that something analogous to the precedence effect (Chapter 6, section 7) operates in judgements of sound quality as well as in the localization of sound. If this were the case, then the perceived quality of a sound would be determined by that part of the sound that reached the ears first, as direct sound from the loudspeaker rather than reflected sound. Thus, changes in signals produced by loudspeaker imperfections would be noticed much more than changes produced by room reflections. This is not to deny that room acoustics have an effect, but their effect is less noticeable than might be predicted from physical measurements. As far as loudspeakers are concerned, a frequency response of 50–15 000 Hz ±3 dB would be exceptionally good and, provided other aspects of its performance were also good, a loudspeaker with this response would add little of its own quality to the reproduced sound; it would be an accurate transducer.

One aspect of loudspeaker performance which has been largely neglected until recently is the phase response. In order for a waveform to be reproduced accurately, not only should all the frequency components be reproduced at the correct relative amplitudes, but also the relative phases of the components should be preserved. This is equivalent to saying that at the listener's ear the time delay of all frequency components should be equal. Changes in the relative phases of the components can produce marked changes in a waveform. Loudspeaker manufacturers have not paid much attention to this, because it has generally been assumed that the ear is insensitive to changes in relative phase. The statement that the ear is 'phase deaf' is often ascribed to Helmholtz (1863), who experimented with harmonic complex tones containing eight successive harmonics, including the fundamental. In fact, Helmholtz did not exclude the possibility that phase changes were detectable for high harmonics, beyond the sixth to eighth, and more recent work has shown that phase changes produce both changes in timbre (Plomp and Steeneken, 1969; Patterson, 1987a) and changes in the clarity of pitch (Bilsen, 1973; Moore, 1977). The effects for steady tones are, however, rather small. This is not particularly surprising, since, for steady sounds, room reflections produce marked alterations in the relative phases of components, and we have already noted that room acoustics have relatively little effect on the perceived quality of reproduced sounds.

The situation is rather different for transient or short-duration sounds, which are, of course, common in music. The results of a number of experiments have indicated that we can discriminate between sounds differing only in the relative phases of the components (and not in the amplitudes of the components), even when those sounds have durations as small as 2–3 ms (Patterson and Green, 1970; see also Chapter 4). When such sounds are reproduced by loudspeakers, any given sound is completed before any reflected sounds (echoes) reach the ears, provided the head of the listener is more than 60–90 cm from any room surface and the loudspeaker is not too close to a wall. Thus, room reflections have little effect on our ability to discriminate between short-duration sounds differing in the relative phases of the components. This has been confirmed by Hansen and Madsen (1974).

What these results mean is that the phase response of a loudspeaker can be important in determining the subjective quality of the reproduced sound. Changes in the relative phases of components are much more noticeable when those components are close together in frequency than when they are widely separated (see Chapter 3, section 2E), so that phase changes which occur abruptly as a function of frequency have a larger subjective effect than phase changes which occur gradually over a wide frequency range. Unfortunately, the former is the more common situation. Most modern 'high fidelity' loudspeakers contain two or more transducers to deal with different parts of the frequency range. A 'woofer' is used for low frequencies and a 'tweeter' for high. The electronic input to the loudspeaker is split into high- and low-frequency bands by electronic filters known as crossover networks, and the transition frequency between a high and a low band is known as the crossover frequency. It is in the region of the crossover frequency that rapid phase changes often occur, and thus the crossover network is a source of phase distortion. In addition, certain cabinet designs, such as the vented enclosure or reflex cabinet, introduce marked phase changes in particular frequency regions. It is noteworthy that loudspeakers which avoid rapid changes in phase as a function of frequency, such as the Quad electrostatic, tend to be judged as reproducing sounds with a greater clarity and realism than those which have a rapidly changing or irregular phase response. Unfortunately, it is difficult to isolate this aspect of performance from other differences between loudspeakers, so it has not yet been conclusively demonstrated that a given loudspeaker sounds better because of its superior phase response.

Blauert and Laws (1978) investigated the audibility of phase distortion by taking a variety of complex sounds, including speech, music, noise and brief impulses, and delaying a group of frequency components with respect to the remainder. They found that the minimum detectable delay was about 400 μs when the frequencies delayed were in the range 1–4 kHz. They also measured the delays which actually occurred for several loudspeakers and headphones. For the headphones the worst case corresponded to a delay of 500 μs, which is only just above the threshold for detection. For the loudspeakers delays up to 1500 μs were found. These are well above the threshold for detection, and might therefore have a significant effect on the perceived quality of the sound reproduced by the loudspeakers. It is to be hoped that in the future the aspects of phase response which are subjectively important will become more clearly defined.

The frequency response of a loudspeaker is usually measured with a microphone directly in front of the loudspeaker, a position known as 'on axis'. If the microphone is placed 'off axis', at some angle to the loudspeaker but at the same distance from it, the measured output generally falls. This is because the sound is 'beamed' forward by the loudspeaker, rather than being propagated equally in all directions. A very narrow beam at any given frequency is undesirable, since the character of the reproduced sound would be strongly influenced by listening position. On the other hand the exceptionally wide beam in 'omnidirectional' loudspeakers also has undesirable effects. With such loudspeakers the perceived sound quality is relatively independent of listening position, but at the listener's ear the ratio of reflected sounds from wall and ceilings to direct sound is much greater than for conventional loudspeakers. This makes sound localization very difficult, since the precedence effect (Chapter 6, section 7) may break down when this ratio is too high. A further result is that the room echoes are not perceptually suppressed, as is normally the case when the precedence effect operates. Thus, the changes in amplitude and phase response produced by room reflections become subjectively more noticeable, and the clarity of the sound is impaired.

Although there is a paucity of research in this area, it is generally held that most listeners prefer a directional characteristic in which some beaming occurs, but where the response is reasonably uniform over an angle of about 45° on either side of the axis. In conventional loudspeakers the degree of beaming depends on the size of the transducer (the vibrating area) relative to the wavelength of the sound being reproduced. The smaller the transducer, and the lower the frequency, the wider is the beam. Thus, for a single transducer the beam gets narrower as the frequency increases. Most manufacturers have dealt with this problem by using more than one transducer (the woofers and tweeters mentioned above) each of which produces a reasonably wide beam over the range of frequencies it reproduces. However, because the angle of dispersion for each transducer varies with frequency, the response off axis tends to be a lot less regular than the response on axis. It is difficult to determine how successful a manufacturer has been in dealing with this problem, since this aspect of performance is usually poorly specified. Sometimes it is possible to obtain polar diagrams which indicate the response as a function of angle at various selected frequencies. Ideally the polar diagrams at different frequencies should be as similar as possible.

An ingenious solution to the problem of achieving a uniform angle of dispersion over a wide range of frequencies is incorporated in the Quad ESL-63 loudspeaker. This has a plane radiating surface, but it is made to behave like a point source situated centrally behind the plane. For such a point source, a given wavefront would reach the centre of the plane surface before it reaches the edges. Thus, the plane surface can be made to mimic the point source by introducing a progressive time delay between sounds radiated from the centre and sounds radiated from the edge. The amount of delay affects the distance of the 'virtual' source from the plane, and thus the angle of dispersion. Thus, the delay can be chosen to optimize the angle of dispersion, and this angle can be maintained over a wide frequency range.

Finally, there is one myth about loudspeaker performance which should be laid to rest. Occasionally in technical and hi-fi magazines the phrase 'Doppler distortion' is used. This distortion arises because the cone in a loudspeaker has to reproduce more than one frequency simultaneously. Consider a high-frequency tone together with a low one. When the phase of the low tone is such that the cone is moving towards the listener, this produces an upward shift in the apparent frequency of the high tone. Conversely, when the phase of the low tone is such that the cone is moving away from the listener, the apparent frequency of the high tone is lowered. These Doppler shifts are similar to the shift in pitch of a train whistle as the train passes you at a station. In principle, therefore, the low-frequency tone produces a slight frequency modulation of the high tone, which might be heard as a distortion. In fact, Villchur and Allison (1980) have shown, both by listening tests and by a theoretical analysis, that Doppler distortion is completely inaudible for any practical cone velocity.

D Pickups

We have dealt at some length on the characteristics of loudspeakers, since loudspeakers are usually the 'weakest link' in a sound-reproducing chain, and so they have the largest effect on how the system sounds. However, the signal source at the start of the chain (e.g. record player or cassette player) can also have a significant effect on the overall sound. In general, top-class pickups are capable of excellent performance, superior to that of most loudspeakers, in terms of frequency response, transient response and phase response, but this is not always true of cheaper models. However, even high quality pickups produce non-negligible amounts of harmonic and intermodulation distortion, the latter being typically 2–5%. The level of intermodulation distortion may well contribute significantly to the overall sound quality of a pickup, high levels of distortion being accompanied by a loss of clarity and by a loss of the definition of individual instruments.

Several important aspects of performance are unique to pickups. One of these, called tracking, refers to the ability of the stylus to maintain contact with the record grooves in highly modulated (i.e. high amplitude) passages of the record. In modern recordings the stylus may be subject to accelerations 1000 times the acceleration due to gravity, so it is something of a miracle that good groove contact can be maintained with downward forces on the stylus of one gram or less. When groove contact is partially lost, a condition known as mistracking, the sound may become fuzzy or distorted, or severe crackling may occur. The cure is usually to *increase* the playing weight, provided it is within the range specified by the manufacturer. Pickups vary considerably in their tracking ability, and few manufacturers (except for Shure) give accurate specifications of this factor; the best that the prospective buyer can do is to rely on test reports. It is worth noting that the tracking ability of a pickup will only be fully realized if it is used with an arm of appropriate quality. A high quality pickup, tracking at one gram or less, requires an arm with very low pivot friction and very low mass.

When stereophonic, or two-channel, reproduction is required, the pickup must be capable of providing two electrical signals, each one derived from the movement of just one wall of the groove. Two factors are of relevance here: the channel separation and the channel balance. Channel separation is usually measured using a signal recorded so that ideally it would be reproduced in one channel only. The ratio of the output in the desired channel to that in the unwanted channel, expressed in decibels, gives a measure of the extent to which the pickup can separate the two channels. A figure of 15–20 dB is generally considered adequate, and many pickups can easily exceed this. It is important, however, that the separation be maintained over a wide frequency range.

Channel balance is measured by recording signals which should be reproduced with equal amplitude on both channels. The ratio of the output levels of the two channels, expressed in decibels, is used as the measure of balance. A difference in level between the two channels which is independent of signal frequency is not important, since it can be corrected using the balance control on the amplifier. However, a difference in level which varies as a function of frequency is more serious. The subjective location of any given instrument in a stereo recording is determined by the relative levels at which the instrument is reproduced by the two loudspeakers. A sound produced equally by the two loudspeakers, and heard by a listener equally distant from them, will be located midway between the two loudspeakers. If the sound coming from the left-hand loudspeaker is slightly higher in level than that from the right, then the sound image is displaced slightly to the left. If the sound from the left-hand loudspeaker is 10–15 dB higher in level than that from the right, the sound is heard entirely at the left-hand loudspeaker. Clearly, then, channel balance is important in determining the subjective location of individual instruments. If the balance varies as a function of frequency, then different frequency components produced by the same instrument will be subjectively located in different places. Thus, there will not be a well-defined 'stereo image'. Instead the 'image' corresponding to any given instrument will be diffuse, and the separation of individual instruments will be reduced. Similar considerations apply to the two loudspeakers of a stereo pair; these should be matched as closely as possible in terms of frequency and phase response, otherwise the 'stereo image' will suffer.

E Turntables

The fluctuations in the speed of a turntable produce corresponding fluctuations in the frequencies of the reproduced sounds. Slow fluctuations, called wow, produce pitch changes which are particularly noticeable on steady piano tones, while rapid fluctuations, called flutter, give the sound a 'rough' quality. There are two standards for specifying wow and flutter. One, the European DIN standard, is based mainly on the peak values of the wow and flutter. The other standard, the American NAB standard, is based on the mean value of the wow and flutter. Wow and flutter is usually undetectable if its value is less than about 0.2% (DIN) or 0.1% (NAB). The values are usually easily achieved by good modern turntables.

Mechanical vibrations in the turntable itself may be detected by the pickup and reproduced as a rumbling sound. Rumble is usually specified by measuring its level relative to that of a tone recorded at a particular reference level, most often a 1 kHz pure tone at a groove velocity (in the lateral direction) of 10 cm/s. A good signal-to-noise ratio for a high quality turntable would be 50 dB unweighted or 70 dB weighted. The extent to which rumble is audible will, of course, depend on the ability of the loudspeakers to reproduce low frequencies. Consequently, high quality loudspeakers, with a good low-frequency response, should be accompanied by a turntable with minimal rumble.

F Cassette players and recorders

The compact cassette was not originally intended to be a medium for hi-fi recording, but tapes and recorders/players ('tape decks') have been developed remarkably in order to overcome the limitations of the medium. The inherent signal-to-noise ratio of the cassette is only about 55 dB. This is far too low for hi-fi reproduction. Hence, a number of 'noise reduction' systems have been developed, with the objective of reducing the effects of the 'hiss' inherent in cassette recordings. The most widely used systems are Dolby B and Dolby C (Dolby A is a comparable but more complex system mainly used in professional recording studios). These systems boost high frequency components in the input signal prior to recording. On playback, these high frequency components are reduced in level, restoring the original balance between high and low frequencies, while reducing hiss emanating from the tape. Unfortunately, when the input signal contains intense high frequencies, a further boost would result in overloading of the tape, giving considerable distortion. To avoid this, the boost to high frequencies is only applied to low level input signals. Consequently, the reduction of high frequencies on playback also has to be level dependent; the level of the signal coming off the tape is used to determine how much the level of the high frequency components should be reduced.

Both Dolby B and Dolby C work in roughly the way described. Dolby B typically improves the signal-to-noise ratio to about 65 dB, while Dolby C improves it to about 73 dB. Both systems only work properly if the circuits are carefully set up so that the boost of high frequencies on recording is exactly matched by the reduction of high frequencies on playback. Unfortunately, different brands of tape vary in their 'sensitivity', which is a measure of the level which is achieved on playback for a given recording level. Since Dolby processing is level dependent, this means that the tape deck has to be set up for use with a particular brand of tape, and will only work properly with that brand, or with brands having essentially the same sensitivity. While Dolby C gives more noise reduction than Dolby B, it is also more affected by inaccuracies in adjustment of the tape deck or variations in tape sensitivity.

Another limitation of the cassette medium is that the tape becomes 'saturated' at high recording levels. As a result, high frequencies are attenuated, and distortion increases. The frequency response of a tape deck is typically quoted at a recording level 20 dB below the maximum. At this level, a response from 30 to 16 000 Hz ±3 dB is typical of a good deck. However, if the recording level is increased, the frequency response usually worsens dramatically; at '0' on the recording level meter, the high-frequency response may be limited to 8000 Hz or even less. One method of improving the frequency response at high levels is Dolby HX (headroom extension). This allows recordings at high levels to be made without noticeable increases in distortion or loss of high frequencies (the technical details of how this is done are beyond the scope of this book).

Finally, it should be noted that wow and flutter can be heard in some inexpensive tape decks. The prospective buyer should look for an amount of wow and flutter less than about 0.2% (DIN) or 0.1% (NAB).

G   Compact disc players and digital audio tape (DAT) players/recorders

Although CD players and DAT players are quite different in the recording medium they use, they are treated together here because their performance is essentially the same. CD and DAT players generally have a specification which is far better than that of other components in a hi-fi system, especially cassette decks and loudspeakers. Essentially, the output signal which they provide is indistinguishable from that which would be obtained from the master tape produced by the recording studio (studio recordings are now usually digital recordings). Thus, *provided a CD or DAT player is working according to specification, it will produce no noticeable degradation in sound quality.* It follows from this that all CD players and DAT players sound the same.

This statement should be qualified by saying that CD and DAT players do differ somewhat in their error-correction capabilities. Thus, it may sometimes be possible to detect slight differences between players in how well they deal with badly damaged or defective discs or tapes. However, most CD and DAT players cope very effectively with the errors which are typically present. It is also possible for CD and DAT players to have faults which can produce very noticeable effects. However, the take home message is: buy the cheapest CD or DAT player which has the facilities you require, but buy from a reputable manufacturer.

H Loudspeaker cable

Some manufacturers have claimed that sound quality can be improved by the use of special cables between the amplifier and the loudspeakers. It is true that some loudspeakers work best if the resistance of the cable is low. However, this does not require the use of special cable. It merely means that if a long cable is used, then it should be thick, so that the overall resistance does not exceed about 0.5 ohm. Ignore claims that exotic cables can give 'fuller bass' or 'brighter highs'; such claims are without foundation.

I General conclusions

In the selection of components for a high-fidelity system it is important that no component be selected in isolation. Rather each component should be chosen so as to be compatible in quality with the other components. If funds are limited, then the best performance will be obtained by buying efficient loudspeakers, which will produce sufficiently high sound levels using an amplifier of moderate power. However, many of the highest quality loudspeakers are relatively inefficient, and if such loudspeakers are to be used, a high-power amplifier may be necessary. An inefficient loudspeaker may require 100 times the power of an efficient loudspeaker to produce the same sound level, so if a 1 W amplifier is sufficient for the former, a 100 W amplifier will be needed for the latter. Record playing equipment (turntable, arm and pickup) and/or a tape deck should be chosen after the loudspeakers. The better the quality of the loudspeakers, the more likely they will be to show up faults in the record player or tape deck. Tape decks with Dolby C and Dolby HX tend to produce less background hiss and have better frequency responses at high recording levels. Apart from minor differences in error correction capability, all CD players sound essentially the same. The loudspeakers are the most critical components of a hi-fi system, but many of the factors which influence sound quality are not specified by manufacturers, or are specified in ways which are not easily related to subjective impressions. Thus, it is difficult to determine from manufacturer's specifications how good a given loudspeaker will sound. If possible, the best way to choose loudspeakers is by listening to them, preferably using a familiar well recorded CD, and preferably in one's own home.

4   THE EVALUATION OF CONCERT HALL ACOUSTICS

This topic is one of great complexity, and it is beyond the scope of this book to cover it in any detail. The interested reader is referred to Beranek (1962) and Ando (1985) for further details. We shall content ourselves with a brief summary of some techniques which go a considerable way towards solving the problems inherent in the comparison of concert hall acoustics.

Judgements of the acoustic quality of concert halls, and comparisons between different concert halls, are difficult because of two major factors. Firstly, the perceived quality at a given performance depends as much on the manner of playing of the musicians and their seating arrangements as on the characteristics of the hall itself. Secondly, long-term acoustical memory is relatively poor, so that many of the subtleties of acoustical quality are not recalled by the time a listener has travelled from one hall to another. Ultimately, the consensus of opinion of a large number of listeners determines whether a hall is 'good' or 'bad', but it is not easy to define the crucial features which influence such judgements, or to derive general rules which could be applied in the design of new halls. Indeed, many new halls are simply modelled on other halls which have been judged as good. While this approach does have some validity, it is also very inflexible.

Schroeder *et al.* (1974) have developed recording and reproduction techniques which make possible immediate comparisons of the acoustic qualities of different halls under realistic free field conditions on the basis of identical musical source material. The first step is to make a recording of an orchestra in an anechoic chamber, so that the acoustics of the recording room are not superimposed on those of the hall which will be evaluated. This ensures that the musical material is always identical. The recording is replayed from the stage of the hall which is to be evaluated. Schroeder *et al.* (1974) used a two-channel recording, replayed via two loudspeakers on the stage of the hall, so as to simulate in a crude way the spatial extent of the orchestra. However, there is no reason why the technique should not be extended to multichannel recordings, which would mimic more accurately the sounds radiated by a live orchestra.

The second step is to record the signals using microphones at the 'ear-drums' of a dummy head. This is a model of a human head with realistic pinnae and ear canals whose acoustical properties match those of an 'average' head as closely as possible. Two different positions were used for each hall, both corresponding to places which would normally be occupied by a listener's head.

The third step is to present the dummy head recordings to listeners for evaluation. One obvious way of doing this is to replay the signals via stereo earphones, but this technique has limitations. One problem which Schroeder and co-workers mention is that "... listening over earphones does not properly recreate the perceived acoustic 'space' or the sense of being sur-rounded by sound, which is one of the important qualities that we wish to describe in an objective way". To overcome this problem the recordings were electronically processed so that, when played back over two selected loud-speakers in an anechoic chamber, the recorded signals were recreated at the eardrums of a human listener. Schroeder *et al.* (1974) explain the technique as follows:

> The sound radiated from each loudspeaker goes into *both* ears and not just the 'near' ear of the listener as would be desired. In other words, there is 'cross-talk' from each loudspeaker to the 'far' ear. However, by radiating properly mixed and filtered compensation signals from the loudspeakers, the unwanted 'crosstalk' can be cancelled out.

The appropriate filter responses in the compensation scheme are computed from measurements obtained by applying short electrical impulses to one of the two loudspeakers and recording the resulting microphone signals from the ears of a dummy head at some distance in front of the loudspeakers. For further details the reader is referred to the original article and to Schroeder and Atal (1963).

The result of this, according to Schroeder *et al.* (1974) is that, when the original dummy head recording is replayed,

> ... the signal from the dummy's right ear will go only to the listener's right ear

and that from the dummy's left ear will go only to the listener's left ear, just as in earphone listening but with the proper free-field coupling of the ear canal and the desired invariance of the perceived acoustical space when the listener's head is rotated around a vertical axis.

Schroeder *et al.* (1974) report that, for head movements up to about ±10°, the externalized sound image remains stationary with respect to the listening room, and does not turn with the head as in earphone listening.

Using this technique, Schroeder and co-workers asked subjects to indicate preferences for different concert halls presented in pairs. For a given pair, the subject was allowed to switch back and forth between recordings made in the two halls as often as desired. The score for a preferred hall was 1, and for the other −1. If there was no preference, both halls were given a score of 0. This was repeated for all subjects and all pairs of halls, and the resulting scores were accumulated in a preference matrix indicating how many times each hall was preferred by each listener.

The results were subjected to a factor analysis (Slater, 1960) which yielded the significant factors accounting for the variance in the data. There was one factor of overriding significance, accounting for 50% of the relative variance, which was called the consensus preference factor. All subjects showed positive weights on this factor. What this means is that if a given hall (say X) has a greater value on this factor than another hall (say Y), then hall X is preferred over hall Y by *all* listeners. The other factors isolated by the analysis seem to represent individual difference preferences. The original recordings were made in unoccupied halls. This has little effect on the acoustics in modern halls, but in older halls with hard wooden seats it can result in excessively long reverberation times. When the analysis was limited to those halls having reverberation times less than 2.2 s, the consensus preference factor became even more important, accounting for 88% of the total variance, while individual preference factors became much less significant.

Schroeder *et al.* (1974) also made various physical measurements in the halls, in order to correlate the consensus preference factor with the geometrical and acoustical parameters of the halls. We will not list all of the measures they considered, but will mention those that appeared to be most significant. For the halls with reverberation times less than 2 s, reverberation time was highly correlated with preference; the greater the reverberation time the greater was the preference. However, for the halls with reverberation times greater than 2 s, the reverberation time was slightly negatively correlated with consensus preference, but showed a fairly large correlation with the first individual difference factor. Thus, in this range of reverberation times, some listeners prefer greater reverberation times and others smaller reverberation times.

One factor which showed a strong negative correlation with preference, for halls with both long and short reverberation times, was the interaural coherence. This is a measure of the correlation of the signals at the two ears. Listeners prefer halls which produce a low interaural coherence, so that the signals at the two ears are relatively independent of one another. Schroeder *et al.* (1974) suggested that "This effect might be mediated by a more pronounced feeling – of being immersed in the sound – that presumably occurs for less coherent ear signals". Interaural coherence can be manipulated by sound diffusers on the walls and ceiling of the concert hall.

Finally, for the halls with longer reverberation times, which also tended to be the larger halls, the volume of the halls showed a strong negative correlation with consensus preference. Thus, once a hall has reached a certain size, further increases in size result in a worsening of the perceived acoustic quality.

5 GENERAL SUMMARY AND CONCLUDING REMARKS

In this chapter we have described some practical applications of auditory research.

Psychoacoustic tests may be of use in the differential diagnosis of hearing disorders, and in predicting the extent to which an impaired person will suffer in everyday life. Measures of frequency selectivity may be particularly useful in this respect. Hearing aids which pre-process sounds prior to delivery to an impaired ear can partially compensate for some of the abnormalities of perception which are associated with the impairment. For example, aids incorporating automatic gain control can help to compensate for loudness recruitment. In patients who are totally deaf, cochlear implants can provide a means of restoring a limited, but useful, form of hearing.

In the reproduction of sounds, particularly music, the transducers in the reproduction system, i.e. loudspeakers, cassette players and pickups, have the greatest influence on the overall sound quality. Unfortunately, the aspects of performance which determine how good a system will sound are often poorly specified. Amplifiers, CD players and DAT players are sufficiently good that they have little or no influence on sound quality.

Recordings made using a dummy head provide a way of comparing the acoustics of different concert halls. The factors correlating most strongly with preference are reverberation time, and interaural coherence.

Our knowledge of the processes involved in the perception of sound has advanced considerably since the pioneering work of Helmholtz (1863) yet the scientific study of hearing is still in its infancy. At the physiological level we now know a good deal about the coding of sounds in the auditory nerve, and the cochlear nucleus, but relatively little is known of how that basic neural information is processed at higher levels in the auditory system. At the perceptual level we know a good deal about peoples' abilities to detect changes in simple stimuli such as pure tones and bands of noise, but we are a long way from understanding how complex auditory patterns such as speech and music are perceived. Unfortunately, the elementary level of our understanding is not accompanied by simplicity in the concepts involved. Many students are deterred by the technical jargon which appears in scientific papers on auditory perception or the neurophysiology or anatomy of the auditory system. For students without a physics background, even the nature of auditory stimuli, and their analysis in terms of Fourier components, may present considerable conceptual difficulties. It is my hope that readers who have reached this point in the book by working through the previous chapters will have overcome these initial difficulties, and that some feeling will have been developed for the fascinating and complex processes that underlie our perception of sound.

References

Abeles, M. and Goldstein, M. H. (1972). Responses of single units in the primary auditory cortex of the cat to tones and to tone pairs. *Brain Res.* 42, 337–352.

American Standards Association (1960). *Acoustical Terminology* SI, 1–1960, American Standards Association, New York.

Anderson, C. M. B. and Whittle, L. S. (1971). Physiological noise and the missing 6 dB. *Acustica* 24, 261–272.

Ando, Y. (1985). *Concert Hall Acoustics*, Springer, New York.

Arthur, R. M., Pfeiffer, R. R. and Suga, N. (1971). Properties of 'two-tone inhibition' in primary auditory neurones. *J. Physiol.* 212, 593–609.

Assmann, P. F. and Summerfield, Q. (1987). Perceptual segregation of concurrent vowels. *J. Acoust. Soc. Am.* 82, S120.

Attneave, F. and Olson, R. K. (1971). Pitch as a medium: a new approach to psychophysical scaling. *Am. J. Psychol.* 84, 147–166.

Bacon, S. P. and Moore, B. C. J. (1986). Temporal effects in masking and their influence on psychophysical tuning curves. *J. Acoust. Soc. Am.* 80, 1638–1654.

Bacon, S. P. and Viemeister, N. F. (1985a). The temporal course of simultaneous tone-on-tone masking. *J. Acoust. Soc. Am.* 78, 1231–1235.

Bacon, S. P. and Viemeister, N. F. (1985b). Temporal modulation transfer functions in normal-hearing and hearing-impaired subjects. *Audiology* 24, 117–134.

Bailey, P. J. (1983). Hearing for speech: the information transmitted in normal and impaired hearing. In *Hearing Science and Hearing Disorders* (eds M. E. Lutman and M. P. Haggard), Academic Press, London.

Bailey, P. J. and Summerfield, Q. (1980). Information in speech: Observations on the perception of [s]-stop clusters. *J. Exp. Psychol.: Human Percept. Perform.* 6, 536–563.

Barford, J. (1978). Multichannel compression hearing aids: Experiments and considerations on clinical applicability. In *Sensorineural Hearing Impairment and Hearing Aids* (eds C. Ludvigsen and J. Barford), *Scand. Audiol.*, Suppl. 6, 315–339.

Batteau, D. W. (1967). The role of the pinna in human localization. *Proc. R. Soc.* B 168, 158–180.

Batteau, D. W. (1968). Listening with the naked ear. In *Neuropsychology of Spatially Oriented Behavior* (ed. S. J. Freedman), Dorsey Press, Illinois.

Beckett, P. and Haggard, M. P. (1973). The psychoacoustical specification of 'tone deafness'. *Speech Perception Ser.* 2, 2, 17–22 (Dept. of Psychology, Queen's University of Belfast).

Békésy, G. von (1928). Zur Theorie des Hörens; die Schwingungsform der Basilar membran. *Phys. Z.* 29, 793–810.

Békésy, G. von (1942). Über die Schwingungen der Schneckentrennwand beim Präparat und Ohrenmodell. *Akust. Z.* 7, 173–186.

Békésy, G. von (1947). The variation of phase along the basilar membrane with sinusoidal vibrations. *J. Acoust. Soc. Am.* 19, 452–460.

Békésy, G. von (1960). *Experiments in Hearing* (trans. and ed. E. G. Wever), McGraw-Hill, New York.

Békésy, G. von and Rosenblith, W. A. (1951). The mechanical properties of the ear. In *Handbook of Experimental Psychology* (ed. S. S. Stevens), Wiley, New York.

Beranek, L. L. (1962). *Music, Acoustics and Architecture*, Wiley, New York.

Best, C. T., Morrongiello, B. and Robson, R. (1981). Perceptual equivalence of acoustic cues in speech and nonspeech perception. *Percept. Psychophys.* 29, 191–211.

Bilger, R. C. and Feldman, R. M. (1968). Frequency dependence in temporal integration. *76th Meeting of the Acoustical Society of America*, paper A1.

Bilsen, F. A. (1973). On the influence of the number and phase of harmonics on the perceptibility of the pitch of complex signals. *Acustica* 28, 60–65.

Bilsen, F. A. and Goldstein, J. L. (1974). Pitch of dichotically delayed noise and its possible spectral basis. *J. Acoust. Soc. Am.* 55, 292–296.

Bilsen, F. A. and Ritsma, R. J. (1967). Repetition pitch mediated by temporal fine structure at dominant spectral regions. *Acustica* 19, 114–116.

Blauert, J. (1969/1970). Sound localization in the median plane. *Acustica* 22, 206–213.

Blauert, J. (1972). On the lag of lateralization caused by interaural time and intensity differences. *Audiology* 11, 265–270.

Blauert, J. (1983). *Spatial Hearing*, MIT Press, Cambridge, Mass.

Blauert, J. and Laws, P. (1978). Group delay distortions in electroacoustical systems. *J. Acoust. Soc. Am.* 63, 1478–1483.

Bloom, P. J. (1977). Creating source elevation illusions by spectral manipulation. *J. Audio. Eng. Soc.* 25, 560–565.

Blumstein, S. E. and Stevens, K. N. (1979). Acoustic invariance in speech production: Evidence from measurements of the spectral characteristics of stop consonants. *J. Acoust. Soc. Am.* 66, 1001–1017.

Blumstein, S. E. and Stevens, K. N. (1980). Perceptual invariance and onset spectra for stop consonants in different vowel environments. *J. Acoust. Soc. Am.* 67, 648–662.

Boer, E. de (1969a). Reverse correlation. II. Initiation of nerve impulses in the inner ear. *Proc. K. Ned. Akad. Wet.* 72, ser. C, 129–151.

Boer, E. de (1969b). Encoding of frequency information in the discharge pattern of auditory nerve fibres. *Int. Audiol.* 8, 547–556.

Boomsliter, P. and Creel, W. (1961). The long pattern hypothesis in harmony and hearing. *J. Music Theory* 5, 2–31.

Boomsliter, P. and Creel, W. (1963). Extended reference: an unrecognized dynamic in melody. *J. Music Theory* 7, 2–22.

Boone, M. M. (1973). Loudness measurements on pure tone and broad band impulsive sounds. *Acustica* 29, 198–204.

Bray, D. A., Dirks, D. D. and Morgan, D. E. (1973). Perstimulatory loudness adaptation. *J. Acoust. Soc. Am.* 53, 1544–1548.

Bregman, A. S. (1978). The formation of auditory streams. In *Attention and Performance* Vol. 7 (ed. J. Requin), Lawrence Erlbaum, New Jersey.

Bregman, A. S. (1987). The meaning of duplex perception: sounds as transparent objects. In *The Psychophysics of Speech Perception* (ed. M. E. H. Schouten), Nijhoff, Dordrecht, The Netherlands.

Bregman, A. S. and Campbell, J. (1971). Primary auditory stream segregation and perception of order in rapid sequences of tones. *J. Exp. Psychol.* 89, 244–249.

Bregman, A. S. and Dannenbring, G. L. (1973). The effect of continuity on auditory stream segregation. *Percept. Psychophys.* 13, 308–312.

Bregman, A. S. and Pinker, S. (1978). Auditory streaming and the building of timbre. *Can. J. Psychol.* 32, 19–31.

Bregman, A. S. and Rudnicky, A. I. (1975). Auditory segregation: Stream or streams? *J. Exp. Psychol.: Human Percept. Perform.* 1, 263–267.

Broadbent, D. E. and Gregory, M. (1964). Accuracy of recognition for speech presented to the right and left ears. *Q. J. Exp. Psychol.* 16, 359–360.

Broadbent, D. E. and Ladefoged, P. C. (1957). On the fusion of sounds reaching different sense organs. *J. Acoust. Soc. Am.* 29, 708–710.

Brugge J. F. and Merzenich, M. M. (1973). Responses of neurones in auditory cortex of macaque monkey to monaural and binaural stimulation. *J. Neurophysiol.* 36, 1138–1158.

Brugge J. F., Anderson D. J., Hind, J. E. and Rose, J. E. (1969). Time structure of discharges in single auditory nerve fibres of the Squirrel Monkey in response to complex periodic sounds. *J. Neurophysiol.* 32, 386–401.

Bucklein, R. (1962). Hörbarkeit von Unregelmässigkeiten in Frequenzgängen bei akustischer Ubertragung. *Frequenz* 16, 103–108. English translation in *J. Audio Eng. Soc.* 29, 126–131 (1981).

Burns, E. M. and Viemeister, N. F. (1976). Nonspectral pitch. *J. Acoust. Soc. Am.* 60, 863–869.

Burns, E. M. and Viemeister, N. F. (1981). Played again SAM: Further observations on the pitch of amplitude-modulated noise. *J. Acoust. Soc. Am.* 70, 1655–1660.

Butler, R. A. (1969). Monaural and binaural localization of noise bursts vertically in the median sagittal plane. *J. Aud. Res.* 3, 230–235.

Butler, R. A. (1971). The monaural localization of tonal stimuli. *Percept. Psychophys.* 9, 99–101.

Buus, S. (1985). Release from masking caused by envelope fluctuations. *J. Acoust. Soc. Am.* 78, 1958–1965.

Buus, S. and Florentine, M. (1985). Gap detection in normal and impaired listeners: the effect of level and frequency. In *Time Resolution in Auditory Systems* (ed. A. Michelsen), Springer-Verlag, Berlin.

Buus, S., Florentine, M. and Redden, R. B. (1982a). The SISI test: A review. Part I. *Audiology* 21, 273–293.

Buus, S., Florentine, M. and Redden, R. B. (1982b). The SISI test: A review. Part II. *Audiology* 21, 365–385.

Carhart, R., Tillman, T. W. and Greetis, E. S. (1969). Release from multiple maskers: effects of interaural time disparities. *J. Acoust. Soc. Am.* 45, 411–418.

Carlyon, R.P. and Moore, B.C.J. (1984). Intensity discrimination: A severe departure from Weber's law. *J. Acoust. Soc. Am.* 76, 1369–1376.

Carter, N. L. (1972). Effects of rise time and repetition rate on the loudness of acoustic transients. *J. Sound Vib.* 21, 227–239.

Christman, R. J. and Victor, G. (1955) The perception of direction as a function of binaural temporal and amplitude disparity. Rome Air Development Center ARDC, USAF, Tech. Note RADC-TH-55-302.

Clark, G. M. *et al.* (1987). *The University of Melbourne-Nucleus Multi-electrode Cochlear Implant*, Karger, Basel.

Cohen, M. F. and Schubert, E. D. (1987). Influence of place synchrony on detection of a sinusoid. *J. Acoust. Soc. Am.* 81, 452–458.

Colburn, H. S. (1977). Theory of binaural interaction based on auditory-nerve data. II. Detection of tones in noise. *J. Acoust. Soc. Am.* 61, 525–533.

Cole, R. A. and Scott, B. (1974). Towards a theory of speech perception. *Psychol. Rev.* 81, 348–374.

Coleman, P. D. (1962). Failure to localize the source distance of an unfamiliar sound. *J. Acoust. Soc. Am.* 34, 345–346.

Coleman, P. D. (1963). An analysis of cues to auditory depth perception in free space. *Psychol. Bull.* 60, 302–315.

Coninx, F. (1978). The detection of combined differences in frequency and intensity. *Acustica* 39, 137–150.

Corliss, E. L. R. (1967). Mechanistic aspects of hearing. *J. Acoust. Soc. Am.* 41, 1500–1516.

Corliss, E. L. R. and Winzer, G. E. (1964). Study of methods of estimating loudness. *J. Acoust. Soc. Am.* 38, 424–428.

Cuddy, L. L. (1968). Practice effects in the absolute judgment of pitch. *J. Acoust. Soc. Am.* 43, 1069–1076.

Dadson, R. S. and King, J. H. (1952). A determination of the normal threshold of hearing and its relation to the standardization of audiometers. *J. Laryngol. Otol.* 66, 366–378.

Darwin, C. J. (1981). Perceptual grouping of speech components differing in fundamental frequency and onset time. *Q. J. Exp. Psychol.* 33A, 185–207.

Darwin, C. J. (1984). Perceiving vowels in the presence of another sound: Constraints on formant perception. *J. Acoust. Soc. Am.* 76, 1636–1647.

Darwin, C. J. and Baddeley, A. D. (1974). Acoustic memory and the perception of speech. *Cognitive Psychol.* 6, 41–60.

Darwin, C. J. and Bethell-Fox, C. E. (1977). Pitch continuity and speech source attribution. *J. Exp. Psychol.: Human Percept. Perform.* 3, 665–672.

Darwin, C. J. and Gardner, R. B. (1986). Mistuning a harmonic of a vowel: Grouping and phase effects on vowel quality. *J. Acoust. Soc. Am.* 79, 838–845.

Deatherage, B. H. and Hirsh, I. J. (1957). Auditory localization of clicks. *J. Acoust. Soc. Am.* 29, 132–137.

Delgutte, B. (1987). Peripheral auditory processing of speech information: Implications from a physiological study of intensity discrimination. In *The Psychophysics of Speech Perception* (ed. M. E. H. Schouten), Nijhoff, Dordrecht, The Netherlands.

Delgutte, B. (1988). Physiological mechanisms of masking. In *Basic Issues in Hearing* (eds H. Duifhuis, J. W. Horst and H. P. Wit), Academic Press, London.

Delgutte, B. and Kiang, N. Y. S. (1984). Speech coding in the auditory nerve: IV. Sounds with consonant-like dynamic characteristics. *J. Acoust. Soc. Am.* 75, 897–907.

Dirks, D. and Bower, D. (1970). Effects of forward and backward masking on speech intelligibility. *J. Acoust. Soc. Am.* 47, 1003–1008.

Divenyi, P. L. and Blauert, J. (1987). On creating a precedent for binaural patterns: When is an echo an echo? In *Auditory Processing of Complex Sounds* (eds W. A. Yost and C. S. Watson), Erlbaum, New Jersey.

Divenyi, P. L. and Hirsh, I. J. (1974). Identification of temporal order in three-tone sequences. *J. Acoust. Soc. Am.* 56, 144–151.

Divenyi, P. L. and Shannon, R. V. (1983). Auditory time constants unified. *J. Acoust. Soc. Am.* Suppl. 1 74, S10.

Dix, M. R. and Hood, J. D. (1973). Symmetrical hearing loss in brain stem lesions. *Acta. Otolaryngol.* 75, 165–177.

Djupesland, G. and Zwislocki, J. J. (1972). Sound pressure distribution in the outer ear. *Scand. Audiol.* 1, 197–203.

Dolan, T. R. and Trahiotis, C. (1972). Binaural interaction in backward masking. *Percept. Psychophys.* 11, 92–94.

Dowling, W. J. (1968). Rhythmic fission and perceptual organization. *J. Acoust. Soc. Am.* 44, 369.

Dowling, W. J. (1973). The perception of interleaved melodies. *Cognitive Psychol.* 5, 322–337.

Duifhuis, H. (1971). Audibility of high harmonics in a periodic pulse II. Time effect. *J. Acoust. Soc. Am.* 49, 1155–1162.

Duifhuis, H. (1972). *Perceptual Analysis of Sound*, Doctoral dissertation, Eindhoven University of Technology.

Duifhuis, H. (1973). Consequences of peripheral frequency selectivity for nonsimultaneous masking. *J. Acoust. Soc. Am.* 54, 1471–1488.

Durlach, N. I. (1963). Equalization and cancellation theory of binaural masking level differences. *J. Acoust. Soc. Am.* 35, 1206–1218.

Durlach, N. I. (1972). Binaural signal detection: equalization and cancellation theory. In *Foundations of Modern Auditory Theory*, Vol. 2 (ed. J. V. Tobias), Academic Press, New York.

Egan, J. P. and Hake, H. W. (1950). On the masking pattern of a simple auditory stimulus. *J. Acoust. Soc. Am.* 22, 622–630.

Elfner, L. F. and Caskey, W. E. (1965). Continuity effects with alternating sounded noise and tone signals as a function of manner of presentation. *J. Acoust. Soc. Am.* 38, 543–547.

Elliot, D. N. and Fraser, W. R. (1970). Fatigue and adaptation. In *Foundations of Modern Auditory Theory*, Vol. 1 (ed. J. V. Tobias), Academic Press, New York.

Elliot, L. L. (1962). Backward and forward masking of probe tones of different frequencies. *J. Acoust. Soc. Am.* 34, 1116–1117.

Emmerich, D. S., Ellermeier, W. and Butensky, B. (1989). A re-examination of the frequency discrimination of random-amplitude tones, and a test of Henning's modified energy-detector model. *J. Acoust. Soc. Am.* 85, 1653–1659.

Evans, E. F. (1968). Cortical Representation. In *Hearing Mechanisms in Vertebrates* (eds A. V. S. de Reuck and J. Knight), Churchill, London.

Evans, E. F. (1975). The sharpening of cochlear frequency selectivity in the normal and abnormal cochlea. *Audiology* 14, 419–442.

Evans, E. F. (1978). Place and time coding of frequency in the peripheral auditory system: some physiological pros and cons. *Audiology* 17, 369–420.

Evans, E. F. and Harrison, R. V. (1976). Correlation between outer hair cell damage and deterioration of cochlear nerve tuning properties in the guinea pig. *J. Physiol.* 252, 43–44P.

Evans, E. F., Pratt, S. R. and Cooper, N. P. (1989). Correspondence between behavioural and physiological frequency selectivity in the guinea pig. *Brit. J. Audiol.* 23, 151–152.

Exner, S (1876). Zur Lehre von den Gehörsempfindungen. *Pflügers Archiv*, 13, 228–253.

Fant, G. C. M. (1960). *Acoustic Theory of Speech Production*. Mouton, The Hague.

Fastl, H. (1976). Temporal masking effects: I. Broad band noise masker. *Acustica*, 35, 287–302.

Fastl, H. and Schorn, K. (1981). Discrimination of level differences by hearing impaired patients. *Audiology*, 20, 488–502.

Feldtkeller, R. and Zwicker, E. (1956). *Das Ohr als Nachrichtenempfänger*, S. Hirzel, Stuttgart.

Feth, L. L. (1972). Combinations of amplitude and frequency difference in auditory discrimination. *Acustica* 26, 67–77.

Filippo, C. L. de and Snell, K. B. (1986). Detection of a temporal gap in low-frequency narrow-band signals by normal-hearing and hearing-impaired subjects. *J. Acoust. Soc. Am.* 80, 1354–1358.

Fischer-Jørgensen, E. (1972). Tape cutting experiments with Danish stop consonants in initial position. *Ann. Rep. VII*, University of Copenhagen, Institute of Phonetics.

Fitzgibbons, P. and Wightman, F. L. (1982). Gap detection in normal and hearing-impaired listeners. *J. Acoust. Soc. Am.* 72, 761–765.

Fletcher, H. (1940). Auditory patterns. *Rev. Mod. Phys.* 12, 47–65.

Fletcher, H. and Munson, W. A. (1933). Loudness, its definition, measurement and calculation. *J. Acoust. Soc. Am.* 5, 82–108.

Florentine, M., Buus, S., Scharf, B. and Zwicker, E. (1980). Frequency selectivity in normally-hearing and hearing-impaired observers. *J. Speech Hear. Res.* 23, 646–669.

Florentine, M. and Buus, S. (1981). An excitation-pattern model for intensity discrimination. *J. Acoust. Soc. Am.* 70, 1646–1654.

Fourcin, A. J. (1970). Central pitch and auditory lateralization. In *Frequency Analysis and Periodicity Detection in Hearing* (eds R. Plomp and G. F. Smoorenburg), A. W. Sijthoff, Leiden.

Fourcin, A. J., Rosen, S. M., Moore, B. C. J., Douek, E. E., Clarke, G. P., Dodson, H. and Bannister, L. H. (1979). External electrical stimulation of the cochlea: clinical, psychophysical, speech-perceptual and histological findings. *Br. J. Audiol.* 13, 85–107.

Fraisse, P. (1982). Rythm and tempo. In *The Psychology of Music* (ed. D. Deutch), Academic Press, New York.

Freedman, S. J. and Fisher, H. G. (1968). The role of the pinna in auditory localization. In *Neuropsychology of Spatially Oriented Behavior* (ed. S. J. Freedman), Dorsey Press, Illinois.

Freedmann S. J., Wilson, L. and Rekosh, J. H. (1967). Compensation for auditory rearrangement in hand-ear coordination. *Percept. Motor Skills* 24, 1207–1210.

Gantz, B. J., McCabe, B. F., Tyler, R. S. and Preece, J. P. (1987). Evaluation of four cochlear implant designs. *Ann. Otol. Rhinol. Laryngol.* Suppl. 128, 145–147.

Gardner, M. B. and Gardner, R. S. (1973). Problem of localization in the median plane: effect of pinnae cavity occlusion. *J. Acoust. Soc. Am.* 53, 400–408.

Gardner, R. B. and Darwin, C. J. (1986). Grouping of vowel harmonics by frequency modulation: Absence of effects on phonemic categorization. *Percept. Psychophys.* 40, 183–187.

Gardner, R. B., Gaskill, S. A. and Darwin, C. J. (1989). Perceptual grouping of formants with static and dynamic differences in fundamental frequency. *J. Acoust. Soc. Am.* 85, 1329–1337.

Garner, W. R. and Miller, G. A. (1947). The masked threshold of pure tones as a function of duration. *J. Exp. Psychol.* 37, 293–303.

Gässler, G. (1954). Über die Hörschwelle für Schallereignisse mit verschieden breitem Frequenzspektrum. *Acustica* 4, 408–414.

Gebhardt, C. J. and Goldstein, D. P. (1972). Frequency discrimination and the M.L.D. *J. Acoust. Soc. Am.* 51, 1228–1232.

Glasberg, B. R. and Moore, B. C. J. (1986). Auditory filter shapes in subjects with unilateral and bilateral cochlear impairments. *J. Acoust. Soc. Am.* 79, 1020–1033.

Glasberg, B. R., Moore, B. C. J., Patterson, R. D. and Nimmo-Smith, I. (1984). Comparison of auditory filter shapes derived with three different maskers. *J. Acoust. Soc. Am.* 75, 536–546.

Goldhor, R. S. (1985). Representation of consonants in the peripheral auditory system: A modeling study of the correspondence between response properties and phonetic features. MIT Res. Lab. of Electronics, Tech. Rep. 505.

Goldstein, J. L. (1967). Auditory nonlinearity. *J. Acoust. Soc. Am.* 41, 676–689.

Goldstein, J. L. (1973). An optimum processor theory for the central formation of the pitch of complex tones. *J. Acoust. Soc. Am.* 54, 1496–1516.

Goldstein, J. L. and Srulovicz, P. (1977). Auditory-nerve spike intervals as an adequate basis for aural frequency measurement. In *Psychophysics and Physiology of Hearing* (eds E. F. Evans and J. P. Wilson), Academic Press, London and New York.

Grantham, D. W. (1986). Detection and discrimination of simulated motion of auditory targets in the horizontal plane. *J. Acoust. Soc. Am.* 79, 1939–1949.

Grantham, D. W. and Wightman, F. L. (1978). Detectability of varying interaural temporal differences. *J. Acoust. Soc. Am.* 63, 511–523.

Grantham, D. W. and Wightman, F. L. (1979). Detectability of a pulsed tone in the presence of a masker with time-varying interaural correlation. *J. Acoust. Soc. Am.* 65, 1509–1517.

Green, D. M. (1960). Auditory detection of a noise signal. *J. Acoust. Soc. Am.* 32, 121–131.

Green, D. M. (1973). Temporal acuity as a function of frequency. *J. Acoust. Soc. Am.* 54, 373–379.

Green, D.M. (1985). Temporal factors in psychoacoustics. In *Time Resolution in Auditory Systems* (ed. A. Michelsen), Springer-Verlag, Berlin.

Green, D. M. (1988). *Profile Analysis.* Oxford University Press, New York.

Green, D. M. and Forrest, T. (1988). Detection of amplitude modulation and gaps in noise. In *Basic Issues in Hearing* (eds H. Duifhuis, J. W. Horst and H. P. Wit), Academic Press, London.

Green, D. M., and Swets, J. A. (1974). *Signal Detection Theory and Psychophysics,* Kreiger, New York.

Green, D. M., Birdsall, T. G. and Tanner, W. P. (1957). Signal detection as a function of signal intensity and duration. *J. Acoust. Soc. Am.* 29, 523–531.

Greenwood, D. D. (1961a). Auditory masking and the critical band. *J. Acoust. Soc. Am.* 33, 484–501.

Greenwood, D. D. (1961b). Critical bandwidth and the frequency coordinates of the basilar membrane. *J. Acoust. Soc. Am.* 33, 1344–1356.

Groen, J. J. (1964). Super- and subliminal binaural beats. *Acta Otolaryngol.* 57, 224–231

Grose, J. H. and Hall, J. W. (1989). Comodulation masking release using SAM tonal complex maskers: Effects of modulation depth and signal position. *J. Acoust. Soc. Am.* 85, 1276–1284.

Gruber, J. and Boerger, G. (1971). Binaurale Verdeckungspegeldifferenzen (BMLD) und Vor- und Rückwärtsverdeckung. *Proc. 7th Int. Congr. on Acoustics,* Budapest, paper 23H5.

Haas, H. (1951). Über den Einfluss eines Einfachechos an die Hörsamkeit von Sprache. *Acustica* 1, 49–58.

Hafter, E. R. and Carrier, S. C. (1972). Binaural interaction in low- frequency stimuli: the inability to trade time and intensity completely. *J. Acoust. Soc. Am.* 51, 1852–1862.

Hafter, E. R. and Jeffress, L. A. (1968). Two-image lateralization of tones and clicks. *J. Acoust. Soc. Am.* 44, 563–569.

Hafter, E. R., Buell, T. N. and Richards, V. M. (1988). Onset-coding in lateralization: Its form, site, and function. In *Auditory Function* (eds G. M. Edelman, W. E. Gall and W. M. Cowan), Wiley, New York.

Hafter, E. R., Dye, R. H. and Wenzel, E. M. (1983). Detection of interaural differences of intensity in trains of high-frequency clicks as a function of interclick interval and number. *J. Acoust. Soc. Am.* 73, 1708–1713.

Haggard, M. P. (1974). Feasibility of rapid critical bandwidth estimates. *J. Acoust. Soc. Am.* 55, 304–308.

Haggard, M. P. and Bates, J. (1974). Changes in auditory perception in the menstrual cycle. *Speech Perception*, ser. 2, no. 3, 55–74 (Dept of Psychology, Queen's University of Belfast).

Hall, J. W. and Fernandes, M. A. (1984). The role of monaural frequency selectivity in binaural analysis. *J. Acoust. Soc. Am.* 76, 435–439.

Hall, J. W. and Grose, J. H. (1988). Comodulation masking release: Evidence for multiple cues. *J. Acoust. Soc. Am.* 84, 1669–1675.

Hall, J. W. and Peters, R. W. (1981). Pitch for nonsimultaneous successive harmonics in quiet and noise. *J. Acoust. Soc. Am.* 69, 509–513.

Hall, J. W., Haggard, M. P. and Fernandes, M. A. (1984). Detection in noise by spectro-temporal pattern analysis. *J. Acoust. Soc. Am.* 76, 50–56.

Hall, J. W., Tyler, R. S. and Fernandes, M. A. (1983). Monaural and binaural frequency resolution measured using bandlimited noise and notched-noise masking. *J. Acoust. Soc. Am.* 73, 894–898.

Hamilton, P. M. (1957). Noise masked threshold as a function of tonal duration and masking noise band width. *J. Acoust. Soc. Am.* 29, 506–511.

Handel, S. (1973). Temporal segmentation of repeating auditory patterns. *J. Exp. Psychol.* 101, 46–54.

Hansen, V. and Madsen, E. R. (1974). On aural phase detection. *J. Audio Engng. Soc.* 22, 10–14.

Harris, G. G. (1960). Binaural interactions of impulsive stimuli and pure tones. *J. Acoust. Soc. Am.* 32, 685–692.

Harris, J. D. (1963). Loudness discrimination. *J. Speech Hear. Dis. Monogr.* Suppl. 11, 1–63.

Harris, J. D. (1972). Audition. *Ann. Rev. Psychol.* 23, 313–346.

Harris, J. D. and Sergeant, R. L. (1971). Monaural/binaural minimum audible angles for a moving sound source. *J. Speech Hear. Res.* 14, 618–629.

Hawkins, J. E. and Stevens, S. S. (1950). The masking of pure tones and of speech by white noise. *J. Acoust. Soc. Am.* 22, 6–13.

Held, R. (1955). Shifts in binaural localization after prolonged exposures to atypical combinations of stimuli. *Am. J. Psychol.* 68, 526–548.

Helmholtz, H. L. F. von (1863). *Die Lehre von den Tonempfindungen als physiologische Grundlage für die Theorie der Musik*, 1st edn, F. Vieweg, Braunschweig.

Henning, G. B. (1966). Frequency discrimination of random amplitude tones. *J. Acoust. Soc. Am.* 39, 336–339.

Henning, G. B. (1967). A model for auditory discrimination and detection. *J. Acoust. Soc. Am.* 42, 1325–1334.

Henning, G. B. (1974). Detectability of interaural delay with high-frequency complex waveforms. *J. Acoust. Soc. Am.* 55, 84–90.

Henning, G. B. and Gaskell, H. (1981). Monaural phase sensitivity measured with Ronken's paradigm. *J. Acoust. Soc. Am.* 70, 1673.

Hind, J. E., Rose, J. E., Brugge, J. F. and Anderson, D. J. (1967). Coding of information pertaining to paired low-frequency tones in single auditory nerve fibers of the squirrel monkey. *J. Neurophysiol.* 30, 794–816.

Hirsh, I. J. (1950). The relation between localization and intelligibility. *J. Acoust. Soc. Am.* 22, 196–200.

Hirsh, I. J.(1959). Auditory perception of temporal order. *J. Acoust. Soc. Am.* 31, 759–767.

Hirsh, I. J. (1971). Masking of speech and auditory localization. *Audiology* 10, 110–114.

Hirsh, I. J. and Bilger, R. C. (1955). Auditory-threshold recovery after exposures to pure tones. *J. Acoust. Soc. Am.* 27, 1186–1194.

Hirsh, I. J. and Ward, W. D. (1952). Recovery of the auditory threshold after strong acoustic stimulation. *J. Acoust. Soc. Am.* 24, 131–141.

Hochmair, E. S. and Hochmair-Desoyer, E. J. (1983). Percepts elicited by different speech coding strategies. In *Cochlear Prostheses – An International Symposium* (eds C. W. Parkins and S. W. Anderson), Annals of the New York Academy of Sciences, Vol. 405.

Holmes, J. (1988). *Speech Synthesis and Recognition*, Van Nostrand Reinhold, London.

Hood, J. D. (1950). Studies in auditory fatigue and adaptation. *Acta Otolaryngol.* Suppl. 92.

Hood, J. D. (1972). Fundamentals of identification of sensorineural hearing loss. *Sound* 6, 21–26.

House, A. S., Stevens, K. N., Sandel, T. T. and Arnold, J. B. (1962). On the learning of speechlike vocabularies. *J. Verb. Learn. Verb. Behav.* 1, 133–143.

House, W. F. (1976). Cochlear Implants. *Ann. Otol. Rhinol. Laryngol.* 85, Suppl. 27, 1–93.

Houtgast, T. (1972). Psychophysical evidence for lateral inhibition in hearing. *J. Acoust. Soc. Am.* 51, 1885–1894.

Houtgast, T. (1973). Psychophysical experiments on 'tuning curves' and 'two-tone inhibition'. *Acustica* 29, 168–179.

Houtgast, T. (1974). Lateral suppression in hearing. Thesis, Free University of Amsterdam, Academische Pers. BV, Amsterdam.

Houtgast, T. (1976). Subharmonic pitches of a pure tone at low S/N ratio. *J. Acoust. Soc. Am.* 60, 405–409.

Houtsma A. J. M. and Goldstein, J. L. (1972). The central origin of the pitch of complex tones: evidence from musical interval recognition. *J. Acoust. Soc. Am.* 51, 520–529.

Howes, W. L. (1971). Loudness determined by power summation. *Acustica* 25, 343–349.

Hubel, D. H. and Wiesel, T. N. (1968). Receptive fields and functional architecture of monkey striate cortex. *J. Physiol.* 195, 215–243.

Huggins, W. H. and Cramer, E. M. (1958). Creation of pitch through binaural interaction. *J. Acoust. Soc. Am.* 30, 413–417.

Hughes, J. W. (1946). The threshold of audition for short periods of stimulation. *Proc. R. Soc.* B 133, 486–490.

Jakobson, R., Fant, G. and Halle, M. (1963). *Preliminaries to Speech Analysis: the Distinctive Features and Their Correlates*, MIT Press, Cambridge, Mass.

Javel, E. (1980). Coding of AM tones in the chinchilla auditory nerve: implications for the pitch of complex tones. *J. Acoust. Soc. Am.* 68, 133–146.

Jeffress, L. A. (1948). A place theory of sound localization. *J. Comp. Physiol. Psychol.* 41, 35–39.

Jeffress, L. A. (1964). Stimulus-oriented approach to detection. *J. Acoust. Soc. Am.* 36, 766–774.

Jeffress, L. A. (1971). Detection and lateralization of binaural signals. *Audiology* 10, 77–84.

Jerger, J. F. (1957). Auditory adaptation. *J. Acoust. Soc. Am.* 29, 357–363.

Jerger, J. and Jerger, S. (1975). A simplified tone decay test. *Arch. Otolaryngol.* 102, 403–407.

Jerger, J. F., Shedd, J. L. and Harford, E. (1959). On the detection of extremely small changes in sound intensity. *Arch. Otolaryngol.* 69, 200–211.

Jesteadt, W., Wier, C. C. and Green, D. M. (1977). Intensity discrimination as a function of frequency and sensation level. *J. Acoust. Soc. Am.* 61, 169–177.

Johnson, D. L. and Gierke, H. von (1974). Audibility of infrasound. *J. Acoust. Soc. Am.* 56, Suppl., S37.

Johnson-Davies, D. B. and Patterson, R. D. (1979). Psychophysical tuning curves: Restricting the listening band to the signal region. *J. Acoust. Soc. Am.* 65, 765–770.

Kalil, R. and Freedman, S. J. (1967) Compensation for auditory rearrangement in the absence of observer movements. *Percept. Motor Skills* 24, 475–478.

Katz, S. J. and Berry, R. C. (1971) Speech modulated noise. Paper presented at the 81st Meeting of the Acoustical Society of America.

Kellog, W. N. (1962). Sonar system of the blind. *Science*, N. Y. 137, 399–404.

Kemp, D. T. (1978). Stimulated acoustic emissions from within the human auditory system. *J. Acoust. Soc. Am.* 64, 1386–1391.

Kewley-Port, D., Pisoni, D. B. and Studdert-Kennedy, M. (1983). Perception of static and dynamic cues to place of articulation in initial stop consonants. *J. Acoust. Soc. Am.* 73, 1779–1793.

Khanna, S. M. and Leonard, D. G. B. (1982). Basilar membrane tuning in the cat cochlea. *Science* 215, 305–306.

Kiang, N. Y.-S. (1968). A survey of recent developments in the study of auditory physiology. *Ann. Otol. Rhinol. Laryngol.* 77, 656–675.

Kiang, N. Y.-S., Watanabe, T., Thomas, E. C. and Clark, L. F. (1965). *Discharge Patterns of Single Fibers in the Cat's Auditory Nerve*, MIT Press, Cambridge, Mass.

Kidd, G. and Feth, L. L. (1982). Effects of masker duration in pure-tone forward masking. *J. Acoust. Soc. Am.* 72, 1384–1386.

Kim, D. O. and Molnar, C. E. (1979). A population study of cochlear nerve fibres: comparison of spatial distributions of average-rate and phase-locking measures of responses to single tones. *J. Neurophysiol.* 42, 16–30.

Kim, D. O., Molnar, C. E. and Matthews, J. W. (1980). Cochlear mechanics: nonlinear behavior in two–tone responses as reflected in cochlear-nerve-fiber responses and in ear-canal sound pressure. *J. Acoust. Soc. Am.* 67, 1704–1721.

Kimura, D. (1961). Some effects of temporal lobe damage on auditory perception. *Can. J. Psychol.* 15, 156–165.

Kimura, D. (1964). Left-right differences in the perception of melodies. *Q. J. Exp. Psychol.* 16, 355–358.

Klatt, D. (1982). Speech processing strategies based on auditory models. In *The Representation of Speech in the Peripheral Auditory System* (eds R. Carlson and B. Granstrom), Elsevier, Amsterdam.

Klatt, D. (1989). Review of selected models of speech perception. In *Lexical Representation and Process* (ed. W. D. Marslen-Wilson), MIT Press, Cambridge, Mass.

Klump, R. G. and Eady, H. R. (1956). Some measurements of interaural time difference thresholds. *J. Acoust. Soc. Am.* 28, 859–860.

Koffka, K. (1935). *Principles of Gestalt Psychology*, Harcourt and Brace, New York.

Kohlrausch, A. (1988). Auditory filter shape derived from binaural masking experiments. *J. Acoust. Soc. Am.* 84, 573–583.

Kruskal, J. B. (1964). Nonmetric multidimensional scaling: a numerical method. *Psychometrika* 29, 115–129.

Kubovy, M., Cutting, J. E. and McGuire, R. M. (1974). Hearing with the third ear: dichotic perception of a melody without monaural familiarity cues. *Science, N. Y.* 186, 272–274.

Ladefoged, P. and Broadbent, D. E. (1960). Perception of sequence in auditory events. *Q. J. Exp. Psychol.* 12, 162–170.

Lamore, P. J. J. (1975). Perception of two-tone octave complexes. *Acustica* 34, 1–14.

Lamore, P. J. J. and Rodenburg, M. (1980). Significance of the SISI test and its relation to recruitment. *Audiology* 19, 75–85.

Laurence, R. F., Moore, B. C. J. and Glasberg, B. R. (1983). A comparison of behind-the-ear high-fidelity linear hearing aids and two-channel compression aids, in the laboratory and in everyday life. *Brit. J. Audiol.* 17, 31–48.

Legouix, P. J., Remond, M. C. and Greenbaum, H. B. (1973). Interference and two-tone inhibition. *J. Acoust. Soc. Am.* 53, 409–419.

Leonard, D. G. B. and Khanna, S. M. (1984). Histological evaluation of damage in cat cochleas used for measurement of basilar membrane mechanics. *J. Acoust. Soc. Am.* 75, 515–527.

Leshowitz, B. (1971). Measurement of the two-click threshold. *J. Acoust. Soc. Am.* 49, 462–466.

Liberman, A. M. (1982). On finding that speech is special. *Am. Psychologist* 37, 148–167.

Liberman, A. M. and Mattingly, I. G. (1985). The motor theory of speech perception revised. *Cognition* 21, 1–36.

Liberman, A. M., Cooper, F. S., Shankweiler, D. P. and Studdert-Kennedy, M. (1967). Perception of the speech code. *Psychol. Rev.* 74, 431–461.

Liberman, M. C. (1978). Auditory-nerve response from cats raised in a low-noise chamber. *J. Acoust. Soc. Am.* 63, 442–455.

Liberman, M. C. (1982). The cochlear frequency map for the cat: Labeling auditory-nerve fibers of known characteristic frequency. *J. Acoust. Soc. Am.* 72, 1441–1449.

Licklider, J. C. R. (1956). Auditory frequency analysis. In *Information Theory* (ed. C. Cherry), Academic Press, New York.

Licklider, J. C. R., Webster, J. C. and Hedlun, J. M. (1950). On the frequency limits of binaural beats. *J. Acoust. Soc. Am.* 22, 468–473.

Lim, J. S. (1983). *Speech Enhancement*, Prentice-Hall, New Jersey.

Lippmann, R. P., Braida, L. D. and Durlach, N. I. (1981). Study of multichannel amplitude compression and linear amplification for persons with sensorineural hearing loss. *J. Acoust. Soc. Am. 69*, 524–534.

Locke, S. and Kellar, L. (1973). Categorical perception in a nonlinguistic mode. *Cortex 9*, 353–369.

Maiwald, D. (1967). Die Berechnung von Modulationsschwellen mit Hilfe eines Funktionsschemas. *Acustica 18*, 193–207.

Mann, V. A. and Liberman, A. M. (1983). Some differences between phonetic and auditory modes of perception. *Cognition 14*, 211–235.

Mayer, A. M. (1894). Researches in acoustics. *Lond. Edinb. Dubl. Phil. Mag. 37*, ser. 5, 259–288.

McAdams, S. (1982). Spectral fusion and the creation of auditory images. In *Music, Mind and Brain* (ed. M. Clynes), Plenum, New York.

McAdams, S. (1989). Segregation of concurrent sounds, I. Effects of frequency modulation coherence and fixed resonance structure. *J. Acoust. Soc. Am.* (in press).

McFadden, D. (1986). The curious half-octave shift: Evidence for a basalward migration of the travelling-wave envelope with increasing intensity. In *Basic and Applied Aspects of Noise-Induced Hearing Loss* (eds. R. J. Salvi, D. Henderson, R. P. Hamernik and V. Colletti), Plenum, New York.

McFadden, D., Jeffress, L. A. and Ermey, H. L. (1971). Differences of interaural phase and level in detection and lateralization: 250 Hz. *J. Acoust. Soc. Am. 50*, 1484–1493.

McFadden, D., Jeffress, L. A. and Ermey, H. L. (1972). Differences of interaural phase and level in detection and lateralization: 1000 and 2000 Hz. *J. Acoust. Soc. Am. 52*, 1197–1206.

McGurk, H. and Macdonald, J. (1976). Hearing lips and seeing voices. *Nature 264*, 746–748.

Meddis, R. and Hewitt, M. (1988). A computational model of low pitch judgement. In *Basic Issues in Hearing* (eds H. Duifhuis, J. W. Horst and H. P. Wit), Academic Press, London.

Mehler, J. (1981). The role of syllables in speech processing: infant and adult data. *Phil. Trans. Roy. Soc. B295*, 333–352.

Mershon, D. H. and Bowers, J. N. (1979). Absolute and relative cues for the auditory perception of egocentric distance. *Perception 8*, 311–322.

Mershon, D. H. and King, L. E. (1975). Intensity and reverberation as factors in the auditory perception of egocentric distance. *Percept. Psychophys. 18*, 409–415.

Mersenne, M. (1636). *Traite des Instrumens*, Book IV, Sebastian Cramoisy, Paris.

Merzenich, M. (1983). Coding of sound in a cochlear prosthesis: Some theoretical and practical considerations. In *Cochlear Prostheses—An International Symposium* (eds C. W. Parkins and S. W. Anderson), Annals of the New York Academy of Sciences, Vol. 405.

Merzenich, M. M., Knight, P. L. and Roth, G. L. (1973a). Cochleotopic organization of primary auditory cortex in the cat. *Brain Res. 63*, 343–346.

Merzenich, M. M., Michelson, R. P., Schindler, R. A., Pettit, C. R. and Reid, M. (1973b). Neural encoding of sound sensation evoked by electrical stimulation of the acoustic nerve. *Ann. Otol. 82*, 486–503.

Merzenich, M. M., Schindler, D. N. and White, M. W. (1974). Symposium on cochlear implants. II. Feasibility of multichannel scala tympani stimulation. *Laryngoscope 84*, 1887–1893.

Meyer, M. (1898). Zur Theorie der Differenztöne und der Gehörsempfindungen überhaupt. *Beitr. Akust. Musikwiss. 2*, 25–65.

Miller, G. A. (1947). Sensitivity to changes in the intensity of white noise and its relation to masking and loudness. *J. Acoust. Soc. Am.* 191, 609–619.

Miller, G. A. and Licklider, J. C. R. (1950). The intelligibility of interrupted speech. *J. Acoust. Soc. Am.* 22, 167–173.

Miller, G. A. and Taylor, W. (1948). The perception of repeated bursts of noise. *J. Acoust. Soc. Am.* 20, 171–182.

Miller, J. D., Wier, C. C., Pastore R., Kelly, W. J. and Dooling, R. J. (1976). Discrimination and labelling of noise-burst sequences with varying noise-lead times: An example of categorical perception. *J. Acoust. Soc. Am.* 60, 410–417.

Mills, A. W. (1960). Lateralization of high-frequency tones. *J. Acoust. Soc. Am.* 32, 132–134.

Mills, A. W. (1972). Auditory localization. In *Foundations of Modern Auditory Theory*, Vol. 2 (ed. J. V. Tobias), Academic Press, New York.

Moore, B. C. J. (1972). Some experiments relating to the perception of pure tones: possible clinical applications. *Sound* 6, 73–79.

Moore, B. C. J. (1973a). Frequency difference limens for short-duration tones. *J. Acoust. Soc. Am.* 54, 610–619.

Moore, B. C. J. (1973b). Some experiments relating to the perception of complex tones. *Q. J. Exp. Psychol.* 25, 451–475.

Moore, B. C. J. (1977). Effects of relative phase of the components on the pitch of three-component complex tones. In *Psychophysics and Physiology of Hearing* (eds E. F. Evans and J. P. Wilson), Academic Press, London.

Moore, B. C. J. (1978). Psychophysical tuning curves measured in simultaneous and forward masking. *J. Acoust. Soc. Am.* 63, 524–532.

Moore, B. C. J. (1986). Parallels between frequency selectivity measured psychophysically and in cochlear mechanics. *Scand. Audiol.* Suppl. 25, 139–152.

Moore, B. C. J. (1989). How much do we gain by gain control in hearing aids? *Acta Otolaryngol.* (in press)

Moore, B. C. J. and Glasberg, B. R. (1981). Auditory filter shapes derived in simultaneous and forward masking. *J. Acoust. Soc. Am.* 70, 1003–1014.

Moore, B. C. J. and Glasberg, B. R. (1983a). Suggested formulae for calculating auditory-filter bandwidths and excitation patterns. *J. Acoust. Soc. Am.* 74, 750–753.

Moore, B. C. J. and Glasberg, B. R. (1983b). Growth of forward masking for sinusoidal and noise maskers as a function of signal delay: Implications for suppression in noise. *J. Acoust. Soc. Am.* 73, 1249–1259.

Moore, B. C. J. and Glasberg, B. R. (1986). The role of frequency selectivity in the perception of loudness, pitch and time. In *Frequency Selectivity in Hearing* (ed. B. C. J. Moore), Academic Press, London and New York.

Moore, B. C. J. and Glasberg, B. R. (1987). Formulae describing frequency selectivity as a function of frequency and level, and their use in calculating excitation patterns. *Hearing Res.* 28, 209–225.

Moore, B. C. J. and Glasberg, B. R. (1988a). Gap detection with sinusoids and noise in normal, impaired and electrically stimulated ears. *J. Acoust. Soc. Am.* 83, 1093–1101.

Moore, B. C. J. and Glasberg, B. R. (1988b). Effects of the relative phase of the components on the pitch discrimination of complex tones by subjects with unilateral cochlear impairments. In *Basic Issues in Hearing* (eds H. Duifhuis, J. W. Horst and H. P. Wit), Academic Press, London.

Moore, B. C. J. and Glasberg, B. R. (1988c). A comparison of four methods of implementing automatic gain control (AGC) in hearing aids. *Brit. J. Audiol.* 22, 93–104.

Moore, B. C. J. and Glasberg, B. R. (1989). Mechanisms underlying the frequency discrimination of pulsed tones and the detection of frequency modulation. *J. Acoust. Soc. Am.* (in press).

Moore, B. C. J. and Raab, D. H. (1974). Pure-tone intensity discrimination: some experiments relating to the 'near–miss' to Weber's law. *J. Acoust. Soc. Am.* 55, 1049–1054.

Moore, B. C. J. and Rosen, S. M. (1979). Tune recognition with reduced pitch and interval information. *Q. J. Exp. Psychol.* 31, 229–240.

Moore, B. C. J., Fourcin, A. J., Rosen, S. *et al.* (1985). Extraction and presentation of speech features. In *Cochlear Implants* (eds R. A. Schindler and M. M. Merzenich), Raven Press, New York.

Moore, B. C. J., Glasberg, B. R., Hess, R. F. and Birchall, J. P. (1985b). Effects of flanking noise bands on the rate of growth of loudness of tones in normal and recruiting ears. *J. Acoust. Soc. Am.* 77, 1505–1513.

Moore, B. C. J., Glasberg, B. R. and Peters, R. W. (1985c). Relative dominance of individual partials in determining the pitch of complex tones. *J. Acoust. Soc. Am.* 77, 1853–1860.

Moore, B. C. J., Glasberg, B. R. and Peters, R. W. (1986). Thresholds for hearing mistuned partials as separate tones in harmonic complexes. *J. Acoust. Soc. Am.* 80, 479–483.

Moore, B. C. J., Glasberg, B. R., Plack, C. J. and Biswas, A. K. (1988). The shape of the ear's temporal window. *J. Acoust. Soc. Am.* 83, 1102–1116.

Moore, B. C. J., Glasberg, B. R. and Shailer, M. J. (1984). Frequency and intensity difference limens for harmonics within complex tones. *J. Acoust. Soc. Am.* 75, 550–561.

Moore, B. C. J., Oldfield, S. R. and Dooley, G. J. (1989). Detection and discrimination of spectral peaks and notches at 1 and 8 kHz. *J. Acoust. Soc. Am.* 85, 820–836.

Moore, B. C. J., Poon, P. W. F., Bacon, S. P. and Glasberg, B.R. (1987). The temporal course of masking and the auditory filter shape. *J. Acoust. Soc. Am.* 81, 1873–1880.

Munson, W. A. (1947). The growth of auditory sensation. *J. Acoust. Soc. Am.* 19, 584–591.

Neisser, U. (1967). *Cognitive Psychology*, Appleton-Century-Crofts, New York.

Newman, E. B. (1948). Chapter 14 in *Foundations of Psychology* (eds E. G. Boring, H. S. Langfeld and H. P. Weld), Wiley, New York.

Noorden, L. P. A. S. van (1971). Rhythmic fission as a function of tone rate. *IPO Annual Progress Rep.* 6, 9–12, Eindhoven, The Netherlands.

Noorden, L. P. A. S. van (1975). Temporal coherence in the perception of tone sequences. Thesis, Technical University Eindhoven.

Noorden, L. P. A. S. van (1982). Two channel pitch perception. In *Music, Mind and Brain* (ed. M. Clynes), Plenum, New York.

Nordmark, J. O. (1970). Time and frequency analysis. In *Foundations of Modern Auditory Theory*, Vol. 1 (ed. J. V. Tobias), Academic Press, New York.

Ohgushi, K. (1984). Recent research on hearing in Japan. *J. Acoust. Soc. Jpn.* (E) 5, 127–133.

Ohm, G. S. (1843). Über die Definition des Tones, nebst daran geknüpfter Theorie der Sirene und ähnlicher tonbildender Vorrichtungen. *Ann. Phys. Chem.* 59, 513–565.

Oldfield, S. R. and Parker, S. P. A. (1984). Acuity of sound localization: a topography of auditory space. I. Normal hearing conditions. *Perception* 13, 581–600.

O'Loughlin, B. J. and Moore, B. C. J. (1981). Off-frequency listening: Effects on psychoacoustical tuning curves obtained in simultaneous and forward masking. *J. Acoust. Soc. Am.* 69, 1119–1125.

Olson, W. O. and Carhart, R. (1966). Integration of acoustic power at threshold by normal hearers. *J. Acoust. Soc. Am.* 40, 591–599.

Palmer, A. R. and Evans, E. F. (1979). On the peripheral coding of the level of individual frequency components of complex sounds at high sound levels. In *Hearing Mechanisms and Speech* (eds O. Creutzfeldt, H. Scheich and C. Schreiner), Springer-Verlag, Berlin.

Parker, E. M., Diehl, R. L. and Kluender, K. R. (1986). Trading relations in speech and nonspeech. *Percept. Psychophys.* 39, 129–142.

Patterson, J. H. (1971). Additivity of forward and backward masking as a function of signal frequency. *J. Acoust. Soc. Am.* 50, 1123–1125.

Patterson, J. H. and Green, D. M. (1970). Discrimination of transient signals having identical energy spectra. *J. Acoust. Soc. Am.* 48, 894–905.

Patterson, R. D. (1976). Auditory filter shapes derived with noise stimuli. *J. Acoust. Soc. Am.* 59, 640–654.

Patterson, R. D. (1987a). A pulse ribbon model of monaural phase perception. *J. Acoust. Soc. Am.* 82, 1560–1586.

Patterson, R. D. (1987b). A pulse ribbon model of peripheral auditory processing. In *Auditory Processing of Complex Sounds* (eds. W. A. Yost and C. S. Watson), Erlbaum, New Jersey.

Patterson, R. D. and Henning, G. B. (1977). Stimulus variability and auditory filter shape. *J. Acoust. Soc. Am.* 62, 649–664.

Patterson, R. D. and Milroy, R. (1980). The appropriate sound level for auditory warnings on civil aircraft. *J. Acoust. Soc. Am.* 67, S58.

Patterson, R. D. and Moore, B. C. J. (1986). Auditory filters and excitation patterns as representations of frequency resolution. In *Frequency Selectivity in Hearing* (ed. B. C. J. Moore), Academic Press, London and New York.

Patterson, R. D. and Nimmo-Smith, I. (1980). Off-frequency listening and auditory-filter asymmetry. *J. Acoust. Soc. Am.* 67, 229–245.

Patterson, R. D. and Wightman, F. L. (1976). Residue pitch as a function of component spacing. *J. Acoust. Soc. Am.* 59, 1450–1459.

Penner, M. J. (1977). Detection of temporal gaps in noise as a measure of the decay of auditory sensation. *J. Acoust. Soc. Am.* 61, 552–557.

Penner, M. J. (1980). The coding of intensity and the interaction of forward and backward masking. *J. Acoust. Soc. Am.* 67, 608–616.

Penner, M. J. and Shiffrin, R. M. (1980). Nonlinearities in the coding of intensity within the context of a temporal summation model. *J. Acoust. Soc. Am.* 67, 617–627.

Perrott, D. R., Marlborough, K. and Merrill, P. (1989). Minimum audible angle thresholds obtained under conditions in which the precedence effect is assumed to operate. *J. Acoust. Soc. Am.* 85, 282–288.

Perrott, D. R. and Musicant, A. D. (1977). Minimum auditory movement angle: Binaural localization of moving sound sources. *J. Acoust. Soc. Am.* 62, 1463–1466.

Pfeiffer, R. R. and Kim, D. O. (1975). Cochlear nerve fiber responses: Distribution along the cochlear partition. *J. Acoust. Soc. Am.* 58, 867–869.

Pick, G. F., Evans, E. F. and Wilson, J. P.(1977). Frequency resolution in patients with hearing loss of cochlear origin. In *Psychophysics and Physiology of Hearing* (eds E. F. Evans and J. P. Wilson), Academic Press, London and New York.

Pickett, J. M. (1980). *The Sounds of Speech Communication*, University Park Press, Baltimore.

Pickles, J. O. (1986). The neurophysiological basis of frequency selectivity. In *Frequency Selectivity in Hearing* (ed. B. C. J. Moore), Academic Press, London.

Pickles, J. O. (1988). *An Introduction to the Physiology of Hearing*, Second Edition, Academic Press, London.

Pisoni, D. B. (1973). Auditory and phonetic memory codes in the discrimination of consonants and vowels. *Percept. Psychophys.* 13, 253–260.

Plack, C. J. and Moore, B. C. J. (1989). Temporal window shape as a function of frequency and level. *J. Acoust. Soc. Am.* (Submitted).

Plenge, G. (1972). Über das Problem der Im-Kopf-Lokalisation. *Acustica* 26, 213–221.

Plenge, G. (1974). On the differences between localization and lateralization. *J. Acoust. Soc. Am.* 56, 944–951.

Plomp, R. (1964a). The ear as a frequency analyser. *J. Acoust. Soc. Am.* 36, 1628–1636.

Plomp, R. (1964b). Rate of decay of auditory sensation. *J. Acoust. Soc. Am.* 36, 277–282

Plomp, R. (1965). Detectability threshold for combination tones. *J. Acoust. Soc. Am.* 37, 1110–1123.

Plomp, R. (1967). Pitch of complex tones. *J. Acoust. Soc. Am.* 41, 1526–1533.

Plomp, R. (1968). Pitch, timbre and hearing theory. *Int. Audiol.* 7, 322–344.

Plomp, R. (1970). Timbre as a multidimensional attribute of complex tones. In *Frequency Analysis and Periodicity Detection in Hearing* (eds R. Plomp and G. F. Smoorenburg), Sijthoff, Leiden.

Plomp, R. (1988). The negative effect of amplitude compression in multichannel hearing aids in the light of the modulation-transfer function. *J. Acoust. Soc. Am.* 83, 2322–2327.

Plomp, R. and Bouman, M. A. (1959). Relation between hearing threshold and duration for tone pulses. *J. Acoust. Soc. Am.* 31, 749–758.

Plomp, R. and Levelt, W. J. M. (1965). Tonal consonance and critical bandwidth. *J. Acoust. Soc. Am.* 38, 548–560.

Plomp, R. and Steeneken, H. J. M. (1969). Effect of phase on the timbre of complex tones. *J. Acoust. Soc. Am.* 46, 409–421.

Plomp, R., Pols, L. C. W. and Geer, J. P. van de (1967). Dimensional analysis of vowel spectra. *J. Acoust. Soc. Am.* 41, 707–712.

Pollack, I. (1952). The information of elementary auditory displays. *J. Acoust. Soc. Am.* 24, 745–749.

Pollack, I. (1969). Periodicity pitch for white noise—fact or artifact? *J. Acoust. Soc. Am.* 45, 237–238.

Pols, L. C. W., Kamp, L. J. Th. van der and Plomp, R. (1969). Perceptual and physical space of vowel sounds. *J. Acoust. Soc. Am.* 46, 458–467.

Port, E. (1963). Über die Lautstärke einzelner kurzer Schallimpulse. *Acustica* 13, 212–223.

Poulton, E. C. (1979). Models for the biases in judging sensory magnitude. *Psych. Bull.* 86, 777–803.

Raab, D. H. and Goldberg, I. A. (1975). Auditory intensity discrimination with bursts of reproducible noise. *J. Acoust. Soc. Am.* 57, 437–447.

Rabinowitz, W. M., Bilger, R. C., Trahiotis, C. and Neutzel, J. (1980). Two-tone masking in normal hearing listeners. *J. Acoust. Soc. Am.* 68, 1096–1106.

Raiford, C. A. and Schubert, E. D. (1971). Recognition of phase changes in octave complexes. *J. Acoust. Soc. Am.* 50, 559–567.

Rakowski, A. (1972). Direct comparison of absolute and relative pitch. In *Hearing Theory 1972*, IPO Eindhoven, The Netherlands.

Rand, T. C. (1974). Dichotic release from masking for speech. *J. Acoust. Soc. Am.* 55, 678–680.

Rasch, R. A. (1978). The perception of simultaneous notes such as in polyphonic music. *Acustica* 40, 21–33.

Rayleigh, Lord (1907). On our perception of sound direction. *Phil. Mag.* 13, 214–232.

Remez, R. E., Rubin, P. E., Pisoni, D. B. and Carrell, T. D. (1981). Speech perception without traditional speech cues. *Science* 212, 947–950.

Repp, B. H. (1982). Phonetic trading relations and context effects: new experimental evidence for a speech mode of perception. *Psych. Bull.* 92, 81–110.

Resnick, S. B. and Feth, L. L. (1975). Discriminability of time-reversed click pairs: intensity effects. *J. Acoust. Soc. Am.* 57, 1493–1499.

Rhode, W. S. (1971). Observations of the vibration of the basilar membrane in squirrel monkeys using the Mössbauer technique. *J. Acoust. Soc. Am.* 49, 1218–1231.

Rhode, W. S. and Robles, L. (1974). Evidence from Mössbauer experiments for non-linear vibration in the cochlea. *J. Acoust. Soc. Am.* 55, 588–596.

Rice, C. E. (1967). Human echo perception. *Science*, N. Y. 155, 656–664.

Richards, V. M. (1987). Monaural envelope correlation perception. *J. Acoust. Soc. Am.* 82, 1621–1630.

Riesz, R. R.(1928). Differential intensity sensitivity of the ear for pure tones. *Phys. Rev.* 31, ser 2, 867–875.

Risset, J. C. and Wessel, D. L. (1982). Exploration of timbre by analysis and synthesis. In *The Psychology of Music* (ed. D. Deutch), Academic Press, New York.

Ritsma, R. J. (1962). Existence region of the tonal residue. I. *J. Acoust. Soc. Am.* 34, 1224–1229.

Ritsma, R. J. (1963). Existence region of the tonal residue. II. *J. Acoust. Soc. Am.* 35, 1241–1245.

Ritsma, R. J. (1967a). Frequencies dominant in the perception of the pitch of complex sounds. *J. Acoust. Soc. Am.* 42, 191–198.

Ritsma, R. J. (1967b). Frequencies dominant in the perception of periodic pulses of alternating polarity. *IPO Annual Prog. Rep. Eindhoven*, 2, 14–24.

Ritsma, R. J. (1970). Periodicity detection. In *Frequency Analysis and Periodicity Detection in Hearing* (eds R. Plomp and G. F. Smoorenburg), Sijthoff, Leiden.

Robertson, D. and Manley, G. A. (1974). Manipulation of frequency analysis in the cochlear ganglion of the guinea pig. *J. Comp. Physiol.* 91, 363–375.

Robinson, D. W. and Dadson, R. S. (1956). A redetermination of the equal-loudness relations for pure tones. *Br. J. Appl. Phys.* 7, 166–181.

Robles, L., Ruggero, M. A. and Rich, N. C. (1986). Basilar membrane mechanics at the base of the chinchilla cochlea. I. Input–output functions, tuning curves, and response phases. *J. Acoust. Soc. Am.* 80, 1364–1374.

Rodenburg, M. (1972). Sensitivity of the Auditory System to Differences in Intensity, Unpublished PhD Thesis, Medical Faculty, Rotterdam.

Rodenburg, M. (1977). Investigation of temporal effects with amplitude modulated signals. In *Psychophysics and Physiology of Hearing* (eds E. F. Evans and J. P. Wilson), Academic Press, London.

Ronken, D. A. (1970). Monaural detection of a phase difference in clicks. *J. Acoust. Soc. Am.* 47, 1091–1099.

Rose, J. E., Brugge, J. F., Anderson, D. J. and Hind, J. E. (1968). Patterns of activity in single auditory nerve fibers of the squirrel monkey. In *Hearing Mechanisms in Vertebrates* (eds A. V. S. de Reuck and J. Knight), Churchill, London.

Rose, J. E., Hind, J. E., Anderson, D. J. and Brugge, J. F. (1971). Some effects of stimulus intensity on response of auditory nerve fibers in the squirrel monkey. *J. Neurophysiol.* 34, 685–699.

Royer, F. L. and Garner, W. R. (1966). Response uncertainty and perceptual difficulty of auditory temporal patterns. *Percept. Psychophys.* 1, 41–47.

Royer, F. L. and Garner, W. R. (1970). Perceptual organization of nine-element auditory temporal patterns. *Percept. Psychophys.* 7, 115–120.

Ruggero, M. A., Robles, L., Rich, N. C. and Costalupes, J.A. (1986). Basilar membrane motion and spike initiation in the cochlear nerve. In *Auditory Frequency Selectivity* (ed. B. C. J. Moore and R. D. Patterson), Plenum, New York.

Russell. I. J. and Sellick, P.M. (1978). Intracellular studies of hair cells in the mammalian cochlea. *J. Physiol.* (Lond.) 284, 261–290.

Sachs, M. B. and Abbas. P. J. (1974). Rate versus level functions for auditory-nerve fibers in cats: tone-burst stimuli. *J. Acoust. Soc. Am.* 56, 1835–1847.

Sachs, M. B. and Kiang, N. Y.-S. (1968). Two-tone inhibition in auditory-nerve fibers. *J. Acoust. Soc. Am.* 43, 1100–1128.

Sachs. M. B. and Young, E. D. (1980). Effects of nonlinearities on speech encoding in the auditory nerve. *J. Acoust. Soc. Am.* 68, 858–875.

Sandel, T. T., Teas. D. C., Feddersen, W. E. and Jeffress, L. A. (1955). Localization of sound from single and paired sources. *J. Acoust. Soc. Am.* 27, 842–852.

Scharf, B. (1961). Complex sounds and critical bands. *Psychol. Bull.* 58, 205–217.

Scharf, B. (1970). Critical bands. In *Foundations of Modern Auditory Theory*, Vol. 1 (ed. J. V. Tobias), Academic Press, New York.

Scharf, B. (1981). Loudness adaptation. In *Hearing Research and Theory* (eds J. V. Tobias and E. D. Schubert), Academic Press, New York.

Scheffers, M. T. M. (1983). Sifting vowels: Auditory pitch analysis and sound segregation. Ph. D. Thesis, University of Groningen, The Netherlands.

Schooneveldt, G. P. and Moore, B. C. J. (1987). Comodulation masking release (CMR): Effects of signal frequency, flanking-band frequency, masker bandwidth, flanking-band level, and monotic versus dichotic presentation of the flanking band. *J. Acoust. Soc. Am.* 82, 1944–1956.

Schooneveldt, G. P. and Moore, B. C. J. (1989). Comodulation masking release as a function of masker bandwidth, modulator bandwidth and signal duration. *J. Acoust. Soc. Am.* 85, 273–281.

Schorer, E. (1986). Critical modulation frequency based on detection of AM versus FM tones. *J. Acoust. Soc. Am.* 79, 1054–1057.

Schouten, J. F. (1940). The residue and the mechanism of hearing. *Proc. K. Ned. Akad. Wet.* 43, 991–999.

Schouten, J. F. (1968). The perception of timbre. In *Reports 6th International Congress on Acoustics*, Tokyo, Japan, Vol. 1, GP-6-2.

Schouten, J. F. (1970). The residue revisited. In *Frequency Analysis and Periodicity Detection in Hearing* (eds. R. Plomp and G. F. Smoorenburg), Sijthoff, Leiden.

Schouten, J. F., Ritsma, R. J. and Cardozo, B. L. (1962). Pitch of the residue. *J. Acoust. Soc. Am.* 34, 1418–1424.

Schroeder, M. R. and Atal, B. S. (1963). Computer simulation of sound transmission in rooms. *IEEE Int. Conv. Rec.* 7, 150–155.

Schroeder, M. R., Gottlob, D. and Siebrasse, K. F. (1974). Comparative study of European concert halls: correlation of subjective preference with geometric and acoustic parameters. *J. Acoust. Soc. Am.* 56, 1195–1201.

Schubert, E. D. (1969). On estimating aural harmonics. *J. Acoust. Soc. Am.* 45, 790–791.

Sellick, P. M. and Russell, I. J. (1979). Two-tone suppression in cochlear hair cells. *Hearing Res.* 1, 227–236.

Sellick, P. M., Patuzzi, R. and Johnstone, B. M. (1982). Measurement of basilar membrane motion in the guinea pig using the Mössbauer technique. *J. Acoust. Soc. Am.* 72, 131–141.

Shailer, M. J. and Moore B. C. J. (1983). Gap detection as a function of frequency, bandwidth and level. *J. Acoust. Soc. Am.* 74, 467–473.

Shailer, M. J. and Moore B. C. J. (1985). Detection of temporal gaps in bandlimited noise: Effects of variations in bandwidth and signal-to-masker ratio. *J. Acoust. Soc. Am.* 77, 635–639.

Shailer, M. J. and Moore B. C. J. (1987). Gap detection and the auditory filter: Phase effects using sinusoidal signals. *J. Acoust. Soc. Am.* 81, 1110–1117.

Shannon, R. V. (1976). Two-tone unmasking and suppression in a forward-masking situation. *J. Acoust. Soc. Am.* 59, 1460–1470.

Shannon, R. V. (1986). Temporal processing in cochlear implants. In *The Scott Reger Memorial Conference*, Iowa U.P., Iowa City, IA, U.S.A.

Shaxby, J. H. and Gage, F. H. (1932). Studies in the localization of sound. *Med. Res. Council Spec. Rept. Ser.* No. 166, 1–32.

Sheeley, E. C. and Bilger, R. C. (1964). Temporal integration as a function of frequency. *J. Acoust. Soc. Am.* 36, 1850–1857.

Shepard, R. N. (1962). The analysis of proximities: multidimensional scaling with an unknown distance function. *Psychometrika* 27, 125–140.

Shepard, R. N. (1964). Circularity in judgments of relative pitch. *J. Acoust. Soc. Am.* 36, 2346–2353.

Shower, E. G. and Biddulph, R. (1931). Differential pitch sensitivity of the ear. *J. Acoust. Soc. Am.* 2, 275–287.

Siebert, W. M. (1968). Stimulus transformations in the peripheral auditory system. In *Recognizing Patterns* (eds P. A. Kolers and M. Eden), MIT Press, Cambridge, Massachusetts.

Siebert, W. M. (1970). Frequency discrimination in the auditory system: place or periodicity mechanisms. *Proc. IEEE* 58, 723–730.

Simpson, A.M., Moore, B.C.J. and Glasberg, B.R. (1989). Spectral enhancement to improve the intelligibility of speech in noise for hearing-impaired listeners. *Acta Otolaryngol.* (in press).

Slater P. (1960). The analysis of personal preferences. *Br. J. Stat. Psychol.* 8, 119.

Small, A. M., Boggess, J., Klich, R., Kuehn, D., Thelin, J. and Wiley, T. (1972). MLD's in forward and backward masking. *J. Acoust. Soc. Am.* 51, 1365–1367.

Smoorenburg, G. F. (1970). Pitch perception of two-frequency stimuli. *J. Acoust. Soc. Am.* 48, 924–941.

Soderquist, D. R. (1970). Frequency analysis and the critical band. *Psychol. Sci.* 21, 117–119.

Soderquist, D. R. and Lindsey, J. W. (1972). Physiological noise as a masker of low frequencies: the cardiac cycle. *J. Acoust. Soc. Am.* 52, 1216–1220.

Spiegel, M. F. (1981). Thresholds for tones in maskers of various bandwidths and for signals of various bandwidths as a function of signal frequency. *J. Acoust. Soc. Am.* 69, 791–795.

Spillman, T. and Dillier, N. (1989). Comparison of single-channel extracochlear and multichannel intracochlear electrodes in the same patient. *Brit. J. Audiol.* 23, 25–31.

Spoendlin, H. (1970). Structural basis of peripheral frequency analysis. In *Frequency Analysis and Periodicity Detection in Hearing* (eds R. Plomp and G. F. Smoorenburg), Sijthoff, Leiden.

Srinivasan, R. (1971). Auditory critical bandwidth for short duration signals. *J. Acoust. Soc. Am.* 50, 616–622.

Stephens, S. D. G. (1973). Auditory temporal integration as a function of intensity. *J. Sound Vib.* 30, 109–126.

Stephens, S. D. G. (1974). Methodological factors influencing loudness of short duration sounds. *J. Sound Vib.* 37, 235–246.

Stevens, K. N. (1968). On the relations between speech movements and speech perception. *Z. Phonetik Sprachwiss. Kommunikationsforsch.* 21, 102–106.

Stevens, K. N. (1980). Acoustic correlates of some phonetic categories. *J. Acoust. Soc. Am.* 68, 836–842.

Stevens, K. N. (1981). Constraints imposed by the auditory system on the properties used to classify speech sounds. In *The Cognitive Representation of Speech* (eds T. F. Myers, J. Laver and J. Anderson), North-Holland, Amsterdam.

Stevens, K. N. (1986). Models of phonetic recognition II: A feature-based model of speech recognition. In *Proceedings Montreal Satellite Symposium on Speech Recognition* (ed. P. Mermelstein), 12th Int. Cong. Acoust., 66–67.

Stevens, K. N. (1989). On the quantal nature of speech. *J. Phonetics* (in press).

Stevens, K. N. and House, A. S. (1972). Speech perception. In *Foundations of Modern Auditory Theory*, Vol. 2 (ed. J. V. Tobias), Academic Press, New York.

Stevens, S. S. (1935). The relation of pitch to intensity. *J. Acoust. Soc. Am.* 6, 150–154.

Stevens, S. S. (1957). On the psychophysical law. *Psychol. Rev.* 64, 153–181.

Stevens, S. S. (1972). Perceived level of noise by Mark VII and decibels (E). *J. Acoust. Soc. Am.* 51, 575–601.

Stevens, S. S. and Newman, E. B. (1936). The localization of actual sources of sound. *Am. J. Psychol.* 48, 297–306.

Sturges, P. T. and Martin, J. F. (1974). Rhythmic structure in auditory temporal pattern perception and immediate memory. *J. Exp. Psychol.* 102, 377–383.

Summerfield, Q. (1987). Some preliminaries to a comprehensive account of audio-visual speech perception. In *Hearing by Eye: The Psychology of Lipreading* (eds B. Dodd and R. Campbell), Erlbaum, New Jersey.

Summerfield, A. Q., Sidwell, A. S. and Nelson, T. (1987). Auditory enhancement of changes in spectral amplitude. *J. Acoust. Soc. Am.* 81, 700–708.

Supa, M., Cotzin, M. and Dallenbach, K. M. (1944). 'Facial vision': The perception of obstacles by the blind. *Am. J. Psychol.* 57, 133–183.

Swets, J. A., Green, D. M. and Tanner, W. P., Jr. (1962). On the width of critical bands. *J. Acoust. Soc. Am.* 34, 108–113.

Tanner, W. P. and Sorkin, R. D. (1972). The theory of signal detectability. In *Foundations of Modern Auditory Theory*, Vol. 2 (ed. J. V. Tobias), Academic Press London and New York.

Tasell, D. J. van, Soli, S. D., Kirby, V. M and Widin, G. P. (1987). Speech waveform cues for consonant recognition. *J. Acoust. Soc. Am.* 82, 1152–1161.

Teich, M. C. and Khanna, S.M. (1985). Pulse-number distribution for the neural spike train in the cat's auditory nerve. *J. Acoust. Soc. Am.* 77, 1110–1128.

Terhardt, E. (1972a). Zur Tonhöhenwahrnehmung von Klängen. I. Psychoakustische Grundlagen. *Acustica* 26, 173–186.

Terhardt, E. (1972b). Zur Tonhöhenwahrnehmung von Klängen. II. Ein Funktionsschema. *Acustica* 26, 187–199.

Terhardt, E. (1974). Pitch, consonance and harmony. *J. Acoust. Soc. Am.* 55, 1061–1069.

Thurlow, W. R. (1963). Perception of low auditory pitch: a multicue mediation theory. *Psychol. Rev.* 70, 515–519.

Thwing, E. J, (1955). Spread of perstimulatory fatigue of a pure tone to neighboring frequencies. *J. Acoust. Soc. Am.* 27, 741–748.

Tobias, J. V. (1963). Application of a 'relative' procedure to a problem in binaural-beat perception. *J. Acoust. Soc. Am.* 35, 1442–1447.

Tobias, J. V. (1965). Consistency of sex differences in binaural-beat perception. *Int. Audiol.* 4, 179–182.

Tobias, J. V. (1972). Curious binaural phenomena. In *Foundations of Modern Auditory Theory*, Vol. 2 (ed. J. V. Tobias), Academic Press, New York.

Tobias, J. V. and Schubert, E. D. (1959). Effective onset duration of auditory stimuli. *J. Acoust. Soc. Am.* 31, 1595–1605.

Tobias, J. V. and Zerlin, S. (1959). Lateralization threshold as a function of stimulus duration. *J. Acoust. Soc. Am.* 31, 1591–1594.

Treisman, M. (1964). Sensory scaling and the psychophysical law. *Q. J. Exp. Psychol.* 16, 11–22.

Tyler, R. S., Moore, B. C. J. and Kuk, F. K. (1989). Performance of some of the better cochlear-implant patients. *J. Speech Hear. Res.* (in press).

Tumarkin, A. (1972). A biologist looks at psycho-acoustics. *J. Sound Vib.* 21, 115–126.

Verschuure, J. and van Meeteren, A. A. (1975). The effect of intensity on pitch. *Acustica* 32, 33–44.

Viemeister, N. F. (1972). Intensity discrimination of pulsed sinusoids: the effects of filtered noise. *J. Acoust. Soc. Am.* 51, 1265–1269.

Viemeister, N. F. (1974). Intensity discrimination of noise in the presence of band reject noise. *J. Acoust. Soc. Am.* 56, 1594–1600.

Viemeister, N. F. (1979). Temporal modulation transfer functions based on modulation thresholds. *J. Acoust. Soc. Am.* 66, 1364–1380.

Viemeister, N. F. (1983). Auditory intensity discrimination at high frequencies in the presence of noise. *Science* 221, 1206–1208.

Viemeister, N. F. (1988). Psychophysical aspects of auditory intensity coding. In *Auditory Function—Neurobiological Bases of Hearing* (eds. G. M. Edelman, W. E. Gall and W. M. Cowan), Wiley, New York.

Viemeister, N. F. and Bacon, S. P. (1988). Intensity discrimination, increment detection, and magnitude estimation for 1-kHz tones. *J. Acoust. Soc. Am.* 84, 172–178.

Villchur, E. (1973). Signal processing to improve speech intelligibility in perceptive deafness. *J. Acoust. Soc. Am.* 53, 1646–1657.

Villchur, E. and Allison, R. F. (1980). The audibility of Doppler distortion in loudspeakers. *J. Acoust. Soc. Am.* 68, 1561–1569.

Vogten, L. L. M. (1974). Pure tone masking: a new result from a new method. In *Facts and Models in Hearing* (eds E. Zwicker and E. Terhardt), Springer-Verlag, Berlin.

Wallach, H. (1940). The role of head movements and vestibular and visual cues in sound localization. *J. Exp. Psychol.* 27, 339–368.

Wallach, H., Newman, E. B. and Rosenzweig, M. R. (1949). The precedence effect in sound localization. *Am. J. Psychol.* 62, 315–336.

Walliser, K. (1968). *Zusammenwirken von Hüllkurvenperiode und Tonheit bei der Bildung der Periodentonhöhe*, Doctoral dissertation. Technische Hochschule, München.

Walliser, K. (1969a). Zusammenhänge zwischen dem Schallreiz und der Periodentonhöhe. *Acustica* 21, 319–328.

Walliser, K, (1969b). Zur Unterschiedsschwelle der Periodentonhöhe. *Acustica* 21, 329–336.

Walliser, K. (1969c). Über ein Funktionsschema für die Bildung der Periodentonhöhe aus dem Schallreiz. *Kybernetik* 6, 65–72.

Ward, W. D. (1963). Auditory fatigue and masking. In *Modern Developments in Audiology* (ed. J. F. Jerger), Academic Press, New York.

Ward. W. D. (1963a). Absolute pitch. Part I. *Sound* 2, 14–21.

Ward. W. D. (1963b). Absolute pitch. Part II. *Sound* 2, 33–41.

Ward, W. D. (1970). Musical perception. In *Foundations of Modern Auditory Theory*, Vol 1 (ed J. V. Tobias), Academic Press, New York.

Ward, W. D., Glorig, A. and Sklar, D. L. (1958). Dependence of temporary threshold shift at 4 kc on intensity and time. *J. Acoust. Soc. Am.* 30, 944–954.

Warren, R. M. (1970a). Elimination of biases in loudness judgments for tones. *J. Acoust. Soc. Am.* 48, 1397–1413.

Warren, R. M. (1970b). Perceptual restoration of missing speech sounds. *Science*, N.Y. 167, 392–393.

Warren, R. M. (1974). Auditory temporal discrimination by trained listeners. *Cognitive Psychol.* 6, 237–256.

Warren, R. M. (1976). Auditory perception and speech evolution. *Ann. N. Y. Acad. Sci.* 280, 708–717.

Warren, R. M. (1981). Measurement of sensory intensity. *Behav. Brain Sci.* 4, 175–189.

Warren. R. M., Obusek, C. J., Farmer, R. M. and Warren, R. P. (1969). Auditory sequence: confusion of patterns other than speech or music. *Science*, N.Y. 164, 586–587.

Watkins, A. J. (1978). Psychoacoustical aspects of synthesized vertical locale cues. *J. Acoust. Soc. Am.* 63, 1152–1165.

Watson. C. S. and Gengel, R. W. (1968). Time-intensity trading relations as a function of signal frequency. *76th Meeting of the Acoustical Society of America*, paper A7.

Webster, F. A. (1951). Influence of interaural phase on masked thresholds. *J. Acoust. Soc. Am.* 23, 452–462.

Weerts, T. C. and Thurlow, W. R. (1971). The effects of eye position and expectation on sound localization. *Percept. Psychophys.* 9, 35–39.

Wegel, R. L. and Lane, C. E. (1924). The auditory masking of one sound by another and its probable relation to the dynamics of the inner ear. *Phys. Rev.* 23, 266–285.

Weiler, M. and Friedman, L. (1973). Monaural heterophonic auditory adaptation. *J. Acoust. Soc. Am.* 54, Suppl. 23.

Welford, A. T. (1968). *Fundamentals of Skill*, Methuen, London.

Whitfield, I. C. (1967). *The Auditory Pathway*, Arnold, London.

Whitfield, I. C. (1970). Central nervous processing in relation to spatiotemporal discrimination of auditory patterns. In *Frequency Analysis and Periodicity Detection in Hearing* (ed. R. Plomp and G. F. Smoorenburg), Sijthoff, Leiden.

Whitfield, I. C. and Evans, E. F. (1965). Responses of auditory cortical neurones to stimuli of changing frequency. *J. Neurophysiol.* 28, 655–672.

Whittle, L. S., Collins, S. J. and Robinson, D. W. (1972). The audibility of low-frequency sounds. *J. Sound Vib.* 21, 431–448.

Whitworth, R. H. and Jeffress, L. A. (1961). Time vs intensity in the localization of tones. *J. Acoust. Soc. Am.* 33, 925–929.

Wiener, F. M. and Ross, D. A. (1946). The pressure distribution in the auditory canal in a progressive sound field. *J. Acoust. Soc. Am.* 18, 401—408.

Wier, C. C., Jesteadt, W. and Green, D. M. (1977). Frequency discrimination as a function of frequency and sensation level. *J. Acoust. Soc. Am.* 61, 178–184.

Willey, C. F., Inglis, E. and Pearce, C. H. (1937). Reversal of auditory localization. *J. Exp. Psychol.* 20, 114–130.

Wilson, J. P. (1967). Psychoacoustics of obstacle detection using ambient or self generated noise. In *Animal Sonar Systems* (ed. R. G. Busnel), Gap, Hautes-Alpes, France.

Wilson, J. P. and Johnstone, J. R. (1972). Capacitive probe measures of basilar membrane vibrations. In *Hearing Theory 1972*, IPO, Eindhoven.

Winckel, F. (1967). *Music, Sound and Sensation*, Dover, New York.

Yates, G. K. (1986). Frequency selectivity in the auditory periphery. In *Frequency Selectivity in Hearing* (ed. B. C. J. Moore), Academic Press, London.

Yost, W. A., Wightman, F. L. and Green, D. M. (1971). Lateralization of filtered clicks. *J. Acoust. Soc. Am.* 50, 1526–1531.

Young, P. T. (1928). Auditory localization with acoustical transposition of the ears. *J. Exp. Psychol.* 11, 399–429.

Zurek, P. M. (1980). The precedence effect and its possible role in the avoidance of interaural ambiguities. *J. Acoust. Soc. Am.* 67, 952–964.

Zurek, P. M. (1981). Spontaneous narrowband acoustic signal emitted by human ears. *J. Acoust. Soc. Am.* 69, 514–523.

Zurek, P. M. and Durlach, N. I. (1987). Masker-bandwidth dependence in homophasic and antiphasic tone detection. *J. Acoust. Soc. Am.* 81, 459–464.

Zwicker, E. (1952). Die Grenzen der Hörbarkeit der Amplitudenmodulation und der Frequenzmodulation eines Tones. *Acustica* 2, 125–133.

Zwicker, E. (1954). Die Verdeckung von Schmalbandgeräuschen durch Sinustöne. *Acustica* 4, 415–420.

Zwicker E. (1956). Die elementaren Grundlagen zur Bestimmung der Informations-kapazität des Gehörs. *Acustica* 6, 365–381.

Zwickern E. (1958). Über psychologische und methodische Grundlagen der Lautheit. *Acustica* 8, 237–258.

Zwicker, E. (1964). 'Negative afterimage' in hearing. *J. Acoust. Soc. Am.* 36, 2413–2415.

Zwicker, E. (1965a). Temporal effects in simultaneous masking by white-noise bursts. *J. Acoust. Soc. Am.* 37, 653–663.

Zwicker, E. (1965b). Temporal effects in simultaneous masking and loudness. *J. Acoust. Soc. Am.* 38, 132–141.

Zwicker, E. (1970). Masking and psychological excitation as consequences of the ear's frequency analysis. In *Frequency Analysis and Periodicity Detection in Hearing* (eds R. Plomp and G. F. Smoorenburg), Sijthoff, Leiden.

Zwicker, E. and Fastl, H. (1972). On the development of the critical band. *J. Acoust. Soc. Am.* 52, 699–702.

Zwicker, E. and Scharf, B. (1965). A model of loudness summation. *Psychol. Rev.* 72, 3–26.

Zwicker, E. and Schorn, K. (1978). Psychoacoustical tuning curves in audiology. *Audiology* 17, 120–140.

Zwicker, E., Flottorp, G. and Stevens, S. S. (1957). Critical bandwidth in loudness summation. *J. Acoust. Soc. Am.* 29, 548–557.

Zwislocki, J. J. (1969). Temporal summation of loudness: An analysis. *J. Acoust. Soc. Am.* 46, 431–441.

Zwislocki, J. J. and Jordan, H. N. (1986). On the relations of intensity jnds to loudness and neural noise. *J. Acoust. Soc. Am.* 79, 772–780.

Glossary

This glossary defines most of the technical terms which appear in the text. Sometimes the definitions are specific to the context of the book and do not apply to everyday usage of the terms. The glossary also defines some terms not used in the text, but which may be found in the literature on hearing.

Absolute threshold The minimum detectable level of a sound in the absence of any other external sounds. The manner of presentation of the sound and the method of determining detectability must be specified.

Amplitude The instantaneous amplitude of an oscillating quantity (e.g. sound pressure) is its value at any instant, while the peak amplitude is the maximum value that the quantity attains. Sometimes the word peak is omitted when the meaning is clear from the context.

Audiogram A graph showing absolute threshold for pure tones as a function of frequency. It is usually plotted as hearing loss (deviation from the average threshold for young normally hearing people) in dB as a function of frequency, with increasing loss plotted in the downward direction.

Aural harmonic A harmonic generated in the auditory system.

Bandwidth A term used to refer to a range of frequencies. The bandwidth of a bandpass filter is often defined as the difference between the two frequencies at which the response of the filter has fallen by 3 dB (i.e. to half power).

Basilar membrane A membrane inside the cochlea which vibrates in response to sound and whose vibrations lead to activity in the auditory pathways (see Chapter 1).

Beats Periodic fluctuations in peak amplitude which occur when two sinusoids with slightly different frequencies are superimposed.

Bel A unit for expressing the ratio of two powers. The number of Bels is the logarithm to the base 10 of the power ratio.

Best frequency See *Characteristic frequency*.

Binaural A situation involving listening with two ears.

Binaural masking level difference (BMLD or MLD) This is a measure of the improvement in detectability of a signal which can occur under binaural listening conditions. It is the difference in threshold of the signal (in dB) for the case where the signal and masker have the same phase and level relationships at the two ears and the case where the interaural phase and/or level relationships of the signal and masker are different.

Categorical perception A type of perception where stimuli can only be distinguished if they are identified as belonging to a different category. It occurs commonly for speech sounds, but is not unique to speech.

Characteristic frequency (CF), Best frequency The frequency at which the threshold of a given single neurone is lowest, i.e. the frequency at which it is most sensitive.

Combination tone A tone perceived as a component of a complex stimulus which is not present in the sensations produced by the constituent components of the complex when they are presented alone.

Complex tone A tone composed of a number of sinusoids of different frequencies.

Co-modulation masking release (CMR) The release from masking which can occur when the components of a masker have the same amplitude modulation pattern in different frequency regions.

Component One of the sinusoids composing a complex sound. Also called a frequency component. In Chapter 9, the section on hi-fi uses the word component to describe one of the pieces of equipment making up a hi-fi system.

Cycle That portion of a periodic function that occurs in one period.

Decibel One-tenth of a Bel, abbreviated dB. The number of dB is equal to ten times the logarithm of the ratio of two intensities, or 20 times the logarithm of the ratio of two amplitudes or pressures.

Dichotic A situation in which the sounds reaching the two ears are not the same.

Difference limen (DL) Also called the just-noticeable difference (JND) or the differential threshold. The smallest detectable change in a stimulus. The method of determining detectability must be specified.

Diotic A situation in which the sounds reaching the two ears are the same.

Diplacusis Binaural diplacusis describes the case when a tone of fixed frequency evokes different pitches in the left and right ear.

Envelope The envelope of any function is the smooth curve passing through the peaks of the function.

Equal-loudness contours Curves plotted as a function of frequency showing the sound pressure level required to produce a given loudness level.

Equivalent rectangular bandwidth (ERB) The ERB of a filter is the bandwidth of a rectangular filter which has the same peak transmission as that filter and which passes the same total power for a white noise input.

Excitation pattern A term used to describe the pattern of neural activity evoked by a given sound as a function of the characteristic frequency (CF) of the neurones being excited. Sometimes the term is used to describe the effective level of excitation (in dB) at each CF. Psychoacoustically, the excitation pattern of a sound can be defined as the output of the auditory filters as a function of centre frequency.

Filter A device which modifies the frequency spectrum of a signal, usually while it is in electrical form.

Formant A resonance in the vocal tract which is usually manifested as a peak in the spectral envelope of a speech sound.

Free field A field or system of waves free from the effects of boundaries.

Frequency For a sine wave the frequency is the number of periods occurring in one second. The unit is cycles per second, or Hz. For a complex periodic sound the term 'repetition rate' is used to describe the number of periods per second (p.p.s.).

Frequency threshold curve See *Tuning curve.*

Fundamental frequency The fundamental frequency of a periodic sound is the frequency of that sinusoidal component of the sound that has the same period as the periodic sound.

Harmonic A harmonic is a component of a complex tone whose frequency is an integral multiple of the fundamental frequency of the complex.

Hz See *Frequency.*

Intensity Intensity is the sound power transmitted through a given area in a sound field. Units such as watts per square metre are used. The term is also used as a generic name for any quantity relating to amount of sound, such as power or energy, although this is not technically correct.

Level The level of a sound is specified in dB in relation to some reference level. See *Sensation level* and *Sound pressure level.*

Linear A linear system is a system which satisfies the conditions of superposition and homogeneity (see Chapter 1, section 3).

Loudness This is the intensive attribute of an auditory sensation, in terms of which sounds may be ordered on a scale extending from quiet to loud.

Loudness level The loudness level of a sound, in phons, is the sound pressure level in dB of a pure tone of frequency 1 kHz which is judged by the listener to be equivalent in loudness.

Masked audiogram See *Masking pattern.*

Masking Masking is the amount (or the process) by which the threshold of audibility for one sound is raised by the presence of another (masking) sound.

Masking level difference (MLD) See *Binaural masking level difference.*

Masking pattern, masked audiogram This is a graph of the amount of masking (in dB) produced by a given sound as a function of the frequency of the masked sound.

Modulation Modulation refers to a periodic change in a particular dimension of a stimulus. Thus, a sinusoid may be modulated in frequency or in amplitude.

Monaural A situation in which sounds are presented to one ear only.

Noise Noise in general refers to any unwanted sound. White noise is a sound whose power per unit bandwidth is constant, on average, over the range of audible frequencies. It usually has a normal (Gaussian) distribution of instantaneous amplitudes.

Octave An octave is the interval between two tones when their frequencies are in the ratio 2:1.

Partial A partial is any sinusoidal frequency component in a complex tone. It may or may not be a harmonic.

Period The period of a periodic function is the smallest time interval over which the function repeats itself.

Periodic sound A periodic sound is one whose waveform repeats itself regularly as a function of time.

Phase The phase of a periodic waveform is the fractional part of a period through which the waveform has advanced, measured from some arbitrary point in time.

Phase-locking This is the tendency for nerve firings to occur at a particular phase of the stimulating waveform on the basilar membrane.

Phon The unit of loudness level.

Pitch Pitch is that attribute of auditory sensation in terms of which sounds may be ordered on a musical scale.

Psychophysical tuning curve (PTC) A curve showing the level of a narrow-band masker needed to mask a fixed sinusoidal signal, plotted as a function of masker frequency.

Pure tone A sound wave whose instantaneous pressure variation as a function of time is a sinusoidal function. Also called a simple tone.

Recruitment This refers to a more rapid than usual growth of loudness with increase in stimulus level, which occurs in certain types of hearing disorder.

Residue pitch Also known as virtual pitch, low pitch and periodicity pitch. The low pitch heard when a group of partials is perceived as a coherent whole. For a harmonic complex tone, the residue pitch is usually close to the pitch of the fundamental component, but that component does not have to be present for a residue pitch to be heard.

Sensation level This is the level of a sound in decibels relative to the threshold level for that sound for the individual listener.

Simple tone See *Pure tone*.

Sine wave, Sinusoidal vibration A waveform whose variation as a function of time is a sine function. This is the function relating the sine of an angle to the size of the angle.

Sound pressure level This is the level of a sound in decibels relative to an internationally defined reference level. The latter corresponds to an intensity of 10^{-12} W/m^2, which is equivalent to a sound pressure of 20 μPa.

Spectrum The spectrum of a sound wave is the distribution in frequency of the magnitudes (and sometimes the phases) of the components of the wave. It can be represented by plotting power, or amplitude, or level as a function of frequency.

Spike A single nerve impulse or action potential.

Timbre Timbre is that attribute of auditory sensation in terms of which a listener can judge that two sounds similarly presented and having the same loudness and pitch are dissimilar. Put more simply, it relates to the quality of a sound.

Tone A tone is a sound wave capable of evoking an auditory sensation having pitch.

Tuning curve For a single nerve fibre this is a graph of the lowest sound level at which the fibre will respond, plotted as a function of frequency. Also called a frequency threshold curve (FTC). See also *Psychophysical tuning curve*.

Virtual pitch See *Residue pitch*.

Waveform Waveform is a term used to describe the form or shape of a wave. It may be represented graphically by plotting instantaneous amplitude or pressure as a function of time.

Index